Person-centred Approaches in Healthcare

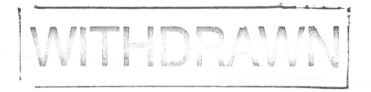

Person-centred Approaches in Healthcare

A handbook for nurses and midwives

Edited by Stephen Tee

Open University Press

Open University Press
McGraw-Hill Education
8th Floor
338 Euston Road
London
NW1 3BT

email: enquiries@openup.co.uk
world wide web: www.openup.co.uk

and Two Penn Plaza, New York, NY 10121-2289, USA

First published 2016

A catalogue record of this book is available from the British Library

ISBN-13: 978-0-33-526358-5
ISBN-10: 0-33-526358-5
eISBN: 978-0-33-526359-2

Library of Congress Cataloging-in-Publication Data
CIP data applied for

Typeset by Transforma Pvt. Ltd., Chennai, India

Printed and bound by CPI Group (UK) Ltd, Croydon, CR0 4YY

Praise Page

"This book offers an innovative, creative and fresh approach to understanding the heart of patient centred care. Its partnership approach has meant that the voices of national experts and patients are represented, and together they share their expertise and experience based insights, which has resulted in a text that illuminates the evidence base for nurses, midwifes and other health care professionals. Never has there been a more significant time to focus on patient centred care and this book makes a meaningful and bold contribution to constructively expanding the concepts of patient centred care and providing an applicable approach for practitioners.

This text helpfully covers the life span of individuals from a range of care settings and as such offers a unique and crisp approach. I would suggest that whether you are a student nurse or an experienced practitioner, this book would provide you with clear, informative and robust evidence to enhance the care you provide. This is a must read for students, health care professionals and academics – an excellent addition to the knowledge base."

Brian J Webster-Henderson, Professor of Nursing and
University Dean of Learning and Teaching,
Edinburgh Napier University, UK

"Evident throughout the book is the collaboration of its contributors, providing a real sense of compassion in care. The service users' 'voice' positively speaks to the reader and together with other contributors inspires a practice of care and compassion, professionally as well as personally. It is easy to read and follow and the activities encourage thinking and debate and reflective practice. The opening chapter introduces person-centeredness well, where its philosophy appears to be embedded within each chapter. It reads as supportive and developmental for practitioners."

Tracey Harding, Lecturer and Programme Lead,
Doctorate in Clinical Practice,
University of Southampton, UK

"This excellent book offers a number of things to the reader: the theory for person-centred care; a structured approach to the development of that knowledge across the lifespan; and, most importantly, people's experiences – these jump off the page bringing life to the theory. For me, it was the 'voices' that were gripping as I grappled with the issues (many of which are challenging and from which the authors did not shy away).

Some of these were hard to read as I wished that the healthcare professionals in those situations had taken the time to really hear what the concerns were. The book is steeped in the realities of practice and helps to make sense of the challenges – and opportunities – that exist in healthcare practice as person-centred care continues to go to the heart of practice."

Ruth Taylor, Pro Vice Chancellor and Dean,
Faculty of Health, Social Care and Education,
Anglia Ruskin University, UK

Contents

Contributors

Stephen Tee is a Professor and Executive Dean of the Faculty of Health and Social Sciences at Bournemouth University, UK.

Andrew Newman is a lawyer who was diagnosed with Parkinsons in 2000.

Glenn Robert is a professor in organizational studies and organizational sociology at King's College London, UK.

Sophie French is a lecturer at King's College London, UK and a registered midwife.

Ruth Adekoya works as a lay auditor for the London Local Supervising Authority, UK.

Dr Sara Donetto is a research fellow at the Florence Nightingale Faculty of Nursing and Midwifery, King's College London, UK.

Andrea Cockett is a tutor in children's nursing at the Florence Nightingale Faculty of Nursing and Midwifery, King's College London, UK.

Joan Walters is a senior practitioner lecturer in children and young people and haemoglobinopathies at the Florence Nightingale Faculty of Nursing and Midwifery, King's College, London, UK.

Dr Suzanne Bench is a lecturer working in the Faculty of Nursing and Midwifery, King's College London, UK.

Annie Holme is a lecturer in the Department of Adult Nursing in the Faculty of Nursing and Midwifery, King's College London, UK.

Jakki Berry is lecturer/practitioner in diabetes nursing working at King's College London and University College Hospitals London, UK.

Julie Bliss is an RGN and district nurse currently working as a senior lecturer at the Florence Nightingale Faculty of Nursing and Midwifery, King's College London, UK.

Nicola Wilson is a mother, wife and part-time postal clerk living with Rheumatoid Arthritis who has lived longer with this disease than without it.

Angela Parry is a registered nurse and Principal Fellow of the Higher Education Academy, UK.

Professor Michael Brown is a consultant nurse in specialist learning disability services in NHS Lothian and Professor of Health and Social Care Research at Edinburgh Napier University, UK.

Dr Zoë Chouliara, Associate Professor in Person-Centred Care is a clinical academic practitioner counselling and health psychologist and a psychotherapist/counsellor.

Professor Alison Metcalfe is Professor of Health Care Research and Dean for Research at the Florence Nightingale Faculty for Nursing and Midwifery, King's College London, UK.

Ian Noonan is a mental health nurse, lecturer in nursing and teaching fellow at The Florence Nightingale Faculty of Nursing and Midwifery, King's College London, UK.

Louise L. Clark is a lecturer at King's College London, UK and leads mental health programmes.

Jimmy Cangy is the ward manager of the male PICU at South West London and St George's Mental Health NHS Trust, UK.

Dr Corina Naughton is a senior lecturer in the Florence Nightingale Faculty of Nursing and Midwifery, King's College London, UK.

Nicky Hayes is currently Consultant Nurse for Older People at King's College Hospital NHS Foundation Trust, and Clinical Lecturer, King's College London, UK.

Ms Bridgit A. Sam-Bailey retired from her Head of Business post in 1995, and is currently Chairperson of the Lewisham Pensioners' Forum.

Fiona Clark originally studied law and worked part-time in the book world while bringing up her four children, and later ran a charity.

Dr Julia E. Pelle is a qualified mental health and general nurse who has previously worked as a nurse educator at both Kingston University/St George's University London and University of Southampton, UK.

Foreword

Person-centred care (PCC) is an oft uttered mantra but much harder to achieve in practice. The chapters in this book provide a critical and kaleidoscopic view of its multifaceted nature and a set of frameworks within which to understand and reflect upon its component parts and practice in a rich range of care settings and care groups. Definitions are central to the meaning of PCC and it becomes apparent that this is a nuanced concept with not one but many meanings, reflecting a constellation of attributes from attitudes, values and beliefs as much as the care environment.

The ascendancy of PCC is not a new phenomenon. Those familiar with Hildegard Peplau's seminal writings in the 1950s will recognize its pedigree as belonging to a much longer line of thinking stretching from Peplau's interactionist approach to the Evidence Based Co-Design thinking of today. But PCC is not taken for granted here but rather interrogated through an evidence-based approach which asks: what does PCC mean in a variety of contexts? We discover the 'what and why' in a broad spectrum of settings, specialties and care groups across the age cycle from intensive care, genetics, maternity care, mental health, learning disabilities, medicine's management, older people's care to long term conditions such as rheumatology, and care groups such as children and adolescents.

Authors are careful not to duck the difficult questions. Different dynamics emerge from different services e.g., lessons from maternity care where engagement with women and families has a longer track record compared with the relational network in which children are cared for in the case of health visiting. It is also recognized that the path of engagement does not always run smoothly, leading to differences and conflict between the different parties involved. PCC therefore requires training and investment in support for skills to develop and manage eventualities effectively.

Chapters contain not only exercises for the reader but engaging vignettes to bring illustrations and examples alive. PCC is not presented as a panacea but it does seem to bear practical benefits in optimizing services. We live in a society where patients and their carers expect personalization. This book provides an invaluable guide to navigating the complex coordinates of PCC.

This book provides strong evidence and inspiring examples of 'what works' in PCC and a welcome antidote to cynicism, connecting – as the accounts in the chapter on EBCD so vividly illustrate – nurses to the 'why we do what we do'. For that reason alone it should be applauded.

Anne Marie Rafferty, Professor of Nursing Policy, King's College London, UK

Introduction

This is a book about the people who use health services, written for nurses and midwives to enhance their practice. It has been written by experienced practitioners, academics and service users with the aim of achieving fusion between theory, evidence from research, the lived experience of healthcare and the everyday practice of nurses and midwives.

The book has been structured around the human lifespan, starting with birth, moving through childhood and adolescence and on toward adulthood and old age. A unique aspect of this text is the 'voice' of those that use services running through each chapter. The book seeks to be an emancipatory vehicle giving voice to people in vulnerable or disadvantaged situations. Through these narratives, that are at times challenging, this book seeks to prompt the reader to think about their role as caregiver in the delivery of evidence-based interventions.

In preparing the text we have sought to remain true to the experience of each patient and service user. We have followed good ethical practice to ensure each account is replicated authentically and honestly. However, the nature and type of contribution necessarily varies according to age, capacity and circumstance. Broadly speaking four approaches were used:

1 Interviews with people –their story has been pieced together by carefully structured questioning
2 Focus groups – with small groups of children and young people
3 Written accounts of experience presented as case studies which are weaved throughout the text
4 Whole chapters written jointly by academics and people receiving healthcare

Whilst the primary aim of this book is to include accounts that emphasize good practice some people encountered practice that was below acceptable standards. We believe that it is often by including accounts of poor practice that readers can learn the most.

Throughout each chapter there are simple exercises for the reader to complete which will prompt reflection and deepen learning. By encouraging reflection we aim to develop empathy and compassion in the reader. At the very least we want to achieve 'reciprocal illumination' between those that use services and those that provide services. In other words by sharing the experience of the person receiving care alongside those delivering care we will illuminate both worlds leading to mutual (reciprocal) learning.

The justification for such an approach is provided by leading writers such as Ronald Barnett and Kelly Coats (2005), who suggest that learning in practice disciplines such as nursing and midwifery requires engagement with the three elements of knowing, acting and being: the knowledge underpinning practice (knowing), the professional skills to deliver evidence-based care (acting) and good insight into who we are as people (being). To achieve this balance this book emphasizes the humanistic elements of caring by seeing the encounters with individuals' health problems as encounters with real people. By including the narratives of patients and service users we aim to encourage readers to see the lives beyond the diagnosis, consider their own values and beliefs about people and acknowledge the funda-mental personhood of the individual.

In taking this approach we do not exhaustively cover every condition encountered in practice or every circumstance, but examine the principles and concepts that can be applied across a range of contexts. Typically nurses and midwives need to support people with complex and multiple needs. For example, the midwife may care for an expectant mother with a mental health problem, a nurse may care for a man with an acute cardiac condition with an intellectual disability and a health visitor may work with a young child in a family with a grandparent who has dementia. To reflect the mix of midwifery practice and the fields of nursing (adult, mental health, learning disability and children's) extra effort has been made in each chapter to ensure multiple health needs are addressed.

By emphasizing the lifecycle we intend to avoid an exclusive focus on diagnostic catego-ries, which arguably place greater emphasis on the knowing and acting at the expense of the being. However the clinical reality is that individuals' referral to, and contact with, healthcare is often on the basis of a diagnosis and illness classification and so in the adult section we have focused on two long-term conditions, diabetes and rheumatoid arthritis, to address the diversity of caring for adults with long-term conditions.

To aid the reader the book has been structured into five sections, the first of which con-tains two chapters that set the scene by discussing the principles of person-centred care and how such principles can be extended to service design as well as individual care. The second section examines practice in caring for women undergoing maternity care, families receiv-ing support from health visitors and the special considerations in caring for children and adolescents. The third section looks at the context of adult care across acute and long-term conditions and includes a chapter on medicines management, which is a source of consider-able challenge in practice. The fourth section contains three chapters examining issues for people with intellectual disability, genetic disorder and mental health problems that tend to transcend all age categories. The two chapters in the final section consider care for older adults and the particular circumstances faced by carers.

We very much hope you enjoy reading this book and undertaking the exercises through-out each chapter. Perhaps more importantly we hope that it will support you in your journey to develop the knowledge, skills and values that will enable you to become a highly capable practitioner with the ability to deliver the best person-centred care possible.

INTRODUCTION TO PERSON-CENTRED APPROACHES

Principles of person-centred approaches to modern healthcare

Stephen Tee and Andrew Newman

Introduction

> Be kind, for everyone you meet is fighting a harder battle.
>
> Plato

Plato's quote will no doubt provoke a range of reactions, but seems to say something profound about the nature of human relationships. Each encounter with another person creates an opportunity, through what we do and say, to build people up physically and psychologically, but equally by making assumptions we can inadvertently leave the person feeling hurt and more vulnerable.

The nature of healthcare typically involves helping people at their most vulnerable, due to illness or injury, disability or disadvantage, and providing a whole range of interventions, care and treatment. It is at these times that the vulnerable person is most in need of the type of help that will lift them up, not put them down.

We know from decades of research what helps a person at vulnerable times in their lives. Whether it's aiding childbirth, recovery after an illness, integrating into society with a disability or managing a long-term condition, it can be summed up in the term 'individualized personal care', in other words an approach that seeks to understand personal circumstances and tailor interventions to that person's needs.

This is essentially what this chapter is all about. It will provide you, the reader, with a broad understanding of person-centred care (PCC) and on completion you will be able to achieve the following learning outcomes:

- Appreciate the nature and scope of PCC
- Identify the origins of the philosophy of PCC

- Specify and practice the skills required to deliver PCC
- Articulate the evidence for PCC
- Discuss common models of person-centred care used in practice

This chapter also aims to set the scene for subsequent chapters that explore and provide a more detailed analysis of PCC within a particular context. This may include a particular stage in the person's life – childhood, old age and so on – or care of people who are managing a particular condition such as diabetes or mental illness. Collectively the book will provide the reader with a deep appreciation of the foundations of PCC and will provide an essential toolkit for the effective practitioner.

About this chapter

This chapter is written by two people: Stephen, who has been a nurse for almost thirty years and Andrew, a regular user of national health services:

> Hello, I am Andrew. I am in my early 50s. I am married. I have two wonderful daughters who pre-occupy my thoughts. I love sport, especially cricket. Oh yes, I have Parkinson's Disease – but it does not define me.

We believe that to convey the best understanding of PCC it seems essential to integrate the words of those that use or receive healthcare services, in order to draw on and learn from their experiences. We are not saying their professional healthcare workers do not have anything important to say: quite the contrary, they routinely deliver excellent care to millions of people every day and have a lot of valuable contributions to make. However we want the patient/person's voice to resonate throughout this chapter to act as balance to more theoretical work and to keep our feet firmly rooted in experience.

What is person-centred care?

Person-centred care in nursing can be defined as care that is designed and delivered through an equal partnership between the nurse, the person (patient) and their family and carers. It is seen as the hallmark of good practice across the world and is enshrined in the standards for professional competence in the UK (NMC 2015):

> All nurses must act first and foremost to care for and safeguard the public. They must practise autonomously and be responsible and accountable for safe, compassionate, person-centred, evidence-based nursing that respects and maintains dignity and human rights.

It is an approach that puts patients and members of their families at the centre of decision-making. Whether it relates to planning, delivering, assessment or even service design, PCC seeks to ensure that it most appropriately meets individual needs. Person-centred caer also aims to support and encourage partnerships between nurses and their patients and carers, in order to promote participatory decision-making.

An outcome of national and international policy drivers, alongside the political lobbying of patients and users of the service, is that there is now an expectation that all who use health services will be involved in all decisions. For the nurse it is important to realize that care cannot be reduced to a task-oriented, dehumanized, process, driven by just getting things done, but must be 'holistic', that is, focused on the whole person. Person-centred care is also not about fitting patients around services but ensuring services are responsive to individual need, which is a huge challenge in a modern highly fragmented and compartmentalized health system.

Reader activity

Given the above description of PCC, how well do you think health services currently achieve individualized care? What factors contribute to PCC being achieved and what are the barriers?

Listening to the people that use health services

National Voices, a coalition of health and social care charities across England, seeks to: 'strengthen the voice of patients, service users, carers, their families and the voluntary organisations that work for them' (National Voices 2013). In their stated aims National Voices (2013) suggest PCC encapsulates the following: 'I can plan my care with people who work together to understand me and my carer(s), allow me control, and bring together services to achieve the outcomes important to me.' Three important dimensions can be derived from this statement:

1   The need to 'understand' the person and their context – person and context refer to the self, the persons relationships, the environment in which they live or are being cared for and their social world
2   The need to allow the individual 'control'
3   An emphasis on negotiating outcomes that are valued by the individual, rather than outcomes the professional alone thinks are important

Andrew, who has been living with Parkinson's for more than ten years, picks up on the issue of working together in a mutual partnership:

I am not in a unique position. Of course there are those in a worse position, some in a much worse position but also some better off.

I am fighting this thing whatever you tell me. I am determined to get and give the most I can. I may look small in the patient's chair but we are in this together – I'm not sure who is in control?

The statement 'I am fighting this thing whatever you tell me' alludes to tensions around the treatment the professional might prescribe and what Andrew might find acceptable and agreeable. Ideally where the two are the same then there is a natural synergy, but so often it seems, healthcare professionals do not take the time to tailor their approach, which can lead to disgruntlement, dissatisfaction and reluctance to follow treatment.

To address this problem, health professionals need to embrace the philosophy that underpins real person-centredness so that it becomes second nature and underpins all their actions and decisions.

The Philosophy of PCC

A philosophy is a theory or set of beliefs and values that guides behaviour. When applied to PCC, it means more than a set of rules or an organization's mission statement. It is about the attitudes and behaviours displayed by caregivers and the principles that inform and support the culture and practices within the clinical environment, whether applied to a hospital, a ward, an outpatient department or a community facility.

On the service provider-side a PCC philosophy should pervade all levels of the organization, transcend disciplinary boundaries and be apparent in all decisions and actions. On the service-receiver side it should be experienced by everyone – patients, carers and family – who has contact with the service and be reflected in positive evaluations of the organization's performance.

To illustrate this point the following motto from a Bombay Hospital, which was adapted from a quotation of Mahatma Gandhi, is a good example of a philosophical statement that seeks to guide the actions of the staff:

> A Patient is the most important person in our Hospital. They are not an interruption to our work. They are the purpose of it. They are not outsiders in our Hospital, they are part of it. We are not doing them a favour by serving them, they are doing us a favour by giving us an opportunity to do so.

Another example is taken from St Michael's Hospital based in Ontario, Canada:

> At St Michael's Hospital we recognize the value of every person and are guided by our commitment to excellence and leadership. We demonstrate this by providing exemplary physical, emotional and spiritual care for each of our patients and their families . . . . where each person is valued, respected and has an opportunity for personal and professional growth.

Such statements seek to set a standard, create a shared vision and articulate the desired values and attitudes that staff are expected to display in their contact with patients. However moving from a vision to reality requires an active engagement with these principles in order to understand how they become apparent in professional practice.

A comment on terminology

The fundamental goal of PCC, which also echoes the National Voices position, is to respect personhood. Kitwood (1997: 8) defines personhood as '*a standing or a status that is bestowed on one human being, by another in the context of relationship and social being*'.

Kitwood further suggests that personhood is both 'sacred and unique' (p.8) and that all people should be treated with respect. Kitwood's (1997) work was focused on the care of people with dementia, and in particular his person-centred approach to people with cognitive impairment. He observed that social context – the environment – influences behaviour and that in turn influences their personhood, as defined above, in other words the degree of recognition, respect and trust that the person experiences. To illustrate this further McCormack (2004) has helpfully connected the key elements of PCC with Kitwood's definition of personhood (see Table 1.1). Whilst this work was conducted in the context of working with people with dementia the principles are highly transferable.

Alongside the terms PCC and personhood the literature makes reference to an array of terms, reflecting the different contexts of care, to describe very similar and overlapping concepts, for example:

- Patient-centred care
- Family-centred care
- Client-centred care
- Women-centred care

It is not the intention of this chapter to provide a detailed analysis of each of these terms, although several are explored in other chapters in this book when discussing the care of a particular client group.

For the purposes of this chapter the definition that captures the essence of PCC is derived from nursing research in the field of older-adult care (McCormack *et al.*, 2010: 13):

> … an approach to practice established through the formation and fostering of therapeutic relationships between all care providers … patients and others significant to them in their lives. It is underpinned by values of respect for persons, individual right to self-determination, mutual respect and understanding. It is enabled by cultures of empowerment that foster continuous approaches to practice development.

This definition stresses the multi-layered nature of PCC by emphasizing the inclusion of carers and family that are, so often, a pivotal feature of an older person's care. What's also appealing about this definition is how it alludes to the impact of organizational culture on

Table 1.1 Links between PCC and Kitwood's definition of personhood

Concepts of person-centred care	Link with Kitwood's definition of personhood
Being in relation with others	People exist in relationships with other people
Being in social world	People are social beings
Being in place	People have a context through which their personhood is articulated
Being with self	Being recognised, respected and trusted as a person impacts on a person's sense of self

Source: McCormack (2004).

whether PCC thrives. Other authors such as Don Berwick (2011) use the term 'patient-centred', which he defines as:

> 'The experience (to the extent the informed, individual patient desires it) of transparency, individualization, recognition, respect, dignity, and choice in all matters, without exception, related to one's person, circumstances, and relationships in health care.'

It's worth noting that the use of the term 'patient' rather than 'person' is challenged in some areas of the literature, particularly within mental health and midwifery. It is seen to suggest an unequal relationship in which the 'patient' becomes subservient to the 'expert' health practitioner.

Whilst having some sympathy with this position, the reality is that the term 'patient' is used widely in healthcare and so a pragmatic position is adopted in this chapter that recognizes the usage of both terms whilst being aware of the risks. The same issues arise in the misuse of diagnostic terms, which can often be used to label a person and further dehumanize the individual. Andrew picks up on this point about language and the need to see the person behind the label:

> Hello again – it's me! Well I should hope that's what you see – me, Andrew, with the condition. And I am not stupid – I know about budgets and compassion fatigue – I appreciate there are many to see. But I would prefer you to know my history. I want continuity and concern. Now that's not pity or sorrow. I want to be treated the same as anyone else. I am human after all!

How do we practise in a more person-centred manner?

As has already been indicated adopting PCC combines a number of philosophical, attitudinal and behavioural components of which an appreciation of nurses acting as therapeutic agents of engagement and support is key. To achieve this it is helpful to have an understanding of power in inter-personal relationships, the nature of anti-oppressive and anti-discriminatory practice and the benefits of immersion in the patient's lived experience through regular contact with people.

Relational power

As professional healthcare practitioners we have a certain degree of 'power' within a therapeutic relationship derived from our professional position and our expertise. The NMC Code of professional conduct makes it clear that nurses must not abuse their privileged position. The NMC Code, revised in 2015, states that all nurses must treat people as individuals and uphold their dignity through kindness, respect and compassion. It requires nurses to avoid making assumptions by recognizing diversity and individual choice as well as respecting and upholding people's human rights. The Code also highlights important boundary issues indicating that nurses should practise in a way that does not take advantage of people's vulnerability or cause them upset or distress, and must stay objective and have clear professional boundaries at all times with people, their families and carers.

Adopting a PCC position is therefore about how we use, and do not misuse, professional power, which determines how 'person centred' we actually are. In all areas we are seeking a position of shared decision-making. This is ideally where conversations occur between the parties to reach a choice together, avoiding any undue influence or coercion but giving sufficient information to make an informed choice.

It is worth reflecting on Arnstein's (1969) seminal text that brought into focus how easy it is to appear to be 'person centred', sharing power with people, but inadvertently getting it so wrong. Working in the context of citizenship and democratic engagement she designed a ladder of participation, which has been adapted for a clinical context (see Figure 1.1).

It can be seen that the ultimate aim of decision-making is to give the power to decide and support autonomy. Therefore as nurses we should be aiming for the top of the ladder, rungs 4 and 5, which involve high levels of shared decision-making and partnership. However the reality is that many interactions take place at the lower rungs with non-participation being contrived to suggest genuine participation.

The lower rungs 1, 2 and 3 could involve high levels of tokenism because the ground rules enable clinicians to inform and consult, but retain for the power-holders the right to decide. These are commonly seen in crude attempts to 'consult' people on changes to services when the decisions have already been made or where a 'token' patient is invited onto a committee or working group dominated by professionals.

This five-rung ladder is of course a simplification, but it does help to illustrate the point that there are significant gradations of participation. When applied to a clinical setting, where one is trying to achieve greater person-centred practice, it is helpful see the partnership as a continuum from paternalistic control, for example of the unconscious patient, through to full independence where responsibility for the self-management of their condition is assumed by the patient.

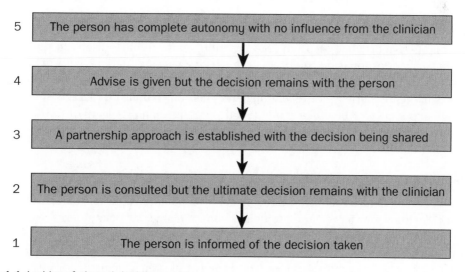

Figure 1.1 Ladder of shared decision-making

(Adpated from Arnstein's Ladder of Participation).

Reader activity

Reflect on one recent experience of patient participation in decision-making:

How did you or others involve the person or family in decisions?
What techniques or skills did you or others use to promote empowerment?
Where would you put this experience on Arnstein's ladder?
What could have been done differently to move further up the ladder?

Adopting an anti-oppressive position in practice

A further helpful position is that adopted in social work, psychology and other helping profes-sions. Known as anti-oppressive practice, Burke and Harrison (2009) suggest it is a dynamic process with the aim to address inequalities in relationships and to challenge oppression and discrimination.

The implication for nurses who seek to adopt an anti-oppressive stance is that nursing problems are seen in the context of the individual's social circumstances and that nurses have a responsibility to challenge practices or policies that may be putting patients or the public at risk. This is a position reinforced by the 2015 NMC Code, which states nurses must:

> raise and, if necessary, escalate any concerns you may have about patient or public safety, or the level of care people are receiving in your workplace or any other health-care setting and use the channels available to you in line with our guidance and your local working practices.

The code also emphasizes the nurse's role as advocate for the vulnerable: *'Act as an advocate for the vulnerable, challenging poor practice and discriminatory attitudes and behaviour relating to their care'*.

Anti-oppressive practice also requires practitioners to avoid presenting themselves as experts but to work alongside and value the service user's experience. To achieve this it is necessary for health practitioners to understand service user perspectives by immersing themselves in their experience of receiving care. This can be done by reading the many texts on people's experience of healthcare but also through listening to users of the service. This brings us to the third point which is the importance of contact.

The value of contact with people

Being truly person centred requires a deep level of personal insight into one's own and oth-ers values. We know our biases and prejudices can influence our behavioural responses and unless revealed to us remain unconscious. Developing an understanding of our own and oth-ers' values and experiences can best be achieved through regular personal and equitable con-tact with people who use health services. This is one of the key arguments for fifty percent of nurse training being in practice, involving many hours of contact with patients.

In the 1950s Gordon Allport proposed the Contact Hypothesis suggesting that if contact between groups of people increases then this can lead to more positive attitudes towards each other. According to Allport (1954) social contact between groups lessens negative prejudice and enhances friendly attitudes and behaviours.

However to be effective contact must be sufficiently close to produce reciprocal knowledge and understanding. In other words there should be equality of status, cooperation, positive expectation and an understanding of difference as well as similarities. This is about developing our cultural intelligence, which is the ability to cross divides and thrive in multiple cultures. As the NMC Code (2015) states nurses must: '*act with honesty and integrity at all times, treating people fairly and without discrimination, bullying or harassment*'.

Andrew picks up on the issues of power, sensitivity to the individual and the need for trust to develop within the relationship:

> Now I have to chip in here. You have power over my treatment. But not 'the' power. I am watching and listening carefully and as much as I love my wife it's me you're treating!
>
> But I do want to trust you and I do need to be told sometimes. I have a strategy but I need your help to get there. You have to listen to what I say and what I don't say. You have to persuade. It's not easy – you know a lot about treatment and medicine but chances are you have not been where I am, where I've been or where I am going – and I don't know that one either!
>
> Power and responsibility – I would not like to be you!

Applying PCC within a modern nursing context

An appreciation of personhood and insight into our own values are important foundations on which to build effective PCC. The emergence of PCC in nursing can be traced back to the 1960s with Virginia Henderson's 1966 definition of nursing being adopted by the International Council of Nursing and being seen as the birth of PCC:

> to assist the individual, sick or well, in the performance of those activities contributing to health or its recovery (or to peaceful death) that he would perform unaided if he had the necessary strength, will, or knowledge. And to do this in such a way as to help him gain independence as rapidly as possible . . . This aspect of her work, this part of her function, she initiates and controls; of this she is master.
>
> (Henderson 1966: 15)

A more contemporary definition is one developed by the Royal College of Nursing in 2003, following a period of consultation with members of the College and a review of the literature. It captures the complexities and the multifaceted nature of the role whatever field of nursing we occupy:

> The use of clinical judgement in the provision of care to enable people to improve, maintain, or recover health, to cope with health problems, and to achieve the best possible quality of life, whatever their disease or disability, until death.
>
> (Royal College of Nursing 2003: 3)

Whilst these are helpful as descriptions of nursing as 'deliverable acts' they do not make reference to the important human qualities, the attributes, values, characteristics and ethics that support PCC. Drawing on the work of another nurse theorist, Hildegard Peplau (1952), she argued that the key to effective nursing was the 'interpersonal bonds' that emerge between the nurse and patient. She believed it was only through these bonds that a positive nurse-patient relationship could be achieved.

To Peplau nursing was not about dependence on the nurse but growth toward independence. She saw nursing not as tick-box task-oriented exercise but as the medium of the art and science of nursing that offered a blend of the nurse's ideals, values, integrity and commitment to wellbeing. In Peplau's eyes nursing was not about hiding behind a box of tools and techniques but was a process of listening, hearing, engaging and responding. She also suggested that nursing occurred in cultures that were either illness maintaining, and by implication unhelpful, or health promoting.

Perhaps more profoundly, she went on to say that the kind of nurse a person becomes makes a huge difference to how the process of care progresses and what each person/client will learn through the experience of care, treatment and illness. The Health Foundation provides a useful history of person-centred care (www.health.org.uk/areas-of-work/topics/person-centred-care/person-centred-care/).

In other words it is not enough just to be aware of the latest technical aspects of nursing, albeit they have their place; it requires a much deeper level of inter-personal connectedness, a set of personal values that enables the nurse to show warmth, compassion and empathy. With society becoming ever more diverse and multi-cultural it also requires the nurse to be able to engage with anyone irrespective of age, ethnicity, religion, gender, sexual orientation or class.

Reader activity

Think about someone you observed receiving care and list the personal characteristics of that individual.

What actions could have been taken to achieve a greater degree of connection with that individual?

What's the evidence for PCC?

Whilst the moral justification for PCC may be strong it is also important to consider the empirical evidence for such an approach. In an environment of budgetary constraint and a culture of performance there is a pressing need to ensure we subject all aspects of practice to empirical examination in order to understand the impact of interventions on areas such as patient symptoms, medication adherence, satisfaction with services, length of stay, discharge planning, mortality and staff performance.

The most comprehensive analysis of the impact of person-centred approaches was reported in a systematic review conducted by Olsson *et al.* (2012). Their aim was to explore the efficacy of PCC as an intervention in controlled trials. Having searched the literature they found eleven studies that fulfilled their inclusion criteria. Whilst there was little homogeneity to the studies, which were carried out in diverse contexts and measure a range of outcomes, they were able to report that PCC as an intervention was successful in eight of the studies. These included improved symptoms, shorter hospital stays, improved functional performance and increased satisfaction. The authors were of course understandably measured in their conclusions, suggesting that whilst the evidence was insufficient, there were indications that PCC may lead to significant improvements but that more research was needed.

In more recent work Clissett *et al.* (2013) undertook a qualitative study involving 72 hours of ward-based non-participant observation of care and 30 hours of formal interviews. Their aim was to employ Kitwood's five dimensions of personhood as a framework for determining ways in which current approaches to care in acute settings had the potential to increase 'personhood' in older adults with dementia. They found examples of good practice but concluded that healthcare professionals were missing opportunities to enhance personhood amongst their patients. They suggested that the concept of PCC needed to be valued at the individual as well as the team/organizational level to be effective. McGilton *et al.* (2012) found that the skills needed to deliver PCC include leadership, facilitation, clinical excellence and critical thinking.

In a further study Tadd *et al.* (2011) conducted an exploration of the care of older adults in acute NHS hospitals. This was an ethnographic study with in-depth interviews undertaken with recently discharged older people (65+) (N = 40) and their relatives/carers (N = 25). This was complemented by evidence from 617 hours of non-participant observation of practices and activities in 16 wards across four acute NHS Trusts. A key finding was that patients who experienced dignified compassionate care, which was interpreted as PCC, were more likely to adhere to treatment and be satisfied with care.

All this evidence resonates with Andrew's experience of what works for him:

> Well I am glad to know it works. Listening not hearing. Informing and guiding. Caring, and interested in me. Rewarding for us both. Yes I need your honesty but mind how you say it! Good things too, please! We don't ask much? Well yes we do ... but then so would you!

Contemporary models of PCC

This final section presents three models drawn from the extensive literature of PCC. These models are multi-dimensional and universal. For illustrative purposes one from the US and two from the UK have been chosen. Each is derived from evidence in the field and taken together reflect the spectrum of care for people across the age span.

The aim is not to suggest one model is superior to another but to illustrate that PCC has a multitude of dimensions and sits within a broader context of interconnected services and agencies which work best when joined up and seamless. The current emphasis on integrated care is an important consideration as future services are designed and shaped by health policy.

Model 1: the Eight Dimensions of Patient-Centred Care

In the US researchers at Harvard and the Picker Institute conducted many thousands of interviews to appreciate what it is that really matters to those that use health services. This resulted in the Eight Dimensions of Patient-Centered Care (National Research Corporation 2015).

Their key observation is that everyone is unique and has a different perspective on what's important to them. Consequently PCC requires an approach: *'that consciously adopts the patient's perspective'* (National Research Corporation 2015). Having analysed and synthesized the data from the many hours of interviews with patients and carers they identified the following eight dimensions, each with its own descriptor:

1. Respect for patients' values, preferences and expressed needs

This dimension involves the need for sensitivity to the individual by those delivering care and treatment. Its about keeping people informed about what's happening particularly about their diagnosis, condition and prognosis. This can only be achieved within an atmosphere of trust and respect that involves the person in decisions and respects the dignity and autonomy of the individual.

2. Coordination and integration of care

The researchers found that people feel vulnerable and powerless when ill or injured and that one way of easing these feelings is by providing reassurance through effective planning, coordination and integration of care. This involves integration between hospital-based clinical services, support services and community and emergency services, in order to ensure joined up, seamless care.

3. Information and education

There is a need to develop trust within the patient/carer relationship as the researchers found that patients can become suspicious that important information is being withheld about their diagnosis and prognosis. Trust can be enhanced and fear reduced by healthcare professionals providing open and honest information about their clinical condition and prognosis and the process of care but also information that will enable autonomous decision-making and self-care and that promotes health.

4. Physical comfort

A very obvious need at a time of illness is the desire for physical comfort as this can have a significant impact on an individual's recovery and their general experience of services. The research revealed three particularly important areas, namely the management of pain, support and help with the activities of daily living and the hospital environment.

5. Emotional support and alleviation of fear and anxiety

Along with physical comfort is the requirement for psychological support, specifically the alleviation of fear and anxiety. Such fear and anxiety can have a very detrimental effect on the individual and be as debilitating as the physical symptoms of illness. The research found that the relief of fear and anxiety can best be achieved by focusing on physical status, the impact of illness on the individual and their family and the financial implications of being unwell.

6. Involvement of family and friends

The effects of illness typically extend well beyond the individual to their family and friends. The researchers found that an effective patient-centred approach should focus on the provision of appropriate information to family and close friends and involving them in the decision-making process. There is also a need to provide support where family and friends will become future caregivers and require their own needs to be recognized.

7. Continuity and transition

One of the biggest concerns expressed by patients is about their ability to care for themselves once they are discharged from hospital. This is particularly important given the proliferation of community providers and agencies that may have a role to play in the provision of follow-up and intervention. The main requirements include patient-friendly information on medicines, dietary needs and physical limitations, the coordination of after-discharge service provision and information on the range of services that can provide ongoing clinical, social and financial support post-discharge.

8. Access to care

The final dimension is to know how care can be accessed in the future should they need it. The focus in the research was mainly on ambulatory care including access and locations of services, transportation availability, follow-up appointments, access to specialists and instructions on referrals. All of this would typically be addressed in a good discharge plan.

Reader activity

Figure 1.2 is a diagrammatic representation of the 8 Dimensions of Patient-Centred Care.

From your experience do you think all dimensions are covered or are there areas missing that would be important to patients/clients you have care for?

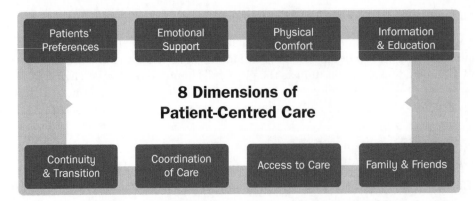

Figure 1.2 8 Dimensions of patient-centred care

Model 2: the Person-Centred Nursing Framework

This second model is known as the Person-Centred Nursing (PCN) Framework, and was developed by McCormack and McCance (2006, 2010). It has been developed from research into older persons-centred practice and nurses experience of caring for older people (McCance 2003; McCormack 2003).

In summary, the Framework comprises four constructs.

1   The first is focused on the attributes of the nurse, which includes their competence, professionalism, interpersonal skills, commitment and self-awareness including the ability to articulate their beliefs and values relating to PCC.
2   The second construct relates to the environmental context in which the care is actually delivered. This will include such elements as the skills and mix of the staff, team working, the systems that operate that support patient involvement in decision-making and power-sharing, the physical environment and whether innovation and risk-taking are encouraged and nurtured.
3   The third construct is focused on processes that support PCC. McCormack and McCance (2010) suggest that certain activities can enhance PCC such as working with the individual values and beliefs of patients through empathic engagement, sharing decision-making and providing holistic care.
4   The fourth construct is arguably the most important, as it focuses on outcomes for patients. This can include measurement of satisfaction, experience of involvement and participation in care decisions, levels of wellbeing amongst patients and what McCormack and McCance describe as creating a therapeutic environment.

Figure 1.3 uses overlapping circles and rings to illustrate the relationship between the four constructs:

Model 3: House of Care

This third model from the UK considers PCC for people with long-term conditions. It is somewhat different to the first two models, which are focused on personal care, in that it takes a broader view of the context in which PCC can be achieved.

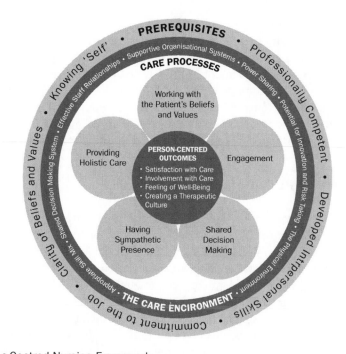

Figure 1.3 Person-Centred Nursing Framework
Source: McCormack and McCance (2010).

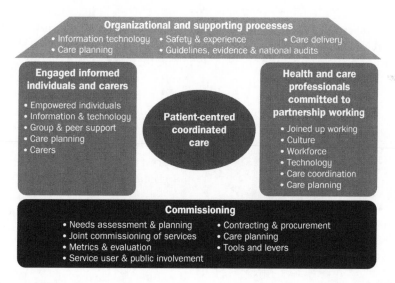

Figure 1.4 House of Care

It uses Callow's House of Care diagnostic tool, which seeks to help practitioners understand how to develop a holistic approach to PCC (see Figure 1.4). The model adopts four inter-dependent components that, it argues, if implemented together: *'will achieve patient centred, coordinated service for people living with long term conditions and their carers'.*

The four components address organizational and supporting processes, engaged and informed individuals and their carers, health and social care professionals committed to partnership working and, perhaps the component absent from other earlier models, commissioners. Commissioners are an important element of the UK health system as they determine where the NHS budget will be spent and on what services.

It is suggested that the 'House of Care' provides an important framework for bringing together policy, evidence and information for the benefit of patients, which in turn can inform the commissioning of new services (see NHS England/Coalition for Collaborative Care 2015).

Moving forward with PCC: from models to reality

Models of care are just that: representations of the inter-relationships between abstract ideas and constructs. They attempt to simplify reality in order to put complex ideas into a form that we can adapt, explain and communicate. It's a way of theorizing through building models that seek to explain theory. However these models are not to be used as rigid dogma, as this will deny the complex reality we encounter every day in clinical practice. However they can and should be used to inform our thinking and guide practice.

Taken together what each of the three models clearly illustrate is that to thrive and evolve in any care setting PCC needs to be more than the direct care delivered by a nurse to the individual patient. It requires acknowledgement and the management of the complex interplay between:

- the nurse, with all the pre-requisite attributes, values, skills and competencies;
- the person receiving care, including their family, close friends and social networks;
- the care processes, which refer to the systems in place in the clinical setting, whether a ward or community environment, including team work and systems of safety;
- the culture of the organization in which care is taking place, including its philosophy and leadership;
- the people making decisions about what services should be in place and how they should be designed, including commissioners.

What seems also very evident is that PCC will thrive when each of these factors are in harmony (see Figure 1.5), but equally if one of these factors are not attended to then PCC is unlikely to thrive.

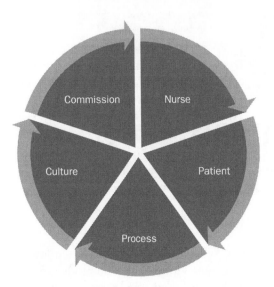

Figure 1.5 Person Centred Care – Five factors in harmony

When things go wrong

Unfortunately, in the UK, nursing has faced considerable criticism in recent years. Sir Robert Francis's report into Mid Staffs,

Sir Bruce Keogh's review of mortality rates and Margaret Flynn's (2012) report on the Winterbourne View hospital abuse in Gloucestershire are just a few that levelled criticism at the quality of nursing care.

This quote is from the Robert Francis Report (Francis 2013) into the terrible care at Mid Staffs:

> There was a lack of care, compassion, humanity and leadership. The most basic standards of care were not observed and fundamental rights to dignity were not respected. Elderly and vulnerable patients were left unwashed, unfed and without fluids. They were deprived of dignity and respect.

What emerges is the failure of services to communicate genuine, meaningful and compassionate engagement with those that receive services: in other words a failure of PCC.

Whilst each cite many reasons for the failures the 2013 report by the Kings Fund entitled *Patient-centred Leadership: Rediscovering Our Purpose* outlines the 'treatment' as essentially bringing services closer to the people that use them from the Board to the Ward. They suggest the following:

- Boards should act on *patient feedback*, hearing patient stories.
- Boards must develop their own *culture* in which patients' needs come first.
- This should be a culture that promotes *openness and honesty*.
- *Patient-centred care* should be understood at all levels, from the board to the ward.
- There should be staff training in the *values* of patient-centred care.

Understanding why compassion and person-centredness seem to thrive in some care environments characterized by sensitivity, tolerance, sympathy, and warmth whereas in others, people are met with a cold indifference at the very least and cruelty at worst, is critical for delivering safer person-centred environments.

In recognition of this need the 2015 'Shape of Caring Review' of nursing led by Lord Willis put as its key recommendation under theme 1 'Enhancing the voice of the patient and the public' the need to: 'commission research to identify the forms of patient and public involvement that best support learning'.

It is arguably only when patients and the public are central to decision-making in staff education and training, as well as service delivery, that authentic PCC will become firmly embedded in the DNA of our health service (Tee 2012).

Summary

As Peplau (1952) said, whatever the context, nursing care is an expression of who we are as people, of the choices we make. Nurses, and the profession as a whole, need to show leadership and stand up for their patients to ensure they get dignity and PCC.

The experience of conducting many engagement exercises with patients and service users reveals some fairly straightforward messages about the care they wish to receive:

1   Seeing me as a whole person within my whole environment – Wholeness
2   Attend to my emotional needs, culture and identity – Uniqueness
3   Take time to negotiate treatment with me – Partnership
4   Integrate my care so that it is joined up – Integration

PCC and the cultures that support such practice stem from the people delivering nursing care, based on our insight and the social skills of self-awareness and self-reflection, reasoning and imagination used in practice. PCC can only be fully developed through exposure to the powerfully transformative voices of the people that use our services that acknowledge the need for shared goals, delivered in partnership. However this must be a meaningful collaborative partnership because patient/service user involvement means cultural challenge and it means change which is likely to produce discomfort.

Perhaps, in the post-Francis era, we are at a tipping point where we need to radically rethink how we work alongside people who use our services toward a more creative and challenging relationship that will allow new PCC models to emerge. As Harry Cayton from the Kings Fund points out: 'When patient leaders arrive, clinical leaders and managerial leaders will have to give way. If they don't want to change their own leadership or style, then don't invite patients in' (Kings Fund 2013).

References

Allport, G.W. (1954) *The Nature of Prejudice*. Reading, MA: Addison-Wesley.

Arnstein, S. (1969) A ladder of participation, *Journal of the American Institute of Planners*, 35(4): 216–24.

Berwick, D. (2009) *What Patient-Centered Should Mean: Confessions of an Extremist*, Health Affairs Web Exclusive. Available at http://content.healthaffairs.org/content/28/4/w555.full(accessed 25 March 2011).

Burke, B. and Harrison, P. (2009) Anti-oppressive approaches, in R. Adams, L. Dominelli, and M. Payne (eds) *Critical Practice in Social Work*, 2nd edn. Basingstoke: Palgrave Macmillian.

Clissett, P., Porock, D., Harwood, R.H. and Gladman, J.R.F (2013) The challenges of achieving person-centred care in acute hospitals: a qualitative study of people with dementia and their families, *International Journal of Nursing Studies*, 50(11): 1495–503.

Flynn, M. (2012) *South Gloucestershire Safeguarding Adults Board Winterbourne View Hospital: A Serious Case Review*. CPEA Ltd. Available at http://hosted.southglos.gov.uk/wv/report.pdf (accessed 4 November 2015).

Francis, R. (2013) *Report of the Mid Staffordshire NHS Foundation Trust Public Inquiry*. London: The Stationery office. Available at www.midstaffspublicinquiry.com/ (accessed 4 November 2015).

Henderson, V. (1966) *The Nature of Nursing: A Definition and its Implications for Practice, Research, and Education.* New York: Macmillan.

Kings Fund (2013) *Patient-centred Leadership: Rediscovering our Purpose.* Available at www.kingsfund.org.uk/sites/files/kf/field/field_publication_file/patient-centred-leadership-rediscovering-our-purpose-may13.pdf (accessed 4 November 2015).

Kitwood, T. (1997) *Dementia Reconsidered: The Person ComesF.* Buckingham: Open University Press.

McCance, T. V. (2003) Caring in nursing practice: the development of a conceptual framework, *Research and Theory for Nursing Practice: An International Journal,* 17(2): 101–116.

McCormack, B. (2003) A conceptual framework for person-centred practice with older people, *International Journal of Nursing Practice,* 9(3): 202–209.

McCormack, B. (2004) Person-centredness in gerontological nursing: An overview of the literature, *International Journal of Older People Nursing,* 13(13a): 31–38.

McCormack, B. and McCance, T. (2006) Developing a conceptual framework for person-centred nursing, *Journal of Advanced Nursing,* 56(5): 472–479.

McCormack, B. and McCance, T. (2010) *Person-centred Nursing: Theory and Practice.* Oxford: Wiley Blackwell.

McCormack, B., Dewing, J., Breslin, L. *et al.* (2010) *The Implementation of a Model of Person-centred Practice in Older Person Settings. Final Report.* Dublin: Office of the Nursing Services Director, Health Services Executive.

McGilton, K.S., Heath, H., Chu, C.H. *et al.* (2012) Moving the agenda forward: a person-centred framework in long-term care. *International Journal of Older People Nursing,* 7(4): 303–9. doi: 10.1111/opn.12010.

National Research Corporation (2015) *Eight Dimensions of Patient-Centered Care.* Available at: www.nationalresearch.com/products-and-solutions/patient-and-family-experience/eight-dimensions-of-patient-centered-care/#sthash.8SSWxqC1.dpuf (accessed 4 November 2015).

National Voices (2013) Who we are and what we do. Available at: www.nationalvoices.org.uk/who-we-are-and-what-we-do (accessd 4 November 2015).

NHS England/Coalition for Collaborative Care (2015) Building the house: the house of care toolkit. Available at: www.nhsiq.nhs.uk/improvement-programmes/long-term-conditions-and-integrated-care/long-term-conditions-improvement-programme/house-of-care-tool-kit.aspx (accessed 5 November 2015).

Nursing and Midwifery Council (2015) *The Code.* Available at: www.nmc.org.uk/standards/code/read-the-code-online/#fivth (accessed 4 November 2015).

Olsson, L., Jakobsson, E., Swedberg, K. and Ekman, I. (2012) Efficacy of person-centred care as an intervention in controlled trials – a systematic review, *Journal of Clinical Nursing,* 22(3–4): 456–65, DOI: 10.1111/jocn.12039

Peplau, H.E. (1952) Interpersonal relations in nursing, in J. George (ed.) *Nursing Theories: The Base for Professional Nursing Practice.* Norwalk, CT: Appleton & Lange.

Royal College of Nursing (2003) Defining Nursing. Available at: www.rcn.org.uk/__data/assets/pdf_file/0003/604038/Defining_Nursing_Web.pdf (accessed 4 November 2015).

St Michael's Hospital Ontario (2015) Mission and values. Available at: www.stmichaelshospital.com/about/values.php (accessed 4 November 2015).

Tadd, W., Hillman, A., Calnan, S. *et al.* (2011) *Dignity in Practice: An Exploration of the Care of Older Adults in Acute NHS Trusts. Preventing Abuse and Neglect in Institutional Care of Older Adults.* London: Department of Health and Comic Relief and HMSO.

Tee, S.R. (2012) Service user involvement – addressing the crisis in confidence in health-care (editorial), *Nurse Education Today*. Available at: http://dx.doi.org/10.1016/j.nedt.2011.12.002

Willis, P. (2015) *Raising the Bar: Shape of Caring: A Review of the Future Education and Training of Registered Nurses and Care Assistants*. London: Health Education England in partnership with the Nursing and Midwifery Council.

Developing person-centred services

The contribution of experience-based co-design to high quality nursing care

Glenn Robert

LEARNING OUTCOMES:

- Understand what it feels like for nurses to take part in person-centred quality improvement 'work'
- Understand the key benefits and challenges of trying to make services more patient centred from a nursing perspective
- Reflect on what it means for person-centred quality improvement 'work' to be 'humanizing'

Introduction

In contrast to the rest of this volume this chapter begins from the perspective – not of patients – but of nurses. Specifically, I explore how individual nurses feel about taking part in a quality improvement intervention aimed at enabling the delivery of person-centred services. In doing so I describe, first, what it means to nurses to actively engage in such endeavours and, secondly, how such participation impacts on their own behaviours and practices in relation to PCC.

The chapter takes as its focus a particular quality improvement intervention called experience-based co-design (EBCD) which is briefly outlined below. It then presents findings from an international survey of EBCD projects to highlight the range of impacts that taking part in such projects has had on nurses. I then review the findings from four published case studies to illustrate these impacts in more detail. The EBCD case studies I shall draw on took place within:

- four services in an Integrated Cancer Centre (Farr 2012, 2013; Tsianakas *et al.*, 2012; Adams *et al.*, 2014)
- two Intensive Care Units (Locock *et al.*, 2014a)
- a cohort of carers of patients receiving outpatient chemotherapy (Ream *et al.*, 2013)
- seven emergency departments (Iedema *et al.*, 2010; Piper *et al.*, 2012).

The chapter concludes with a discussion of the impact on nurses of participating in EBCD projects and the implications this has for the development and delivery of person-centred services. As part of this discussion, I draw on the work of Todres *et al.* (2009) to speculate on the 'humanising' effect on nurses of taking part in such person-centred quality improvement interventions.

Experience-based co-design

Experience-based co-design is an approach to improving healthcare services that combines participatory and user experience design tools and processes to bring about quality improvements in healthcare organizations (Bate and Robert 2007a; Donetto *et al.*, 2014; Robert *et al.*, 2015). Through a 'co-design' process the approach entails staff, patients and carers reflecting on their experiences of a service, working together to identify improvement priorities, devising and implementing changes, and then jointly reflecting on their achievements. As explained elsewhere four overlapping strands of thought have contributed to the development of the EBCD approach (Robert 2013), namely:

- Participatory action research
- User-centred design
- Learning theory
- Narrative-based approaches to change

In particular, user-centred design offers two particular contributions to quality improvement thinking in the healthcare sector: a new lens, or frame of mind, through which to think about approaches to improving patient experiences of healthcare, and methods, tools and techniques (such as modelling and prototyping) which were little used in healthcare improvement work until recently (Robert *et al.*, 2015).

Drawing explicitly on such design theory and practice, an EBCD cycle (see Figure 2.1) typically has six stages (Bate and Robert 2007a; Robert 2013; Robert *et al.*, 2015):

1   setting up the project;
2   engaging staff and gathering their experiences through observation and in-depth interviews;

3   engaging patients and carers and gathering their experiences through 12–15 filmed narrative-based interviews;

4   bringing staff, patients and carers together in a first co-design meeting to share their experiences of a service and identify their shared priorities for improvement, prompted by an edited 30-minute 'trigger' film of the patient narratives;

5   sustained small co-design teamwork over a period of 3–4 months in small groups formed around those priorities (typically 4–6); and

6   a 'celebration' and review event. Importantly, the filmed patient narratives set the process apart from other consultative formats in which anonymity and circumspection can hinder rather than enable quality improvement.

Both a full description of the original pilot work in a head and neck cancer service (Bate and Robert 2007b) and a free-to-access online EBCD toolkit for practitioners to use (King's Fund 2012) are available.

How does participating in an EBCD project impact upon nursing staff?

International survey of EBCD projects

In this section I focus on an international online survey of EBCD projects undertaken in 2013. In carrying out this survey, we also conducted 18 follow-up telephone interviews with a sample of the respondents (Donetto *et al.*, 2014). The survey identified 59 EBCD projects which had been implemented in six countries worldwide during the period 2005–2013;

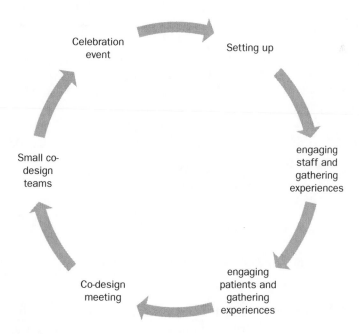

Figure 2.1 The EBCD process

a further 27 projects were in the planning stage at the time of the survey. We found that EBCD has been implemented in a variety of clinical areas (including emergency medicine, drug and alcohol services, a range of cancer services, paediatrics, diabetes care and mental health services). The respondents reported that EBCD projects typically take between 6–12 months to complete and that the free-to-access, online EBCD toolkit is a helpful resource for those leading projects.

The interviewees identified a range of specific impacts on staff of participating in an EBCD project:

Box 2.1   Impacts on staff of participating in an EBCD project

- Emotional impact of hearing the patient voice through films and co-design events
- Changing attitudes about ways of working and towards listening to patients
- Reminding staff why they do what they do, leading to behavioural impacts by changing the way staff do things
- Staff felt listened to
- Staff were encouraged and motivated by hearing from patients what they are doing well (i.e. not just about the negative aspects of the care patients received)
- Gave staff a different outlook/perspective to the way they work
- A desire among staff to work with patients more often in the future
- Increased staff knowledge (e.g. greater understanding of how other departments operate/function).

Source: Donetto *et al.*, 2014

Reader activity

Try this reflective exercise:

Think about the last time you were really engaged and enthused in a project at work.

Did the experience of taking part in that project mirror the type of impacts summarized in Box 2.1 And described in the quotations below?

Why was this?

One interviewee spoke very strongly about the impact participating in an EBCD project had had on her personally:

It was one of the most meaningful things I've ever done in my entire career I think. That sounds really trite, but I really do mean it, it was wonderful. I am glad I had the opportunity even though I felt like an emotional ragdoll by the end of it. It was a great experience. If we could do more of it I think it would really help. It's the level of engagement that we should do, but we just don't invest the time, and the energy, and the money. We wait for complaints . . .

(Interview#05)

Interviewees highlighted how the act of participating in an EBCD project had both affected and changed the way in which nurses thought about their work and interactions with their patients: 'It did help change their [staff] attitude towards really listening . . . and [showed] the value of actually spending some time out of the operational frontline, and that patients had something valuable to say' (Interview#02). Another interviewee commented that taking part in the project had 'brought back her passion for the work that she does' and that a colleague had said that it 'really affected her in a big way; she had never thought about the boxes that we put people in and the impact that has on people' (Interview#14). The sentiment in the latter quotation was echoed in several of the interviews:

. . . that being involved in the whole project gave [the nurses] a different outlook, a different insight into how they're doing their work . . . And, although we always try to be patient focused or whatever, sometimes we think we are, and we're not. And, I think that by doing the [EBCD] project, people are really beginning to realize that maybe we do need to listen to patients and family more . . . we don't know everything as healthcare professionals . . . It's just been an eye-opener.

(Interview#03)

Many of them said, 'Wow, I've never stopped to think of the patient perspective, but hearing it in their voice I can see now . . .' – they just get to see that different viewpoint, and the impact of what they do on patients that they'd sort of stopped, and never had time to consider, it just wasn't in their frame of reference.

(Interview#12)

In the follow-up interviews we also explored in more detail the advantages and disadvantages of filming patient interviews, a key component of the EBCD approach. Eight of the 18 interviewees had used film to gather patient experiences and they spoke about the power of hearing the patient voice and the impact of film on staff members. The majority of those who had used film in their projects confirmed they would use it again in future projects:

Film was a very important part of helping staff take a step back and have a look at what was really going on, and see people they've been treating as patients as just people, as human beings . . . it had a dramatic effect for the staff to suddenly see someone who they only perceive, for example, as a problem . . . seeing somebody's face, hearing their voice, it made a difference. I think if you hadn't seen that, if they had just been written down, it would have just been words. Having that there in front of them made a big difference. You could measure that in the room.

(Interview#02)

Now what we found is by showing the staff the films, just showing them, that that had a really big impact. So when we were evaluating why did we show these films to so many people, and why we have subsequently repeated that exercise, it's because the act of watching the films themselves, actually, the feedback was that they reflected quite a lot themselves about how they communicate with patients as well.

(Interview#09)

Several spoke of how viewing the patient films elicited a strong emotional response from nurses, contrasting the impact with that of just reading patient experience data:

When you see the video and you can see the emotion and you can see what's happened . . . it's very hard to argue with an experience. You can't argue with that; it's their experience. If it's just written down it's easy to dismiss, it's easy to dismiss opinions. When it's in your face and you see it, it has a much deeper psychological impact.

(Interview#03)

Given the strength of the responses, interviewees also cautioned for the need to manage the process of viewing the films:

The power just blows me away because as soon as the story comes up there's a physical change, they go back in their seats and it's quite confronting even though you prepare them for it and say, 'This is what I'm going to show you.' And these are clinicians that see this stuff every day, but just to be taken out of their clinical environment, to sit and be actually talking about the interaction is so powerful. So yes I would use it more, but I would prepare people more too because sometimes it can be too confronting.

(Interview#12)

On the basis of the survey and interview findings we suggested six priorities for the ongoing development of EBCD as a quality improvement intervention that seeks to enhance PCC:

- providing training and support to staff in order to transfer knowledge and skills, and thereby build capacity, for facilitating such projects within healthcare systems;
- the continuing use of non-participant observation (as devoting even short periods of time to sitting and watching seemingly mundane day-to-day activities can provide rich insights into how and why things work – or not – and how they might be redesigned for the better);
- recognizing the use of film as an important catalyst in the co-design process; the visualization of patient experiences helps (re)connect people – including staff – with similar experiences and stories and offers an emotionally and cognitively powerful starting point for the co-design process;
- reinforcing the fundamental importance of co-design itself as lying at the very core of EBCD, underpinning service change as well as the broader impacts on staff well-being and behaviours (whilst recognizing that it is also, in practice, the most challenging aspect of EBCD);

- developing greater understanding of the nature and scale of changes brought into practice through EBCD – whilst EBCD projects are initially more likely to bring about a series of incremental quality improvements rather than radical organizational change, the individual and collaborative work underpinning these small changes lies at the root of deeper changes in staff attitudes and behaviours;
- strengthening the evidence base – research priorities for the future include learning much more about which person-centred quality improvement interventions are most cost-effective and what proportion of an organization's limited resources can justifiably be dedicated to such activities.

Following this broad overview of the 'state of the art' of EBCD around the world, I now move on to describing nurses' experiences of participating in four specific EBCD case studies. For each, I provide a brief overview of the context and aims of the EBCD project – further information can be found in the references provided – before then reviewing the evidence of the impact upon nurses as reported by the authors of the various studies.

Case study 1: Integrated Cancer Centre (Farr 2012; Farr 2013; Tsianakas *et al.*, 2012; Adams *et al.*, 2014)

The primary aim of this project was to use EBCD to identify and implement improvements in the patient experiences of two breast and two lung cancer services that were part of an Integrated Cancer Centre. In addition, one of the studies also sought to explore participants' reflections on the value and key characteristics of this approach to improving patient experiences (Tsianakas *et al.*, 2012). In keeping with the EBCD approach, fieldwork involved 36 filmed narrative patient interviews, 219 hours of ethnographic observation, 63 staff interviews and a facilitated co-design change process involving patient and staff interviewees over a 12-month period. Four of the staff and five patients were interviewed about their views on the value of the approach and its key characteristics. The project setting was a large, inner-city cancer centre in England.

Sixty-two quality improvements (or 'co-design solutions') were identified and implemented across the original four Cancer Centre services as a result of EBCD (Adams *et al.*, 2014). Farr (2012) reports that participants of successful co-design teams felt that their involvement in the project had been very beneficial and it had both significant organizational and personal impact: 'I think the process has been brilliant . . . I think that what we have gained from it is enormous, and I don't think we would have got anywhere near as far in solving some of these issues if we hadn't done this'. It was reported that key to the success of the project was the strong relationship between patients and staff that has been built over time (Tsianakas *et al.*, 2012). This team or community aspect was remarked upon consistently by those staff participants who were interviewed:

[T]he patients are actually very supportive in the way in which they respond to the staff. That's something that I found quite surprising about this as an approach. On paper, it might feel that it's a bit confrontational, but the reality is that it's very much about bringing about understanding between people who are coming at things from a different perspective.

(Tsianakas *et al.*, 2012: 2645) Farr (2012: 31) also reports that viewing the patient film at the co-design event had a powerful effect on staff: 'I just got so overwhelmed with the emotion of it . . . I just had this huge lump in my throat and I remember thinking, "if I feel this way, it must be a really good thing to get involved in" because it stirred me enough to want to change something.' Staff also found the co-design event itself very powerful: 'It felt really good actually because there were all these different groups and to see all the key members of the team actually taking part in it – so there was a feeling, "Gosh, maybe something can really happen here"' (p. 31) However, levels of staff engagement within the projects varied and this became apparent to some patients at these events.

The impact of involvement in the project had the potential to be intense, both for staff and for patients. Staff were concerned about how their services were experienced by patients: 'For the staff, it's shocking, it's like, we're hoping that we have done a really good job and you hear that in some places we are getting it hopelessly wrong. That's just gutting' (p.33); 'Some staff have found it very challenging. I think staff find it very hard to hear they are delivering services badly and I think you have to think about the support in that, because it will never be an individual's fault, it will be some organizational complexity' (p.33) Staff themselves spoke about the impact that the project had had on them or those that they worked closely with:

> It was interesting, because patients were actually giving me feedback on me, all those years ago, I don't mind, people say what they want to say about me, I mean it is quite interesting, even if it is a negative and you think, "well, thanks for that, and I will take it on board and change it". But I think thank goodness I didn't get any negative . . .
>
> (p. 33)

> At first, they seemed to take it as an assault on them, it was just a big attack, saying that you need to work harder. But when we explained that we are doing this because something is wrong, not because you are wrong, we need to look at it and see how we can change it so that it works for us and our patients. So they put in a lot of good ideas actually about changing the way the systems work . . . So it did work out.
>
> (p. 33)

Farr (2012) proposes that the EBCD process is based on the idea of collective action, involving different people in generating 'movements' for change and that this collaborative approach was seen to be highly significant to many of the participants who took part. She reports that people spoke of a sense in which hierarchical relationships were dissolved to some extent within the space of a co-design group and that everybody was working together toward common goals (Farr 2012). Having patients involved and participating in these groups was seen as an important catalyst to change. People spoke about how the conversations that they had in co-design groups were quite different to traditional meetings; there was less of a sense of blame amongst staff and a more active focus. Farr (2012) concludes that in order to enable this process to work effectively, trusting relationships need to be facilitated both between different staff groups and between staff and patients, especially where patients are still receiving treatment and may be reliant on particular services.

Two years after the end of this EBCD project a 'spread and sustainability' study was conducted in the same cancer centre (Adams *et al.*, 2014). Two of the research objectives were to examine: (1) whether specific improvements made in the breast and two lung cancer services as a result of EBCD had been sustained and if further potential areas for improvement continue to be identified and acted upon in these services; and (2) whether the underlying PCC philosophy of EBCD had had a broader impact within the cancer centre.

Adams *et al.* (2014) found that overall, 19–22 months after initial implementation, 39 (66 per cent) of the 56 co-design solutions on which the researchers were able to collate data were sustained. The authors' qualitative findings highlighted the success of the EBCD approach in supporting strategic leaders to promote new approaches to quality improvement in some clinical and operational areas. However, the impact of the EBCD approach in terms of supporting the wider professional workforce were less clear; some subsequent clinician-led attempts to co-design services with patients without wider, formal organizational support and engagement had negative effects on the workforce (and, in some circumstances, on their commitment to future quality improvement work). For example some members of staff felt that the work on decision-making fell beyond their own as well as patients' responsibility and skill:

> I can [say] 'well this is my dream house' but I'm not a builder or an architect [in reality] . . . somebody else needs to put it on paper and come back to me and say 'I'll just check with you that it's alright' and then will go off and do it . . . so with EBCD I don't think that it is our job to be sorting out services.
>
> (Adams *et al.*, 2014: 24)

The impact of EBCD on collaborative decision-making with patients was also found to be highly varied across the four services and, overall, not extensive (although there was positive evidence of impact in terms of individual clinician-patient encounters). Staff, as well as patients, had a range of different understandings of the nature of collaborative decision-making and what was necessary – or 'appropriate' – for patients. Other members of staff reflected on the emotional demands of working alongside patients, for example: '[The co-design group was] nerve wracking, I was sitting across a [meeting] table from a woman that I knew, I'd looked at her scan and I was going to have to tell her that her cancer had come back in the next clinic . . . and she's telling me how brilliant her life is . . .' (p.48).

Adams *et al.* (2014) also report a marked difference between the expectations of senior cancer centre staff and the practices of frontline clinical as well as more junior service improvement staff. Thus, one member of staff remarked that: '[for] the amount of time it takes you need to get some really good stuff out of it . . . changing [things] a little bit . . . that's good, but is that good enough?' (Donetto *et al.*, 2014: 46), whilst a more experienced staff member commented (p. 46): '[People talk about minor but] How minor? If that minor change affects 100 people that year, and it's a better experience for 100 people, how wonderful is that?'. It appeared that frontline staff were convinced by improvement outcomes that were more immediate, tangible and larger scale whilst senior clinical and improvement staff approached improvement as a longer term and incremental process.

Case study 2: Intensive Care Units and lung cancer services in England (Locock *et al.*, 2014a)

This project aimed to evaluate an 'accelerated' form of EBCD in terms of how speeding up the implementation of the approach affected the process and outcomes of the intervention (Locock *et al.*, 2014a; Locock *et al.*, 2014b). Whilst retaining all components of EBCD, the adapted approach:

- replaced local patient interviews with secondary analysis of a national archive of patient experience narratives to create national trigger films;
- shortened the timeframe; and
- employed local improvement facilitators.

This form of EBCD was then tested in the intensive care units (ICU) and lung cancer services in two English National Health Service (NHS) hospitals. A total of 96 clinical staff (primarily nursing and medical), and 63 patients and family members participated in the co-design activities. An ethnographic process evaluation of an adapted form of EBCD was conducted, including observations, interviews, questionnaires and documentary analysis.

The observations of the staff events by the ethnographer, and in interviews with the facilitators and others involved in the process, revealed the positive impact that participating in the projects had on staff (Locock *et al.*, 2014a). As the study authors report the evaluation data suggest that the face-to-face encounters with patients often had a profound effect on staff in making them think differently about their practice and reconnect with their core professional values, resulting in a renewed sense of motivation. A senior manager in one site reported that a member of staff in intensive care had said it was the first time in more than 20 years of practice that he had sat down and talked to patients in this way. A senior lung cancer nurse (unprompted) told a meeting of the project advisory group that it was the most inspiring thing she had done in her professional career. One of the co-design group leads (intensive care) described her experience of the process:

> It was very interesting. It was a light bulb moment, because you had four different groups, nurses, doctors, patients, and relatives. It was one of the first times I've sat down and talked about the same problem and how we all view it, and some of the things other people were concerned about I didn't think anything of that, and then at the same time some of the things I thought were important, other people didn't think they were important. It was very, very interesting. It made me realise what a crazy system we are working in at the moment. People are doing their own things; they are assuming lots of things.
>
> (Locock *et al.*, 2014a: 24)

Staff consistently identified having space and time to reflect on their own practices and how these impacted upon patients as a key benefit of their participation in the EBCD project:

> I think the most important things were that staff really appreciated the time to think about the experience. It became apparent that they perhaps didn't have or make time to reflect on what they do in their daily workings, so I think they actually found it quite cathartic and therapeutic. It actually raised the thinking of experience, and I think the

staff really appreciated that their point of view was being listened to because up until that point the political drive had always been patient experience and now all of a sudden we were interested in staff experience.

(Facilitator, interview; Locock *et al.*, 2014a: 24–5)

Such reflection often led to changes in practice as illustrated by one nurse who commented that 'I have already changed the way I think and care for patients even though we haven't started implementing changes yet. I have a better understanding now of how things are from the patients' perspective'.

As the evaluation of the intervention reported, it is possible that some staff might feel unable to voice major concerns or disagreement with the process without appearing to lack empathy or to place low priority on patient experience (Locock *et al.*, 2014a). The authors note that staff were assured of anonymity in giving their feedback but in a defined service area people may not trust that this will be the case. However, the fieldwork observations suggest genuine enthusiasm rather than socially desirable compliance. There were some comments about the time commitment required, but overall the feedback suggested that staff felt it was a good investment of time compared with some other organizational activities, and one that was likely to improve morale rather than threaten it.

Case study 3: Carers of patients receiving outpatient chemotherapy in London, England (Ream *et al.*, 2013)

The aim of this EBCD project – the third case study in this chapter – was to develop an intervention for carers in the chemotherapy outpatient setting and then test it. A three-phase mixed methods research design was used. Phases I and II addressed the development of the intervention using EBCD; data collection for Phase I comprised 20 hours of non-participant observation, 20 semi-structured interviews with staff members and 20 filmed narrative-based interviews with carers. Healthcare professionals and carers were then given the opportunity in Phase II to co-design an intervention for carers supporting someone through chemotherapy. The process of co-designing the intervention involved two facilitated feedback events where findings from Phase I were fed back to (1) healthcare professionals (Staff) involved in phase I and (2) carers interviewed in phase I. Following these was a third event referred to as a 'co-design event' that was attended by both carers and staff where the elements of the intervention were designed and refined. Phase III of the study aimed to test and evaluate the carer support package developed in Phase II through a small randomized feasibility trial. Finally, two focus groups were conducted at the end of the study – one with carers and the other with staff. These explored the feasibility and acceptability of the intervention. All phases of the study were undertaken in a chemotherapy day unit of a large teaching hospital in London.

As Ream *et al.* (2013) describe the co-design process led to the development of what became known as the 'Take Care' intervention which comprised: a supportive/educative DVD, accompanying booklet and one-hour group consultation facilitated by a chemotherapy nurse after the pre-chemotherapy consultation but prior to beginning first cycle of treatment. 'Take Care' included preparatory information, advice and practical tips from carers and staff about supporting someone through chemotherapy. It addressed topics such as: treatment side effects, the impact of being a carer and dealing with emotions, the importance of taking time out for themselves and accessing support as well as hospital-specific information such as maps and contact numbers. The support package was delivered in one-off consultations by one of two chemotherapy nurses trained in group facilitation. It was provided to groups of no more than five carers. Consultations provided carers opportunity to watch the DVD and engage in conversation facilitated by the chemotherapy nurse about chemotherapy. Carers were provided a copy of both the 'Take Care' DVD and booklet and were encouraged to consult both if and when they needed information and/or support during the patients' treatment. In the feasibility trial (Phase III) the intervention proved acceptable to both carers and Staff and demonstrated considerable promise and utility in practice. The findings suggested that the intervention warranted investigation within the context of a fully powered randomized controlled trial to determine effectiveness and cost effectiveness.

Focus group participants felt the project was worthwhile and felt positive about their involvement in the EBCD process. The most positive aspect of being involved was hearing the carers' voices through the initial film and the co-design events, which as many commented, are not often heard:

> I think we really, really heard the carers' voices, I think that was, for me very, very powerful. And that, they're quite unheard actually, even compared to patients' voices, which I think are getting louder, as it were. But to hear carer's voices was very significant, and very, very moving watching the film of carers talking about their experiences.
>
> (Ream *et al.*, 2013: 154)

Participants said that the events provided a forum for carers to speak honestly and openly with other carers about their experience, as one commented (p.154):

> It was impressive actually. And I thought how it was structured, you know, from the beginning, the introducing the other person. That worked well, in that event. People very much got involved in that. Quite interesting actually, if you think that's often used with staff groups and in training, and I've experienced staff groups being much more reserved . . . these were carers who'd never met the other carers and they were confident actually, and forthcoming in talking . . . people felt at ease, comfortable, they were cared for . . .

The facilitator of the carer, staff and joint events was asked about the difference of working with carers rather than with patients as has been done in the past in other EBCD projects (p.154):

> I think some of the conversations were slightly different, and I think that the carers wouldn't have said a lot of those things in front of patients, because they wouldn't have wanted the patients to feel bad about kind of, almost what they were causing, even though it wasn't the patients causing that, it was the cancer that was causing all of that. I think that was the surprising bit about the carers, and what happened in the event where we brought the carers together, was that they did turn to each other and go, 'blimey you've gone through the same thing as I have', and previous to that they only knew that that's what they were going through.

As Ream *et al.* (2013) reported, staff highlighted the main impacts of the package were to: empower carers and increase their confidence; increase carers' knowledge and awareness; and increase carer support by reducing their anxiety. The legitimization of the carer role was also highlighted. Staff were satisfied with the components of the 'Take Care' support package and considered the DVD and leaflet to be a complementary package. They valued the carer consultations as a useful forum at which carers could receive information and address concerns. The chemotherapy nurses who delivered the consultations spoke about the benefits of group consultations but pointed out the potential difficulties of managing group dynamics. Staff agreed that the intervention should be delivered to carers at the pre-chemotherapy consultation but be followed up to ensure their needs were met at later stages. They agreed that the chemotherapy nurses were best placed to offer this intervention but emphasized the importance of establishing processes for carers and working across hospital disciplines to support them such as linking in with clinical nurse specialists.

Case study 4: emergency departments in New South Wales, Australia (Iedema *et al.*, 2010; Piper *et al.*, 2012)

This final case study encompasses three multisite evaluations of EBCD projects that were conducted in emergency departments (EDs) and associated departments in seven public hospitals in New South Wales, Australia. The data for the evaluations were derived from: EBCD documentation provided by the participating sites; interviews with 117 key informants; performance data and the policy and academic literature on EBCD.

In their evaluation, Piper *et al.* (2012: 167) concluded that:

> For those participating in EBCD, its 'co-production' approach paid off at two levels. First, it gave patients, carers and staff a deeper understanding of each others' experience. It provided an opportunity to work meaningfully together, and this strengthened relationships among those involved in EBCD. Second, EBCD produced change in ways and at levels that mattered to consumers, and this appreciation refracted back onto clinicians.

Aside from the successful implementation of the solutions, the data analysis revealed that interviewees perceived co-design to harbour three main benefits (see Box 2.2):

Box 2.2 Main benefits of EBCD in emergency departments

- The ability of co-design to involve a wide variety of stakeholders, including consumers;
- The potential for the solutions implemented to spread within the hospital and to other sites;
- The implementation of staff and patient and carer interviews in other clinical settings as a tool for promoting and facilitating patient-centred care.

Source: Adapted from Piper *et al.* (2012)

Piper *et al.* (2012) reported that participants commented positively on the experience of deliberating with patients and hearing their experiences. A recurrent theme in their interview responses was we are learning to see our work through the patients' eyes: 'I think that everybody should go on a meeting with consumers . . . because they actually see what's on the other side' (Iedema *et al.*, 2010: 80); 'It [co-design] made us look at things from the patient's perspective much more' (p. 80); 'Listening to the patient experiences does open your eyes. You pick up on things. You think . . . oh my God, how did we do that?' (p. 80). Despite these benefits, interviewees perceived several challenges in sustaining the principles and solutions of co-design (Box 2.3):

Box 2.3   Challenges in sustaining impact

- the uncertain project status of Co-design;
- restricted appointment and role of implementation of officers and clinical leads of working groups;
- the need for improved communication of solutions and project status to project and frontline staff;
- the need for ongoing documentation and measurement of project status and solutions;
- the problem of staff turnover;
- the need for ongoing training and education;
- the need for strong executive commitment, day-to-day leadership and identification of key messengers;
- the importance of site readiness; and
- the challenges of maintaining consumer engagement.

Source: Adapted from Piper *et al.* (2012)

Reader activity

Try this reflective exercise:

Think about a recent project or initiative that you were involved with where any benefits or impact were not sustained over time.

Why do you think this was?
Were there similar challenges to those shown in Box 2.3?
What could have been done to overcome these?

Interviewees therefore saw some aspects of the co-design project as challenging. For instance, the process required them to explain ED processes 'over and over again' to patient and caregiver participants: 'They [consumers] didn't know what was going on. . . I had to tell them over and over again, I had to tell them more from the beginning to the end, that was the biggest impact.' This comment points to the effort involved in bridging clinicians', patients' and caregivers' understanding, and reveals the potential for conflict. As Iedema *et al.* (2010) argue, the difference in stakeholders' knowledge and understanding necessitates not just the giving and receiving of explanations but also the need to keep the conversation going by ensuring that the differences in understanding do not lead to conflict, miscommunication or non-communication. As the authors argue, 'practical solutions are contingent on participants (patients, caregivers and staff) discursively negotiating common ground, both technically and interpersonally, before an improvement solution becomes apparent and can be coarticulated' (p. 81).

Discussion: humanizing healthcare

The brief exploration in this chapter of how nurses react to taking part in a quality improvement intervention aimed at enabling the delivery of person-centred services has sought to illustrate what it means to nurses to actively engage in such endeavours and how such participation impacts on their own behaviours and practices in relation to PCC.

In reviewing studies of EBCD projects – such as those summarized in the preceding pages – one recurring theme from observing and interviewing nursing staff participants is that of 'connection', or rather – as it was often framed by interviewees themselves – the reconnection of nursing staff to the reasons they became nurses in the first place. In the follow-up interviews to the international survey participants reflected on the 'different insights . . . outlooks' the process provided, as well as it 'being the most meaningful thing I've done in my career'. And so it is that nurses in the first case study in a cancer centre talk of being 'stirred enough' to want to change something; those in the second case study speak of 'light bulb moments' and the importance of having time to reflect and think; in the third case study of how 'moving' and 'powerful' it was to hear the carer's voice; and then in the final case study describe the impact of the process in terms of 'opening our eyes'. Such responses are in stark contrast to the way in which staff commonly react (if they react at all) to feedback of anonymous patient survey results (Robert and Cornwell, 2013; Coulter *et al.*, 2014) which remains the dominant form of attempts to influence PCC in contemporary health care systems.

I would like to draw a parallel here with Todres *et al.*'s, (2009) distinction between the 'humanizing' and 'dehumanizing' potential of qualitative research. Todres *et al.* (2009: 68) argue that whilst '[q]ualitative research, through its illumination of people's perspectives and experiences, has contributed a particular kind of useful evidence for caring practices', it has not fulfilled its potential in terms of impacting on behaviours and practices. They proposed that qualitative research needs to be 'translated into practice in ways that place people as human beings at the centre of care' (p. 68) and propose 'eight philosophically informed dimensions of humanization, which together, form a framework that constitutes a comprehensive value base for considering both the potentially humanizing and dehumanizing elements in caring systems and interactions' (p. 68; see Table 2.1).

The adoption of qualitative research methods (non-participant observation, narrative-based interviews) in EBCD or other patient-centred quality improvement interventions do seem to lend themselves to the 'forms of humanization' proposed by Todres *et al.* (2009).

Table 2.1 Conceptual framework of the Dimensions of Humanization

Forms of humanization	Forms of dehumanization
Insiderness	Objectification
Agency	Passivity
Uniqueness	Homogenization
Togetherness	Isolation
Sense-making	Loss of meaning
Personal journey	Loss of personal journey
Sense of place	Dislocation
Embodiment	Reductionist body

Source: Todres *et al.* 2009: 70.

The interviews with staff and observational data of EBCD events and processes point towards feelings of, for example, agency ('to experience oneself as making choices and being generally held accountable for one's actions'), togetherness ('makes possible the experience of empathy in which we can appreciate the suffering and struggles of "the other"'), and sense-making ('an impetus or motivation to bring things together, to find significance and to make wholes out of parts'). In contrast, so much of what is represented as 'person-centred' in health care organizations – the ubiquitous use of surveys, anonymous feedback and reduction of narratives to data 'points' – tends to the right hand column of Table 2.1, leading to the objectification of patient (and staff) experience, and to seeing (and treating) patients and carers as passive, isolated and dislocated.

Reader activity

Try this reflective exercise:

Thinking about Table 2.1, Can you relate your own experiences of taking part in (or leading) different projects to the two columns?

What was it about those projects that made them either 'humanizing' or 'dehumanizing'?

Summary

Even the brief review presented here of the survey results and four case studies attests to the challenges of adopting and implementing quality improvement interventions designed to improve PCC. Simply adopting qualitative research methods and striving to ensure that they are applied within a 'humanizing' process is insufficient; our survey results and case studies also illustrate the challenging contexts in which such methods and processes have to be implemented and, crucially, sustained. It is still the case that much of what is done in the name of improving PCC serves only to dehumanize what should be one of the most humanizing aspects of anyone's life: a shared encounter with healthcare services and the nursing staff that work within them. Experience-based co-design and other such participatory approaches may offer one route to not only over-coming these unplanned consequences but also enriching the experiences of both staff and their patients.

References

Adams, M., Maben, J. and Robert, G. (2014) *Improving Patient-Centred Care through Experience-based Co-design (EBCD). An Evaluation of the Sustainability* and *Spread of EBCD in a Cancer Centre.* London: King's College London.

Bate, S.P. and Robert, G. (2007a) *Bringing User Experience to Health Care Improvement: The Concepts, Methods and Practices of Experience-based Design.* Oxford: Radcliffe Publishing.

Bate, S.P. and Robert, G. (2007b) Towards more user-centric organisational development: lessons from a case study of experience-based design, *The Journal of Applied Behavioural Science*, 43(1): 41–66.

Coulter, A., Locock, L., Ziebland, S. and Calabrese', J. (2014) Collecting data on patient experience is not enough: they must be used to improve care, *British Medical Journal*, 348: g2225.

Donetto, S., Tsianakas, V. and Robert, G. (2014) *Using Experience-based Co-design to Improve the Quality of Healthcare: Mapping Where We are Now and Establishing Future Directions.* London: King's College London.

Farr, M. (2012) *Patient Centred Care and Experience-Based Co-Design. The King's Fund Evaluation Report.* Unpublished report.

Farr, M. (2013) Collaboration in public services: Can service users and staff participate together?, in M. Barnes and P. Cotterell (eds) *Critical Perspective on User Involvement.* Bristol: Policy Press.

Iedema, R., Merrick, E., Piper, D. *et al.* (2010) Co-designing as discursive practice in emergency health services: the architecture of deliberation, *Journal of Applied Behavioral Science*, 46: 73–91.

King's Fund (2012) Experience-based co-design toolkit. London: The King's Fund. Available at www.kingsfund.org.uk/projects/point-care/ebcd (accessed February 2014).

Locock, L., Robert, G., Boaz, A. *et al.* (2014a) Testing accelerated experience-based co-design: a qualitative study of using a national archive of patient experience narrative interviews to promote rapid patient-centred service improvement, *Health Services and Delivery Research*, 2(4): 1–122.

Locock, L., Robert, G., Boaz, A. *et al.* (2014b) Using a national archive of patient experience narratives to promote local patient-centred quality improvement: an ethnographic process evaluation of 'accelerated' Experience-based Co-design, *Journal of Health Services Research* and *Policy*, 19(4): 200–7.

Piper, D., Iedema, R., Gray, J. *et al.* (2012) Utilizing Experience-based Co-design to improve the experience of patients accessing emergency departments in New South Wales public hospitals: an evaluation study, *Health Services Management Research*, 25: 162–72.

Ream, E., Tsianakas, V., Verity, R. *et al.* (2013) *Enhancing the Role of Carers in the Outpatient Chemotherapy Setting: A Participatory Action Research Project.* London: King's College London. Available at: www.dimblebycancercare.org/wp-content/uploads/2013/09/Dimbleby-report-executive-summary-pdf-3rd-Sept.pdf (accessed 4 November 2015).

Robert, G. (2013) Participatory action research: using experience-based co-design (EBCD) to improve health care services, in S. Ziebland, J. Calabrase, A. Coulter and L. Locock (eds) *Understanding and Using Experiences of Health and Illness.* Oxford: Oxford University Press.

Robert, G. and Cornwell, J. (2013) Designing the future: rethinking policy approaches to measuring and improving patient experience, *Journal of Health Services Research* and *Policy*, 18(2): 67–8.

Robert, G., Cornwell, J., Locock, L. *et al.* (2015) Patients and staff as co-designers of health care services, *British Medical Journal*, 350: g7714.

Todres, L., Galvin, T. and Holloway, I. (2009) The humanisation of health care: a value framework for qualitative research, *International Journal of Qualitative Studies on Health and Wellbeing*, 4: 68–77.

Tsianakas, V., Robert, G., Maben, J. *et al.* (2012) Implementing patient centred cancer care: using experience-based co-design to improve patient experience in breast and lung cancer services, *Supportive Care in Cancer*, 20(11): 2639–47.

CHILDREN, YOUNG PEOPLE AND THEIR FAMILIES

Person-centred maternity care

Sophie French and Ruth Adekoya

Every conception, pregnancy and birth is a unique event and there is a fundamentally particular story behind every woman's experience and the start of every baby's life. For women the experiences of motherhood are often profound, bringing a transformation in life circumstances, expectations, relationships and responsibilities. Beliefs as to what is considered 'best' for mothers and their babies often link to complex assumptions around how and why choices should be made. In the light of increasing national and global expenditure on maternity care and affiliated clinical negligence, there is increasing interest in developing and evaluating economically viable partnership care models that balance the rights and choices of individuals with those of wider society.

This chapter will explore PCC perspectives during preconception, antenatal, intra-partum and postnatal maternity care. For the purpose of this chapter a maternity service user is defined as anyone who is currently using or has recent experience of using a maternity service.

This chapter aims to:

- Review contemporary maternity care issues in relation to service user experience
- Learn from service users' experience of maternity care and explore evidence that underpins maternity care recommendations
- Raise awareness of collaborative partnership models of care

Contemporary issues in maternity care

Reader activity

List expectations that women and families might have of maternity care.

What do you think are key issues for maternity services today?

Key priorities in maternity care

The United Kingdom (UK) Public Health Outcome Framework 2014–15 has identified improving effectiveness, safety and service user experience as key priorities for future maternity services (DH 2014a). Service evaluation identifying how to effectively reduce iatrogenic interventions whilst improving care and satisfaction outcomes remains a priority especially during a decade that has seen an annual increase in the national birth rate (ONS 2013).

The development, implementation and evaluation of public and independently funded maternity services is a complex issue, and there is a growing body of evidence exploring relationships between organizational and care outcomes. In the UK, maternity services are commissioned from NHS trusts through Clinical Commissioning Groups (CCGs) whose responsibility it is to address specific demographic needs within a local population. Maternity care costs have been estimated at around £2800 per woman on 'low' risk care pathways (Tyler 2012), although regional variations in tariffs are often reflected in communities with diverse healthcare needs. The Health and Social Care Act 2012 sets out regulation frameworks through the Care Quality Commission (CQC) and outlines maternity performance management structures designed to monitor activity against strategic policy against Standard 11 of the National Service Framework (NSF) for children, young people and maternity services (DH 2004).

Morbidity and mortality outcomes

One of the main concerns for UK maternity care is a persistently higher rate of morbidity and mortality for women and babies relative to other European countries. This is of note for women from non-English speaking backgrounds, those who live in deprivation and those who have mental health or substance misuse issues (Lewis *et al.*, 2011). Although maternal mortality has fallen to 11.39 per 100,000 maternities, there continues to be concerns about the rising incidence of adverse outcomes linked to 'complex' and 'vulnerable' factors. For example, the trend towards older motherhood and choices for women with pre-existing cardiac, obesity, neurological, thromboembolic, endocrinal and psychiatric conditions result in opportunities for healthcare professionals to work in partnership with women so as to collaboratively manage preventable adversities.

Policy review and sources of evidence

Strategic policy outlined in *Maternity Matters* (DH 2007) focuses on strengthening women's experiences by:

- offering choice in where and how they have their baby(ies);
- providing continuity of care;
- ensuring an integrated service through networks and agreed care pathways.

Focus is on strategies to increase transparency of 'low' and 'higher' risk evidence-based pathways of antenatal, intra-partum and postnatal care to assist women and healthcare professionals to plan individualized care and to audit compliance with quality standards.

Scrutiny to ensure policy recommendations are underpinned by reliable evidence remains a priority. Maternity care pathways are based on graded recommendations which arise from synthesis of evidence such as meta-analyses, randomized controlled trials, cohort studies and qualitative methodologies. Sources informing antenatal, intra-partum and postnatal care pathways include national statistics, confidential enquiries, professional reports, primary and secondary research/evidence, and sources are regularly reviewed by the National Institute for Health and Care Excellence (NICE).

Models of care

Attention has focused on evidence that supports the positive benefits to mothers and babies when 'woman centred' continuity models of care are implemented (Sandall 2007). Enhancements of these partnership-oriented philosophies of care include a higher user perception of informed choice and level of satisfaction in addition to more 'normal' clinical outcomes. Equitable implementation can be challenging and dependent on regional complexities in service demand and workplace capacity and the Kirkup Report (Kirkup 2015) indicates there are opportunities to review maternity services organization and professional regulation in order to deliver the NHS Five Year Forward View (DH 2014b).

Women's experiences of care

Despite concerns there is evidence that many women positively rate their maternity experience (NAO 2013). In 2010 the CQC survey indicated that 76 per cent highly rated experiences of pregnancy care and 84 per cent rated care in labour and birth as excellent or very good. The areas demonstrating poorer outcomes relate to postnatal care with only 67 per cent positively rating experiences. The 2013 CQC survey indicates improvements in relation to communication, involvement in care and experiences of kindness, understanding, trust and confidence. Women valued seeing the same midwife during the antenatal and postnatal periods although a troubling finding was access inequality between white women and black and minority ethnic women indicating scope to improve person-centred approaches to care.

Key roles and contexts of care to support women during maternity care

Reader activity

List the people a woman may seek professional and personal support from during childbirth.

> What knowledge, competencies and values do you think healthcare professionals need to care for women, babies and families using the maternity service?

- List the contexts in which a woman may experience maternity care.

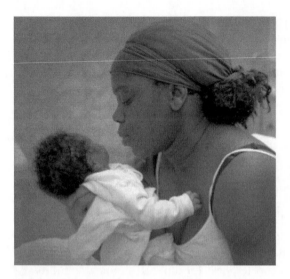

Figure 3.1 Equity of access remains an important area for improvement

Statutory professional roles

By law healthcare practitioners supporting women during childbirth work within frameworks of knowledge, skills and professional values, as defined by regulatory bodies such as the Nursing and Midwifery Council (NMC) and General Medical Council (GMC). Professional codes and standards promote individualized evidence-based PCC and embed collective safeguards in cultures and systems in such a way as to enable practitioners to reflect on care in partnership with clients in order to ensure that care is relevant, acceptable, equitable, accessible and responsive (NMC 2015, 2012).

Figure 3.2 outlines the people who may be involved with women during the childbirth continuum. Most 'low' risk maternity care is provided by midwives and/or GPs with obstetricians and other specialist teams getting involved if problems are identified. Contributors from each sphere may vary according to client circumstances. Some women may have overlapping connections, for example, if they have a supportive personal network, access to

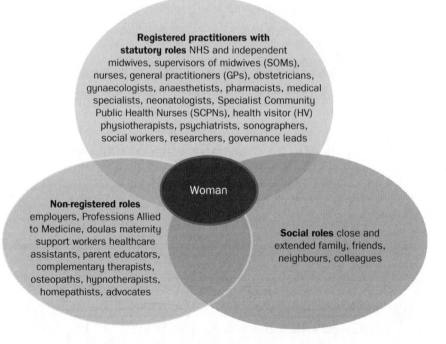

Figure 3.2 People involved with women during the childbirth continuum

complementary therapists and NHS staff. Conversely, others may have limited support access as in the case of homeless or asylum-seeking women. Midwives provide the majority of maternity care in the UK, and play a central advocacy role in mobilizing the inter-professional team disabilities and interpretation needs. The midwife's scope of practice is outlined in Box 3.1.

Box 3.1

The **midwife** is recognized as a **responsible** and **accountable professional** who works in **partnership with women** to give the necessary **support, care and advice** during **pregnancy, labour** and the **post-partum** period, to conduct **births** on the midwife's own responsibility and to provide care for the **newborn** and the **infant**. This care includes **preventative measures**, the **promotion of normal birth**, the **detection of complications** in mother and child, the **accessing of medical** care or other appropriate assistance and the carrying out of **emergency measures**.

International Confederation of Midwives
International Federation of Gynaecology and Obstetrics
World Health Organization

Maternity care settings

Box 3.2 summarizes the care settings in which women and healthcare professionals can meet. Midwives are ideally situated to respond to women's place of care requests as they work across community and hospital settings, and are licensed to provide antenatal, intra-partum and postnatal care.

Box 3.2

- Acute hospitals
- Contraception, fertility and assisted conception centres
- Antenatal, day assessment clinics and antenatal wards
- Labour wards and triage centres
- Obstetric led labour wards
- Midwife led alongside labour wards
- Postnatal wards
- Neonatal units
- Midwifery led and/or standalone centres
- Community health centres
- GP, midwives and health visitor clinics
- Home
- Private obstetric and midwifery units

Service users' experience of preconception care

> ### Reader activity
>
> Reflect on experiences of caring for women and families during the preconception period. using the following comments from a service user as a starting point.
>
> *I have always hoped to have children at some point but have never been able to pin point the exact time as it seems you have to have everything planned out. Finding the right partner, somewhere settled to live, the right job, money to live off, it goes on. Will I be able to get pregnant? Will the baby be alright? It all seemed so simple when my mum had us – somehow it just happened and there wasn't so much to worry about. I remember at school they told us that if you smoked, or drank alcohol or took drugs and got pregnant there might be problems for the baby and that has always made me feel really guilty and really frightened me.*

Parameters of preconception care

Bhutta *et al.* (2011) defines preconception care as 'any intervention provided to women and couples of childbearing age, regardless of pregnancy status or desire, before pregnancy, to improve health outcomes for women, newborns and children'. The World Health Organization (WHO 2012) advocates that preconception care, when integrated from adolescence to menopause, has important contributions to global maternal and neonatal health. It not only empowers women and men in fertility decisions, but also has a direct impact on national and global socio-economic outcomes. Women's fertility choices relate to highly individual personal circumstances and factors underpinning decisions are often complex.

Preconception care strategies and determining the 'right' time to have a baby

Not all women plan pregnancies or formally access preconception services, so it is important that healthcare professionals design flexible ways for prospective parents to use resources. A primary aim of preconception care is to offer opportunities to make informed choices and to explore implications arising from individual genetic, physical, psycho-social, environmental and lifestyle issues. Given the potential sensitivity this raises, it is important to establish respectful partnerships so as to avoid alienating perceptions of surveillance and/or prescriptions. The WHO (2012) puts forward five broad strategies to underpin preconception partnerships, namely:

- Health education and promotion
- Vaccination
- Nutritional supplementation and food fortification
- Provision of contraceptive information and services
- Screening, counselling and management (medical and social)

Conversations around these activities can be daunting for service users who may feel judged, vulnerable or intimidated. It is important that those offering professional advice listen to clients and respect their needs, as perceptions of fertility can, for some, have deep seated associations with self-esteem and/or validation of socio-cultural roles. . It is not just women who should be involved in preconception care as men's health can have important implications for the health of their partners and children.

Preconception care takes time. Being asked numerous questions about health profiles, demographics, employment and lifestyle in addition to disclosing intimate details of sexual activity, histories of infections, family genetics and pre-existing medical issues could be perceived as intrusive. The focus on pathology prevention can also run the risk of 'medicalizing' experiences. NICE (2012a) advice sets out a systematic assessment plan which can assist in supporting pregnancy choices and offers guidance for those with specific considerations such as older motherhood, mental health issues, metabolic disorders, chronic medical disorders and genetic haemaglobinopathies.

Risk factors

A risk history from prospective parents is ideal as factors associated with higher incidences of maternal and perinatal/neonatal morbidity and mortality may have preconception implications. Preconception screening aims to detect pre-existing medical, metabolic, immunological, lifestyle and genetic disorders associated with poor maternal and foetal outcomes. Adverse gynaecological and obstetric outcomes such as miscarriage, stillbirth, premature labour, low/excess birth weight and congenital and neural tube defects (NTD) are often associated with psychological trauma. It is important that care plans that require specialist referral are done in partnership with clients and that consent for routine and specialist assessments are obtained sensitively.

Preconception care may be offered by a range of practitioners such as doctors, midwives, nurses, specialist fertility clinicians and those working in sexual health and contraception services. It does not need to be offered as a 'one stop' package and there are inherent dangers in formulaic targeted care approaches that make assumptions about fertility choices. Ideally, preconception care would link seamlessly to early antenatal services, and strategies to increased service user partnership should be a priority in the development of accessible and equitable pathways of care.

Service users' experience of antenatal care

Reader activity

Reflect on experiences of caring for women and families during the antenatal period using the following comments from a service user as a starting point.

When I discovered I was pregnant I was thrilled as we had been trying for some time. My GP sent me for a scan and they told me the baby was 8 weeks old – I saw the heart beat and I hoped that everything would be alright. I went to the hospital for my booking appointment and it was very busy – the midwife took loads of blood and asked me lots of questions. I was a bit scared to ask why in case they told me something that would burst my bubble of excitement. One of the highlights was seeing my boyfriend's face when he saw the baby at the scan. After that it felt 'real' as we had a photo to show everyone. It made a difference when I discovered I could join a 'group practice' of midwives – it meant I had the same midwives for appointments. It meant I didn't have to tell my story over and over again.

When I was 36 weeks I gave up work and my midwife spent time discussing my birth plan. She explained things like pain relief, birth positions, whether to have an injection to help the placenta come away and how to get breast feeding. It really helped me decide that I wanted a home birth – somehow she inspired me to have confidence. As it happened my waters broke on a Saturday night and the midwife came to our home to check me over. She was there throughout and our son was born in our bedroom.

Parameters of antenatal care

The antenatal phase starts when a conception is confirmed and lasts until onset of labour and therefore spans a range of opportunities to collaboratively design PCC. NICE (2008) antenatal guidelines state that pregnancy is, in the main, a normal physiological process and emphasize that care offered to women should have known benefits. There are standardized antenatal visit schedules that differ for first time and subsequently pregnant mothers and these pathways offer templates for the content and organization of information to be raised in PCC discussions.

Women's experiences of antenatal care

The CQC survey of women's experiences of maternity care (2013) indicates that the majority of women first access GPs although increasing numbers are accessing midwives. With quality standards to encourage women to have the first booking appointment by 10 weeks (NICE 2012b), the fact that only 44 per cent meet any healthcare professional between 7 and 12 weeks indicates that there is scope for further investigation into what is important to women in early pregnancy. It could be that women have confidence in confirming pregnancies using over-the-counter kits and choose not to access care. However, challenges in making first contact could impede discussion on issues which may have significant consequences. For example, benefits of earlier prenatal screening tests, folic acid and vitamin D supplementation, prevention of food-acquired infections may be delayed in addition to opportunities to discuss adverse foetal developmental effects resulting from smoking and recreational drug and alcohol use.

The initial booking appointment

Most booking questionnaires begin with gathering personal details related to demographic factors before eliciting medical, surgical, gynaecological and obstetric histories. Questions designed to assess mood orientation and psychological wellbeing in addition to identifying factors that may raise safeguarding concerns are usually left until a degree of trust is established. This is of particular importance for women who may be living with vulnerabilities such as experiences of sexual abuse (Montgomery 2013) or domestic violence, substance abuse or mental health issues which may benefit from continuity of care/carer or specialist expertise. Common questions that arise at the booking appointment relate to discomforts caused by physiological symptoms of pregnancy changes, maternity entitlements, safety of exercise, travel, sexual and lifestyle activities. Conversations often develop into more specific concerns about foetal development, diet, vitamin or folic acid supplements, promotion of pelvic floor care, infant feeding and access to NHS or lay antenatal education programmes.

Foetal assessments and screening tests

Time to discuss milestones for key antenatal and postnatal screening tests – as outlined by the UK National Screening Committee – is important. Increasingly, foetal dating is reliant on technological interventions and combining this with personal sexual and menstrual histories requires specialist skills in explanation. For example, when estimating the expected date of birth, midwives, doctors and sonographers need to respectfully listen to the woman's account of her menstrual history and consider this alongside foetal crown–rump length and head circumference measurements so as to eliminate false positive/negative findings. Similarly, in preparing women with the information to make an informed choice around foetal anomaly and placental location scans between 18 and 20 weeks, time should be allocated to discuss implications.

In supporting PCC it is important to clarify differences between screening and diagnostic prenatal tests, and to frame statistical information so that women can make informed choices on the basis of their own individualized risk adjustments. This is fundamental when offering screening for Down's syndrome and other abnormalities where gestational age estimations are crucial to test validity and reliability. It is equally important to enable women and their partners to weigh up their own perceptions of risk about positive screen tests and to balance some of the inherent iatrogenic risks of prenatal diagnostic tests, such as chorionic villus sampling and amniocentesis, with the benefits of having a definitive diagnosis.

Maternal assessments

Routine maternal assessments are offered at booking and subsequent appointments and findings can be used to personalize and refine culturally sensitive care plans. Records of discussions, preferred requests, birth plans, test results and referrals must all be clearly documented in maternal notes. In appointments where there are multiple assessments concerning maternal and foetal health, it may help to group interventions into clustered activities so that there is continuity to questions and topics. For example, systematic questions about physical aspects of maternal health could be separated from those exploring psychological wellbeing and specific sensitivity should be implemented when undertaking intimate abdominal/ vaginal and/or psychological assessments. . In providing person-centred antenatal care it is important to consider the timing and experiential aspects of individualized needs and birth plans so as to ensure informed decision-making and access to appropriate specialist referrals pathways should it be required.

Service users' experience of intra-partum care

Reader activity

Reflect on experiences you have had caring for women and families during the intra-partum period using the following comments from a service user as a starting point.

I couldn't exactly say when my labour started. I had been feeling so heavy and "full" for so long especially when I passed my expected date and days rolled by. The night before I was due to have an appointment to discuss an induction of labour, my waters went. The contractions didn't start immediately – I was a bit confused as I hadn't really thought of this in the birth plan. Fortunately my husband got back from work just before it all 'kicked off' big time. By the time I got to the labour ward I was screaming for an epidural – forget the water pool and essential oils! I couldn't believe my luck when the midwife from the surgery walked in. She was on for the night and when she told me that I was eight centimetres dilated and that my baby was fine, I knew that I could do it with just gas and air. Even though it was the hardest and most undignified situation I had ever been in, once the pushing took over I went into a different world. I was worried that my husband would find it all off putting but he was great getting me into a hand and knees position, giving me sips of water and fanning me. The baby came all at once – in one HUGE push and splash. I was completely shocked and dazed and it was the midwife who scooped up my baby and put it in my arms. The afterbirth came away very quickly without any injections and I was tremendously lucky to only have a very small tear which the midwife sewed up whilst I watched my husband cuddle our daughter. I will always be grateful for the calmness and professionalism of the team who supported us that night – they made me believe in myself as a new mother.

Parameters of intra-partum care

Data from the NAO (2013) indicates that most women give birth in hospitals. The majority of pregnant women have uncomplicated pregnancies, go into labour spontaneously and give birth to healthy singleton babies who present in a head first cephalic presentation at term (37 to 42 weeks). However, there is scope for further exploration into person-centred intra-partum care provision and NICE (2007) has identified research priorities into how to assess evidence based information in women's decision-making choices, as well as long-term consequences of offering care in different settings.

The intra-partum period covers a range of physiological and psychological changes and choices for a mother and baby. Traditional knowledge differentiates labour into three stages, however, some would argue that conceptualizing labour as a continuum is a more useful approach (Downe 2004) as it enables caregivers to attune to the experiential aspects of individualized labours rather than superimpose artificial biomedical parameters that potentially lead to unnecessary cascades of intervention.

NICE guidance offers a cluster of clinical guidelines aimed to support intra-partum care for low and high risk conditions and offers an invaluable tool for women and their carers to explore choices. The intra-partum pathway for healthy women and their babies during childbirth (NICE 2014) includes evidence recommendations related to place of birth, latent phase, initial and ongoing intra-partum assessments, transfers of care and pain relief including regional anaesthesia. Guidance addresses foetal monitoring, pre-labour rupture of membranes, first, second and third stage management protocols including the use of oxytocic drugs and care of the mother and baby following birth. 'Low' risk care pathway guidance is complemented with 'higher' risk guidance addressing specific circumstances such as care of a woman having an induction of labour, caesarean section, vaginal birth after caesarean section and other specific conditions requiring the expertise of the multi-professional team.

Place of birth

The Birthplace study (Brocklehurst *et al.*, 2011) has strengthened opportunities for women and healthcare professionals to discuss choices between settings. Evidence shows that there are lower rates of interventions for 'low risk' multiparous women having a baby at home or in a free standing/alongside maternity unit than in an obstetric unit and no differences in outcomes for the babies. Similarly, evidence for 'low risk' primigravid mothers suggests that birthing in midwifery-led units also reduces risks of unnecessary interventions whilst resulting in the same outcomes for babies as compared with obstetric units. With regards birth at home for first time mothers, evidence would suggest that there is a small increase in risk of an adverse outcome for the baby.

Women's experiences of intra-partum care

Findings from the CQC (2013) survey report that at least one in five women felt that concerns during labour were not taken seriously and first time mothers felt more uncertain. There are particular concerns about inconsistent advice especially during labour admission. Some women reported being left alone during early labour and feeling worried about how to establish the onset of labour suggesting that there is still scope for healthcare professionals to clarify processes. It also appears that pain relief is not always adequately explained or that access to labour aids is not equitable.

Birth plans

Many women are keen to outline birth preferences in advance and value opportunities to discuss and document choices. Open and early discussion/review enables women to consider information at their own pace and to formulate, agree and record plans with those involved and from 34 weeks most women welcome discussion to clarify roles of significant persons who will be present at their births. Standard topics the midwife might prepare for relate to benefits of various labouring and birth positions, foetal monitoring methods, pain relief options, perineal management, early skin to skin contact with their baby, third stage management, prolonged pregnancy, induction of labour, breast and infant feeding, vitamin K prophylaxis and newborn screening tests. Sometimes there are specific considerations such as plans for Vaginal Births following Caesarean Section (VBAC), vaginal breech births, multiple birth requests that may require the involvement of the multi-professional team and supervisor of midwives. It remains a priority of PCC to collaboratively explore choices with women so as to enable acceptable informed decision-making in the intra-partum period.

Service users' experience of postnatal care

Reader activity

Reflect on experiences of caring for women and families during the postnatal period using the following comments from a service user as a starting point.

After our baby was born it was all a blur. It was the strangest feeling – total body exhaustion and curiosity about seeing our baby. I wanted to sleep but the ward was noisy and I worried that the baby hadn't fed. My partner went home and I remember thinking what am I going to do without him? I felt stupid asking for help especially as I had gone to classes. Once the anaesthetic had worn off my stitches were painful – I just couldn't get comfortable – every time I moved there was a gush. When the baby woke up I tried to get him onto the breast but I wasn't sure if he was getting anything as he kept snuffling and it hurt. The more I tried he cried – I felt useless as I had imagined that something like breast feeding would be instinctual. In the end a really nice midwife came. I was in tears, the baby was crying and I felt totally overwhelmed. She sat down and suggested that we undress my baby so I could hold him close with his skin against mine – it was lovely feeling of warmth and closeness of his little body. When he opened his eyes to look up at me I knew somehow we would muddle through.

Parameters of postnatal care

The postnatal period is traditionally defined as the time immediately after labour ends until six to eight weeks after birth. Bick *et al.* (2012) argue that physical, emotional and social adaptations to motherhood can extend for a longer timeframe and that trends towards earlier hospital discharge and selective frequency of postnatal visits can fragment services and potentially lead to long-term consequences for maternal and child health. Despite implementation of evidence-based care resulting from recommendations arising from the

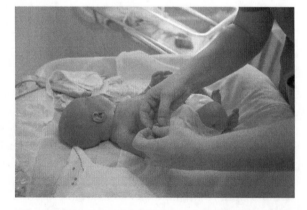

Figure 3.3 Postnatal care – A vital period of adaptation

Implementing Midwifery-Led Postnatal Care Trial (IMPaCT; MacArthur *et al.*, 2003) and NICE postnatal guidelines (NICE 2006), it would appear that many women continue to find raising issues about postnatal health difficult (Bick *et al.*, 2009). Trends indicate that postnatal wards generate more complaints than other services, suggesting that there is further scope for healthcare professionals to strengthen person-centred approaches to care.

Women's experiences of postnatal care

The CQC (2013) report recommends refinements for person-centred approaches to postnatal care. In relation to admission duration, 72 per cent felt postnatal admission duration was 'about right', 16 per cent felt it was 'too long' and 12 per cent felt it was 'too short'. Once home, the majority (97 per cent) had telephone access and 53 per cent received three or four midwifery visits. Women reported higher rates of 'being helped' in postnatal as compared with antenatal care and this was associated with midwifery continuity. Opportunities to strengthen PCC arise as 61 per cent reported not seeing the same midwife despite wanting to. This was especially noted for primiparous mothers who wanted to see midwives 'more often'. Some positive dimensions of PCC were demonstrated in improvements in emotional assessment; however, persistent challenges remain in relation to infant feeding, contraception and ensuring access to acceptable facilities, equipment and food.

The content and delivery of postnatal care

NICE (2006) guidance advocates that culturally sensitive individualized care is a priority at every postnatal contact and that care plans should be developed before or immediately after birth. Traditionally midwives have provided hospital and community postnatal care and although it is within a midwife's scope of practice to offer care to 28 days, this arrangement is the exception rather than the norm. Further research priorities could address gaps in the evidence to explore how different care interventions relate to morbidity detection and to evaluate the impact that access to healthcare professional support has on outcomes.

Maternal postnatal care

Routine postnatal care aims to involve mothers in care decisions related to themselves and their babies, whether in hospital or at home. Postnatal care offers opportunities for healthcare professionals to explore what is important to mothers and to tailor content, delivery and evaluation of care plans. Postnatal contacts are assessment episodes to enable mothers and carers to detect potentially life threatening conditions such as post-partum haemorrhage, infection, pre-eclampsia and thromboembolism. NICE (2006) guidance recommends providing women with information on what to do in the event of pathological signs/symptoms and also what to expect in terms of normal physiological changes for themselves and their babies. The initial assessment review provides a foundation for follow-up discussion on physical and emotional health and specific sensitivity may be required when caring for those at risk or with safeguarding concerns. From a mother's perspective it is important to be informed about different professional roles and how accountabilities link with choices on neonatal screening, immunization and contraception which may span beyond midwifery discharge to the six- to eight-week

GP and HV review. In addition, in accordance with priorities to improve perinatal mental health, regular and sensitive person-centred assessments of emotional wellbeing are recommended. This necessitates careful review designed to differentiate states such as 'baby blues' from more severe states of mood change such as depression, anxiety, suicidal thoughts, delusions and/or hallucinations.

Neonatal postnatal care

NICE (2006) guidance sets out evidence-based standards to ensure that healthcare professionals support parents in their new roles. This includes dissemination to parents of the DH (2014a) *Birth to Five* guide within five days of birth, which outlines information aimed to enable parents to make informed choices on behalf of their babies and children. It covers topics such as parenting and emotional attachment, home and transport safety, prevention of common neonatal health problems such as skin conditions, thrush, nappy rash, fever, colic and digestive disorders. Importantly, NICE guidance sets out standards to inform PCC regarding Vitamin K prophylaxis to prevent deficiency bleeding and prevent incidence of Sudden Infant Death Syndrome (SIDS).

One of the first decisions taken by parents is how to feed their baby. The NICE Postnatal Guidelines (2006) recommend that healthcare professionals implement a structured programme that encourages breastfeeding with the Baby Friendly Initiative standards used as a bench mark for monitoring quality standards. This position underpins recommendations outlined in the Public Health Outcomes Framework (DH 2012).

Findings from the National Infant Feeding Survey (McAndrew *et al.*, 2012) indicate that although UK breastfeeding rates at birth have increased to 81 per cent there is still scope to address the drop to 17 per cent at 4 and 1 per cent at 6 months. The survey highlights demographic characteristics linked to breastfeeding uptake such as being 30 years or over, from ethnic groups, in education up to 18 years, in professional occupations and living in more affluent areas. This indicates there is further scope to explore PCC in infant feeding and to evaluate healthcare interventions which address health inequalities. As acknowledged by the United Nations International Children's Emergency Fund report (UNICEF 2012) significant financial savings could be made through improved maternal and neonatal health outcomes by breastfeeding. Increasing emphasis could be prioritized to support PCC links to staff with required knowledge, skills and professional attitudes to support choices and to collate metrics such as skin-to-skin and early/late feeding outcomes.

Neonatal postnatal care includes opportunities for person-centred approaches to care when parents consider implications of physical examination and screening programmes as recommended by the National Screening Committee. Parents are offered a series of neonatal screening choices starting with an examination within 72 hours of birth to identify major hips, heart, palate and vital organ abnormalities. A blood spot test is offered at five to eight days screening for phenylketonuria, congenital hypothyroidism, sickle cell disease, cystic fibrosis and Medium-Chain Acyl-COA Deyhydrogenase Deficiency (MCADD). Parents are also informed about a neonatal hearing screen by week five and a repeat neonatal physical examination at six to eight weeks. Ongoing immunization choices in relation to preventative programmes against Hepatitis B, Group B strep, diphtheria, tetanus, pertussis, polio and meningitis C raise further opportunities for parents to consider PCC decisions for their babies.

Collaborative partnership models

Example of good practice

The Lewisham and Greenwich NHS Trust Maternity Service Liaison Committee (MSLC) was set up in 2007 and is co-chaired by two lay members. The MSCL comprises of service users, providers and representatives from third sector organizations and has links with Lewisham Refugee and Migrant Network. It meets every two months in a children's centre and at the hospital. The core aims are normalizing childbirth, supporting breastfeeding and supporting women and children in the postnatal period.

One of the achievements of the MSLC in 2013 was leading the fight to save Lewisham Healthcare Trust maternity service. The MSLC worked tirelessly to ensure that women's views were reflected in the Trust Special Administrator (TSA) report submitted to Jeremy Hunt, Secretary for Health. The MSLC submitted two reports to the TSA, met with the Lead for maternity care, coordinated a written bombardment to the DH and staged two dramatic flash-mobs at the DH. The 'battle' culminated in victory for Lewisham's acute services at the High Court where the appeal by the Secretary of State for Health was overthrown.

Other activities undertaken by the MSLC include regular discussions about neonatal care and engagement with women and/or partners in the community in activities such as 'Walking the Patch' – an initiative inviting clients to walk around clinical areas and share experiences. The committee have also forged links with other MSLCs and continue to build links to strengthen the voice and reach of MSLCs at a national level.

Reader activity

List health professional members and organizations who may be involved in providing and developing care.

Explore how maternity healthcare practitioners can encourage staff and users to share and respect opinions and negative feedback.

The National Voices Report (National Voices 2009) suggests that partnership in care development, implementation and evaluation has several distinct role contributions – see Box 3.3.

Box 3.3   Service user contributions

- Acting as a knowledge base
- Participating in event and activities
- Informing decision-making
- Influencing other service users and organizations

- Co-producing frameworks, policies, pathways, consultations
- Representing an authentic 'voice'
- Acting as a strategic lead

Service User Involvement Best Practice Guidelines (check author 2014) also offers a useful model outlining a 'Ladder of Participation' which may benchmark service user involvement and participation – see Box 3.4.

Box 3.4   Ladder of Participation

FULL CONTROL: Service users control decision-making at the highest level.

SHARING POWER: Service users share decisions and responsibility, influencing and determining outcomes.

PARTICIPATION: Service users can make suggestions and influence outcomes.

CONSULTATION: Service users are asked what they think but have limited influence.

INFORMATION: Services users are told what is happening but have no influence.

NO CONTROL: Service users are passive consumers.

Opportunities for partnership arise at various participatory levels and shared views and involvement in decision-making are part of maternity policy evaluation led by the DH and CQC. Professional organizations such as the Royal College of Midwives (RCM) and Royal College of Obstetricians and Gynaecologists (RCOG) regularly consult women in protocol and guideline development. However, there is evidence that although maternity service user representation at strategic CCGs and/or NHS Trust Boards is frequently sought, there can be difficulties in ensuring equality of access for 'harder to reach' groups.

Participation at local Trust MSLCs can be challenging given the transient nature of maternity service use. Even within statutory structures, for example validation of professional programmes leading to registration, there may be challenges recruiting recently birthed women. Development of robust ways to attract maternity service users to work in partnership with providers remains a priority, and possible initiatives include representation at Labour Ward Forums, 'Walking the Patch' and client engagement events. The National Childbirth Trust (NCT 2013) summarizes examples of how MSLCs can develop decision-making through memoranda of understanding with service organizations, universities and research bodies and Box 3.1 identifies healthcare professionals that could be involved.

Benefits of collaborative partnership

The DH (2006) outlines formal arrangements for service users to work with healthcare commissioners, managers and practitioners in such a way as to strengthen collaborative partnerships in line with needs and wishes of local women. Technological advances, medical research, the internet, media, service user perceptions and expectations are factors that impact on service delivery and perceptions of experience and satisfaction. There is significant pressure on maternity healthcare practitioners to meet service user expectations 365 days a year and 24 hours a day. Creating environments that encourage partnership has many advantages – see Box 3.5:

Box 3.5

- Increases client experience and 'being listened to'
- Tailors service provision to client needs
- Empowers healthcare professionals to advocate for women
- Includes involvement from 'seldom heard' and 'vulnerable' groups
- Aligns evidence-based policy development to client expectations
- Ensures the development of realistic and effective solutions

---

Managing service user expectations

Initially, setting up a service user forum that encourages collaborative working can be easy. However, maintaining and motivating practitioners and users can be more challenging. In any patient forum, there are occasions when service users might feel that their healthcare practitioners are not doing enough to improve the service. Practitioners may feel 'beaten down' by service users telling them what they are not doing well without appreciating the pressured environment they work in. Some suggestions to strengthen working relationships are outlined below:

NCT Voices training

This is a workshop that helps to promote team working and effectiveness of MSLCs, labour ward forums and breastfeeding initiative groups.

Terms of Reference and goal setting

Shared partnership creation of group 'Terms of Reference' and goals may be useful.
    Review and action setting is central to measuring progress and effectiveness and encourages innovation.

Feedback and complaints

The creation of clear communication channels for feedback and complaints management helps consolidate respect. The Patient Advisory Liaison Services (PALS) forums and MSLCs are useful forums to discuss complaints trends rather than confidential individual cases.

Communication

Open lines of communication are the foundation of effective collaboration. This includes updates on service development, implementation and evaluation. A major source of conflict amongst maternity service users and practitioners is poor communication and involvement in audit processes including report dissemination outlining recommendations.

Transparency

The need for transparent working relationships cannot be underestimated, and this includes informing maternity service providers of visits and inspections by reviewing and regulatory professional organizations. Since 2014, the Health and Social Care Information Centre (2013) has collected information on local maternity care to inform commissioning, payment and quality assurance monitoring systems.

Setting up a service user initiative – Ready, Set, Go!

Each maternity service provider is unique hence 'one size does not fit all' when it comes to setting up service user forums and creating a culture of collaborative partnership. To support facilitative approaches the following may be useful:

Work smarter not harder

The recruitment of service users is one of the first steps and it is recommended that working with existing groups such as local Patient Experience/Engagement Teams, PALS, Local Health Watch, CCGs and not for profit organizations will avoid isolation. Recruitment through drafted invitation can be a useful strategy to elicit interest from a wider audience within the local community groups. If possible utilize any marketing, communications and personnel resources at the local hospital and/or birth centres. It may be possible to explore the feasibility of designing joint posters, leaflets, newsletters and articles which can be uploaded to websites and printed on demand.

Think outside the box

To create a memorable impact it may be worth considering innovative, creative and unusual ways to disseminate key aims, objectives and messages and this may be a good way to evaluate the impact and reduce unanticipated consequences. There may be opportunities to include user and practitioner testimonials through diaries, reflections on trends on support, counselling, out-reach and follow up services in addition to multi-professional case conferences.

Connect with other user groups

Attending other MSLCs, labour ward and user forums is a useful way of maximizing insights into how similar groups function in relation to agenda, representation, decision-making, consultation and action ratification. There are many MSLCs and other maternity forums demonstrating best practice and the benefits of collaborative partnership working. A Google search may be a good starting point.

GO, don't wait

Effective service user engagement strategies often rely on those leading the initiative to actively approach a target audience by taking the service to them. Although placing posters in waiting areas is a traditional publicity strategy, it is unlikely to be effective in the long run. Publicity targeted to a wider audience through dissemination on supermarket, hair/beauty salons, church, mosque and temple noticeboards in addition to free online adverting spaces such as Netmums, Mumsnet, local Council and Health Watch events pages can be considered. Meeting venues which are convenient and health and safety compliant for pregnant and post-natal mothers are important considerations. Potential venues include local children's centres, surgeries, libraries and community halls.

Summary

This chapter has explored aspects of preconception, antenatal, intra-partum and post-natal care in order to strengthen opportunities to develop person-centred approaches to maternity care. It recognizes that whilst maternity care sits within a complex national and global context of environmental, social, political and economic factors, there is also scope to respect individual lifestyle choices that are important features of holistic care. The promotion of optimal maternity care strategies requires organizational consider-ations with regards who, what, when and where services and resources are available and there continues to be scope to develop collaborative care frameworks that put the experiences of service users at the centre.

References

Bhutta, Z., Dean, S., Imam, A. and Lassi, Z. (2011) *A Systematic Review of Preconception Risks and Interventions*. Karachi: The Aga Khan University. Available at: http://mother-childlink.tghn.org/site_media/media/articles/Preconception_Report.pdf (accessed 5 November 2015).

Bick, D., MacArther, C. and Winter, H. (2009) *Postnatal Care: Evidence and Guidelines for Management*, 2nd Edn. London: Churchill Livingstone Elsevier.

Bick, D., Murrells, T., Weavers, A. *et al.* (2012) Revising acute care systems and processes to improve breastfeeding and maternal postnatal health: a pre and post intervention study in one English maternity unit, *British Medical Council, Pregnancy Childbirth*, 12: 41.

Brocklehurst, P., Hardy, P., Hollowell, J. *et al.* (2011) Perinatal and maternal outcomes by planned place of birth for healthy women with low risk pregnancies: the Birthplace in England national prospective cohort study. Available at: www.bmj.com/content/343/bmj. d7400 . DOI: http://dx.doi.org/10.1136/bmj.d7400

CQC (2013) *National Findings from the 2013 Survey of Women's Experiences of Maternity Care.* Available at: www.cqc.org.uk/sites/default/files/documents/maternity_report_for_publication.pdf (accessed 4 November 2015).

Dean, S., Bhutta, Z., Mason, E.M. *et al.* (2011) Care before and between pregnancy, in WHO *Born Too Soon: The Global Action Report on Preterm Birth.* Available at: www.who.int/pmnch/media/news/2012/borntoosoon_chapter3.pdf (accessed 4 November 2015).

DH (Department of Health) (2004) *National Service Framework for Children, Young People and Maternity Services.* Available at: www.gov.uk/government/uploads/system/uploads/attachment_data/file/199952/National_Service_Framework_for_Children_Young_People_and_Maternity_Services_-_Core_Standards.pdf (accessed 4 November 2015).

DH (2005) *Commissioning a Patient-Led NHS.* Available at: http://webarchive.nationalarchives.gov.uk/+/www.dh.gov.uk/en/publicationsandstatistics/publications/publicationspolicyandguidance/dh_4106506 (accessed 4 November 2015).

DH (2006) *National Guidelines for Maternity Services Liaison Committees (MSLCs).* Available at: www.dhsspsni.gov.uk/guidelines-for-maternity-services-liaison-committees-july-2008.pdf (accessed 4 November 2015).

DH (2007) *Maternity Matters: Choice, Access and Continuity of Care in a Safe Service.* Available at: http://webarchive.nationalarchives.gov.uk/+/www.dh.gov.uk/en/Publicationsandstatistics/Bulletins/Chiefnursingofficerbulletin/Browsable/DH_073728 (accessed 4 November 2015).

DH (2012) *Public Health Outcomes Framework 2013 to 2016.* Available at: www.gov.uk/government/publications/healthy-lives-healthy-people-improving-outcomes-and-supporting-transparency (accessed 5 November 2015).

DH (2014a) *Birth to Five.* Available at: www.publichealth.hscni.net/publications/birth-five (accessed 4 November 2015).

DH (2014b) NHS Five Year Forwards View. Available at: www.england.nhs.uk/ourwork/futurenhs/nhs-five-year-forward-view-web-version/5yfv-exec-sum/ (accessed 5 November 2015).

Downe, S. (2004) *Normal Childbirth: Evidence and Debate.* London: Churchill Livingstone.

Health and Social Care Information Centre (2013) Maternity and Children's Data Sets. Available at: www.hscic.gov.uk/media/11993/Maternity-and-Childrens-Data-Set-Bulletin—Issue-3—May-2013/pdf/MCDS_bulletin_issue3_V0.3.pdf (accessed 4 November 2015).

Kirkup, B. (2015) *The Report of the Morecambe Bay Investigation.* Available at: www.hscic.gov.uk/media/11993/Maternity-and-Childrens-Data-Set-Bulletin—Issue-3—May-2013/pdf/MCDS_bulletin_issue3_V0.3.pdf (accessed 4 November 2015).

Lewis, G.E., Cantwell, R., Clutton-Brock, T. *et al.* (2011) *Saving Mothers' Lives: Reviewing Maternal Deaths to make Motherhood Safer – 2006–08. The Eighth Report of the Confidential Enquiries into Maternal Deaths in the United Kingdom.* DOI: http://onlinelibrary.wiley.com/doi/10.1111/j.1471-0528.2010.02847.x/pdf

MacArthur, C., Winter, H., Bick, D. *et al.* (2003) Redesigning postnatal care: a randomised controlled trial of protocol based midwifery led care focussed on individual women's physical and psychological health needs. Available at: www.journalslibrary.nihr.ac.uk/__ data/assets/pdf_file/0004/59602/ExecutiveSummary-hta7370.pdf (accessed 5 November 2015).

McAndrew. F., Thompson, J., Fellows, L. *et al.* (2012) The Infant Feeding Survey 2010. Available at: www.hscic.gov.uk/catalogue/PUB08694/Infant-Feeding-Survey-2010-Consolidated-Report.pdf (accessed 5 November 2015).

Montgomery, E. (2013) Feeling safe: A metasynthesis of the maternity care needs of women who were sexually abused in childhood, *Birth*, 40(2): 88–95.

National Audit Office (2013) *Maternity services in England*. Available at: www.nao.org.uk/wp-content/uploads/2013/11/10259-001-Maternity-Services-Book-1.pdf (accessed 4 November 2015).

National Voices (2009) *Service User Involvement in Practice: A Summary Report of a Survey of National Voices' Member Organisations*. Available at: www.nationalvoices.org.uk/ (accessed 4 November 2015).

NCT (2013) *MSLCs: A Consensus Statement from NCT, RCM and RCOG*. Available at: www.nct.org.uk/sites/default/files/related_documents/MSLC%20document%20FINAL%20 2013%20V2.pdf (accessed 4 November 2015).

NICE (2006) Postnatal Care: Routine Postnatal Care of Women and their Babies. Available at: www.nice.org.uk/guidance/QS37 (accessed 5 November 2015).

NICE (2007) *Postnatal Care: Routine Postnatal Care of Women and their Babies*. Available at: www.nice.org.uk/guidance/QS37 (accessed 4 November 2015).

NICE (2008) *Antenatal Care: Routine Care for the Health Pregnant Woman*. Available at: www.nice.org.uk/Guidance/CG62 (accessed 4 November 2015).

NICE (2012a) *Pre-conception – Advice and Management*. Available at: http://cks.nice.org.uk/pre-conception-advice-and-management (accessed 4 November 2015).

NICE (2012b) *Quality Standard for Antenatal Care*. Available at: www.nice.org.uk/guidance/qs22 (accessed 4 November 2015).

NICE (2014) *Intrapartum Care: Care of Healthy Women and their Babies in Childbirth*. Available at: www.nice.org.uk/guidance/CG55 (accessed 4 November 2015).

NMC (2012) *Midwives Rules and Standards*. Available at: www.nmc-uk.org/Documents/NMC-publications/Midwives%20Rules%20and%20Standards%202012.pdf (accessed 4 November 2015).

NMC (2015) *The Code*. Available at: www.nmc-uk.org/Publications/Standards/The-code/Introduction/ (accessed 4 November 2015).

ONS (2013) *NHS Maternity Statistics – England, 2012–13*. Available at: http://data.gov.uk/dataset/nhs_maternity_statistics_england (accessed 4 November 2015).

Patients and Information Directorate (2013) *Transforming Participation in Health and Care: 'The NHS belongs to us all'*. Available at: www.england.nhs.uk/wp-content/uploads/2013/09/trans-part-hc-guid1.pdf (accessed 4 November 2015).

Sandall, J. (2007) *The Contribution of Continuity of Midwifery Care to High Quality Maternity Care*. Available at: www.rcm.org.uk/sites/default/files/Continuity%20of%20Care%20A5%20Web.pdf (accessed 4 November 2015).

Service User Involvement Web Resource (2014) *Service User Involvement Best Practice Guidelines*. Available at: www.serviceuserinvolvement.co.uk/whatisit_laderOfP.asp (accessed 4 November 2015).

Tyler, S. (2012) *Commissioning Maternity Services: A Resource Pack to Support Clinical Commissioning Groups.* Available at: www.england.nhs.uk/wp-content/uploads/2012/07/comm-maternity-services.pdf (accessed 4 November 2015).

WHO (2012) *Preconception Care to Reduce Maternal and Childhood Mortality and Morbidity: Meeting Report and Packages of Interventions.* Geneva: WHO.

Person-centred approaches to family care and health visiting

Sara Donetto[1]

LEARNING OUTCOMES

- Understanding some core dimensions of person-centred practice in the context of family support in the community
- Reflecting upon the importance of paying attention to service users' experiences of care to inform and improve community nursing practice
- Being able to think critically about priorities and constraints for person-centredness and family-centredness in the context of child health and care

Introduction

In this chapter I explore person-centred approaches to family care by focusing on health visiting services and the integrated care they offer alongside Children's Centres. The aim of the chapter is to encourage a discussion about what counts as PCC in the context of child and family health. To this aim, I draw upon parents' accounts of their experiences with health visiting services and/or Children's Centres to illustrate what kind of professional practices

---

[1] This chapter draws upon a study which was commissioned and supported by the Department of Health in England as part of the work of the Policy Research Programme. The views expressed are those of the author and not necessarily those of the Department of Health.

make people – especially mothers – feel supported (or not) in their transition and adjustment to parenthood. Of course the examples I use are not representative of all the forms that family care can take in nursing practice; however, they offer a useful platform to begin to think about what counts as person-centredness when it comes to caring for young children and their families. This is because of the breadth of vision – including the preventative, health-promoting character – of health visiting (Cowley *et al.*, 2013) and of the other early years practices that are more or less directly connected with it. To illustrate the complexities of understanding and promoting 'family health and wellbeing' in a child's early years of life and of working with young children and their families in a person-centred way, I draw upon some concrete examples of parents' expressed needs and challenges from the accounts our research team collected for a qualitative study of parents' views of health visiting services (Donetto *et al.*, 2013). I discuss the ways in which feeling 'known' to the service and respected as an individual by professionals, and being able to rely on consistent and well-coordinated care were, for parents, essential aspects of good care. I then problematize the concept of person-centredness in the context of family care and draw on examples from parents' experiences to think critically about the strengths and limitations of person-centredness when caring for the whole family whilst safeguarding the wellbeing of a child. Throughout the chapter I use examples from research interviews to give life to, and highlight the practical relevance of, discussions about PCC.[2] Before I explore these examples in further detail, though, I provide a very brief overview of health visiting and related support services to put my discussion into context.

Health visiting services and integrated care in the community

In the UK health visitors are qualified Specialist Community Public Health Nurses offering support to families with children aged 0–5years with the aim of having a positive impact on the lifelong health and wellbeing of young children and their families. This support is offered through a 'universal service designed to promote the healthy development of pre-school children, whilst improving public health and reducing health inequalities' and through more targeted care packages for families with additional needs (Cowley *et al.*, 2014: 3). As a result of the revitalization of health visiting promoted in 2011 by the Conservative-Liberal democrat coalition government with the *Health Visitor Iimplementation Pplan: A Call to Action* (DH 2011), the service operates across four levels of 'family offer' and focuses on six high impact areas for health outcomes. The four levels reflect a stepped approach to families' support needs and include: a 'community' level, offering support for all families through health visitors' knowledge of community-based resources; a 'universal' level, providing access to a health visitor, essential information about healthy start issues, and child development reviews for all families; a 'universal plus' level offering time-limited additional support to families with specific issues (such as weaning or sleep amongst others); and a 'universal partnership plus' level providing ongoing additional support for families with continuing complex health

---

[2] The examples I use are not intended to represent all possible case-scenarios and refer the reader to the full study report for a discussion of the methodological approach and strengths and limitations of the study in question (Donetto *et al.*, 2013).

needs. Built in these four levels of 'offer' are six areas of focus aimed at maximizing health visitors' impact: transition to parenthood, early weeks maternal mental health, breastfeeding, healthy weight, minor illnesses management and accident reduction, and health and development review at age 2. Across impact areas and levels of service provision, health visitors and their teams deliver the Healthy Child Programme, the early intervention and public health programme that aims to provide a core universal service as well as a number of evidence-based preventive interventions for more vulnerable families (Shribman and Billingham 2009). They also ensure that, across all levels of service, child protection concerns are identified promptly and raised with the relevant agencies.

Health visitors work in teams, the skill mix of which is established in accordance with local needs (Fisher 2009). They also work in close collaboration with midwives and Early Years practitioners in children's centres, although specific work arrangements and degree of integration/overlap between services can vary significantly (Pugh and Duffy 2010; NHS England 2014). Health visiting support is provided through a combination of home visits by health visitors and other members of the team and individual or group consultations within child health clinics and/or group activities in Children's Centres. All mothers should receive at least one home visit by the health visitor soon after the birth of their child (and many trusts are currently in the process of implementing routine antenatal contacts) and then – depending on their specific circumstances – will either attend a local child health clinic (usually situated in a community centre, health centre, or Children's Centre) for routine checks and advice about common baby and toddler issues (for example, breastfeeding, weaning, sleep, toilet training) and/or for support with emotional and practical issues (for example, low mood, financial issues, childcare). Depending on specific circumstances, some mothers will also be offered further visits at home by the health visitor or another practitioner for specific issues or more complex needs (for example, maternal postnatal depression, complex long-term conditions).

Health visitors aim to support families and communities. However, in the vast majority of cases and due largely to practical circumstances and the conventional division of childcare responsibilities within the family, they interact directly with mothers and their children, with limited opportunities for contact with children's other main carers and fathers in particular. This is a crucial aspect of practice when it comes to reflecting upon the limitations of family-centredness and the potential tensions between person-centredness and family-centredness, which I do later in the chapter. The importance of considering the needs of all immediate family members for effective child support is embedded in the Healthy Child Programme (Shribman and Billingham 2009), which constitutes the official guidance underpinning the provision of support for children aged 0 to 5 years and their parents. The Healthy Child Programme highlights the health visitor's role in supporting 'mothers and fathers to provide sensitive and attuned parenting' and 'strong couple relationships and stable positive relationships within families in accordance with The Children's Plan (DCSF 2007),' and of ensuring 'that contact with the family routinely involves and supports fathers, including non-resident fathers' (Shribman and Billingham 2009: 10). Of course, whenever family circumstances pose a threat to the physical and/or emotional safety of a child, health visitors and early years workers have a duty to prioritize the safeguarding of the child's health and wellbeing above all else. To ensure this, in these delicate and often very complex cases, relationships of trust and cooperation between parents and healthcare workers can become strained or even require severing. I flag these particular circumstances here because they point to additional layers of complexity that PCC can present in early years support. However, I do not explore them any further here as they involve complex multi-agency care arrangements, which would need too much space to discuss and distract from the immediate task of painting a picture of what person-centredness looks like in 'normal practice' for health visiting and community support.

Reader activity

Reflection:

What do you think parents and parents-to-be need to know about the role of the health visitor and the health visitor's extended team?

What makes parents feel supported in practice?

It is difficult to outline what parents want, in broad terms, from health visiting and early years support. This is partly due to the fact that people often have a limited understanding of the role of health visitors and other early years workers unless they have had some sustained contact with services or are well acquainted with this area of work for professional or personal reasons (Donetto et al., 2013). The difficulty also stems from the fact that a lot of research within health visiting and maternal and child health (MCH) focuses on specific areas of practice, most often those characterized by high health risk (for example, postnatal depression or immunization) or underserved groups/clinical areas (for example, seldom heard/hard to reach groups such as minority ethnic groups, travelling families, asylum seekers). This makes it very difficult to draw a detailed picture for health visiting practice as a whole (Cowley et al., 2013; Tiitinen et al., 2013). Professional codes of conduct and proficiency standards allude to aspects of nursing practice that sound clearly person centred in nature, although are not necessarily described in these terms.

As nurses, health visitors are expected to 'listen to people and respond to their preferences and concerns', to 'recognise and respect the contribution that people can make to their own health and wellbeing', and to 'respect a person's right to accept or refuse treatment' (NMC 2015: 3–5). They are also expected to provide a service 'which is accessible and does not stigmatize any individual; which maintains an openness to other concepts of health and wellbeing and how others wish to live; and is central to the purpose of specialist community public health practice' (NMC 2004: 6–8). In their work with parents, health visitors are meant to use strengths-based approaches such as motivational interviewing and/or the Solihull approach to 'promote positive lifestyle choices and support positive parenting practices to ensure the best start in life for the child' (NHS England 2014: 10). In the study I draw upon here,[3] which

---

[3] This was a qualitative study exploring in detail the views of parents who had experience of engaging with health visiting services within the 'universal' and/or 'universal plus' level of provision. The study was carried out by a team of researchers at the National Nursing Research Unit, King's College London, in 2012, and a full report can be freely accessed online at the following link: http://www.kcl.ac.uk/nursing/research/nnru/publications/Reports/Voice-of-service-user-report-July-2013-FINAL.pdf. For this study, 44 parents (42 mothers and two fathers) were interviewed across two NHS trusts in England. Full details of the study methods, findings and implications for practice can be found in the study report.

explored parents' views of their engagement with health visiting services, participants gave concrete examples of their experiences of services which had clear resonances with these person-centred service aspirations. The accounts our research team collected from parents shed light on the features of services they found valuable and enabling (as well as off-putting). Below, I report a few examples to illustrate how mothers in our study valued support and advice that made them feel 'known', respected in their choices and free to ask any questions they may have without fear of sounding 'silly'. I also use extracts from the same study to look at how – beyond the interactions with individual professionals – the broader engagement with services contributed to parents' perceptions of care that was reliable and always at hand, thus arguably enabling a person-centred approach on a more systemic level.

Feeling 'known' and respected

Mother of three, Scarlett, pointed out that she listened to her health visitor's recommendations not simply because of her professional role but because of the relationship they had built over time:

> I always listen to good advice, but in a way I only ended up really listening to [my health visitor's] advice. One, because obviously she was my health visitor, but mainly because she knew us and I was going through stages with her . . .
>
> (Scarlett, mother of three)

This 'being known' came through small everyday gestures that gave parents the confidence that healthcare workers genuinely cared about the families with which they worked:

> And it was nice because she [nursery nurse] knew [my daughter] and she knew about what was happening with her [health condition], so when treatment week came she'd remember: 'Oh, how did it go at the hospital?'
>
> (Lydia, mother of one)

In particular, mothers in our study valued receiving support that was tailored to their life circumstances and their approaches to parenting. By contrast, suggestions and recommendations that were seen to be 'by the book' were an important reason for disengaging from services. An example is provided again by Lydia, who talked about the information she received about breastfeeding:

> I saw Justeen [health visiting team member] a few times, and she was the only one really who didn't go on and on about breastfeeding. Because each time I went to get [my daughter] weighed the others seemed to go on and on about the breastfeeding, and she understood how I felt because I was breastfeeding and mixed feeding, and the others tended to be like, 'Knock the bottle off and just carry on with the breastfeeding.' But this was working for me and Justeen understood that. So I was lucky enough to have Justeen each week when I went to take [my daughter] to get weighed.
>
> (Lydia, mother of one)

In the absence of complicating factors, health visitors have the professional responsibility to promote and support exclusive breastfeeding for the first six months of a child's life in view of its benefits for the child's health as well as the mother-child relationship (Ip *et al.*, 2007; NHS Start 4 Life 2012). In practice, mothers' experiences of breastfeeding vary in relation to a range of factors (for example, cultural context, lack of support, latching problems, etc). Mothers who choose not to breastfeed or to stop breastfeeding early or partially really appreciate support that takes into account and respects their choices, as was the case for Lydia above.

In consultations, feeling 'heard' and respected involved being able to express one's concerns and share one's experiences without feeling rushed, judged or pressured in any way. Denise, for example, commented on the health visitor's ability not to make her feel rushed despite the time pressures she must surely have been under, whilst Roxanne referred to the reassurance that came from being able to ask 'silly' questions without fear of wasting professionals' time:

> I suppose you have to remember that they've got lots of other people to see. But she never rushed, no. I never felt rushed. Whether she set aside more time for me or what, I don't know.
>
> (Denise, mother of one)

> Like you don't feel stupid or like you're wasting their time about anything. You know, because with some places you can feel as if you're pestering them almost by ringing. But it's not . . . when you ring, even if you say, 'Oh, this is a stupid question. . .' they'll go, 'Oh, that's not a stupid question'. I think all mums kind of have them, so I think it's really good that you're able to just ring up and ask questions when you need to.
>
> (Roxanne, mother of one)

Reflecting on the factors that helped parents build trusting relationships with health visiting staff, mother of one, Vicky, described what practitioners' listening skills meant to her:

> For somebody to feel comfortable with you and trust you, yes, you have these guidelines, and yes, that's what you're supposed to stick to or whatever, but I think it's having that there but also letting somebody talk about what they want to talk about, and say what they think they want to do and encourage that maybe, as long as they're not doing anything awful.
>
> (Vicky, mother of one)

The aspects of interaction in consultations with health visitors and other early years workers described by these mothers begin to draw a more concrete outline of what parents value in seeking support from services. They help us to pin down how person-centredness can underlie everyday practice. The aspects of interaction described here are not – as it were – the icing on the cake of evidence-based child health advice. On the contrary, they are core to the development of enabling relationships that actively contribute to parents feeling supported and confident that help is at hand when needed. In our study, this was highlighted by the extent to which unsatisfactory interactions with members of the health visiting team could jeopardize future access to services. Especially in the early weeks after the birth of a child, parents – particularly mothers – can feel vulnerable, sensitive or simply emotionally strained. When they feel judged by healthcare professionals or approached with 'one-size-fits-all' advice that does not take into account personal life-stories and family circumstances, they can remain reluctant to engage with services also at later stages (Donetto et al., 2013).

Reader activity

Reflection:

Can you think of a situation (either in the clinical setting or in your personal life) where you had to adapt the support you offered to a person's specific needs and preferences? Did you find that difficult? Why?

Reliable services and coordinated care

Coordination and reliability of services can mean a range of different things within health visiting practice. The mothers we spoke to in our study emphasized the reassurance they drew from knowing that the service existed, that it was easy to access and prompt in responding in the event that they would need it. Knowing that it was possible to access a member of the health visiting team or a Children's Centre worker when issues or queries arose helped mothers to feel more secure in their parental role. Jennifer's comment below captures this perception:

Interviewer: *So what did you find helpful about having your health visiting team?*

Jennifer: *Just kind of having them there if I needed them. It's kind of like reassurance that you're kind of not just left to it, if you like. And if you do need that extra support, like professional extra support, then they are there and you can just call them up or you can just come in, whichever. But I do tell everybody how great they are.*

(Jennifer, mother of two)

Similarly Lorraine and Paula described how they felt they could rely on services being accessible when they needed them:

It's just nice to know that there's people close by that you can . . . if you've got any worries, you can ask. And also they'll say to you, 'Oh no, you need to go and ask the doctor about that.' Sometimes you're not sure whether you need to go to the doctor or not, but they'll always tell you whether you need to or if it's something you can sort out with them.

(Lorraine, mother of one)

> They're all friendly . . . I pretty much know most of the women who work here now, if there's a problem. They say they'll pass the message on. It's quite easy to phone up and say, 'Can I speak to so-and-so,' and they'll phone back.
>
> (Paula, mother of two)

Lorraine also alluded to one of the pivotal roles that health visitors can have in mediating contact with other services. She referred to health visitors being able to assess when a concern should be discussed with a doctor; however, this mediating and connecting role was also described in other situations. For example, Adele referred to her health visitor actually contacting the GP herself:

> [My son] went to hospital a few times and we were at the doctors' a few times, but my health visitor . . . when she came out, she saw he wasn't a hundred per cent, so she actually got on to the doctors to phone me . . . . Obviously because it was the health visitor who got in touch, they phoned me in a matter of half an hour after my health visitor left. Straight back in touch with me, and then [my son] ended up in hospital for a week, so it could have been a lot worse if my health visitor didn't [phone].
>
> (Adele, mother of three)

The accounts of mothers of children with complex and ongoing health needs also highlighted the important coordination work that health visitors can do behind the scenes: work which contributes to making parents' experiences relatively seamless and consistent. For children who need to attend a range of different services and who have several professionals involved in their care, health visitors can be in a key position and have the knowledge and skills to ensure that all the necessary steps happen and they do so in the right sequence. In less complex cases, health visitors and their team colleagues had the local knowledge and contacts to link parents to the right community services and resources, or even simply to ensure parents could access and benefit from services they were entitled to, for example claiming benefits or linking with social care services. In Denise's case, having moved to the area only recently, social isolation was a challenge when her first baby was born; the health visiting team helped her to find the right support for her family within the local community:

> So I went up there for [baby's] 12 week check and it was then that I broke down to [the health visitor] and told her exactly how lonely I was feeling because I didn't have any friends, because I'd only moved up here literally three weeks before he was born. . . . And that's when she helped me, and put me in touch with the [Children's Centre] and got me a [family support worker], and helped me integrate a little bit better. . . . Because I went through a stage where I didn't want to go out of the house. . . . I was nervous to come down here on my own to the [baby class]. . . . [The family support worker] met me at my house and actually walked me down here . . . and she came in with me. . . . Without that I would never have got out and I wouldn't have got the friends that I've got now so . . .
>
> (Denise, mother of one)

Coordination of antenatal and postnatal care with a relatively seamless transition from midwife-led to health visitor-led care also plays a part in making parents feel supported and linked in an effective network to which they can turn for help and advice. Whilst this transition is usually relatively straightforward (although not always fully explained) for uncomplicated births and healthy parents and babies, it can also take a significant amount of 'backstage' work when circumstances are more complex, for example when a baby has a longer hospital stay due to premature birth or other complications.

Why all this emphasis on the various aspects of coordination of care within health visiting provision? Because, just as with unsatisfactory interactions with individual practitioners, poor coordination – which often translates into lack of or inconsistent information, gaps in care, missed routine developmental checks – can have a significant impact on parents' experiences of care, leading to feelings of distress, abandonment or being overwhelmed by having to manage too vast an amount of information and interactions. The accounts above also underline the importance – for a service to be seen as accessible and reliable – of interactions in which staff's attitudes and behaviours convey approachability and genuine concern, echoing the examples described in the previous section. All these professional practices, however, are embedded within and shaped by organizational contexts that can support and/or erode them to varying degrees, as I go on to discuss in the following section.

Reader activity

Reflection:

In your experience as a user of NHS services, what forms of communication/information gave you the impression that the system was reliable and up to speed (or not)?

Person-centredness for the health and wellbeing of young children and their families

The examples illustrated above provide an initial picture of what person-centredness might look like when caring for young children and their families. Looking more closely at what parents value – even if it is *some* parents rather than a statistically representative sample of the overall population – can help us think about what approaches to practice actually enact principles of PCC and support. Before doing this, however, it might be worth reminding ourselves of the meaning of person-centredness in its most common uses. The concept of person-centredness (or patient-centredness as it was initially referred to) has evolved over time but remains characterized by ambiguity in relation to the different frameworks that can be used to make sense of it and/or operationalize it. In general terms person-centredness can be thought of as an overarching organizing principle for professional practice that takes into account issues of choice and responsibility in health and lifestyle matters (Mead and Bower 2000). A recent review of the core elements of PCC featuring in the discourses circulated via the medical, nursing, and health policy literature identifies three themes that prove relatively more consistent across these different bodies of work: degree and nature of patient participation and involvement in care, characteristics of the relationship between patient and health professional, and systemic features of the context in which care takes place

(Kitson *et al.*, 2012). However, the review also points out the lack of a shared framework that can apply across professional boundaries and be shared by users of healthcare services as well (Kitson *et al.*, 2013) Recent work has also drawn attention to the persistent difficulties in defining and measuring the *activities* that exemplify PCC principles – summarized as (1) affording people dignity, respect and compassion; (2) affording people coordinated care, support or treatment; (3) offering personalized care; and (4) enabling people to develop their capabilities – in practice (de Silva 2014; Collins 2014). Berwick's conceptualization of PCC as 'the experience (to the extent the informed, individual patient desires it) of transparency, individualization, recognition, respect, dignity, and choice in all matters, without exception, related to one's person, circumstances, and relationships in health care' (2009: 560) is also useful here as it conveys the inherent complexity of this approach to clinical care (Donetto 2012).

The examples from parents' accounts reported above illuminate the practical ways in which – in line with a person-centred approach to care as broadly defined here – support can be individualized to take into account personal circumstances and relationships, respect for beliefs and choices can be conveyed in interaction, and coordination of services can be effectively choreographed to help parents feel enabled in looking after their health and that of their child/children. Some of the features illustrated may seem 'common sense': listening to parents, understanding their views, becoming familiar with their circumstances – who would practise any differently in a healthcare environment? And yet we know from research, and often from personal experience of engaging with NHS services as patients or carers, that in the real world things are often less ideal and much more complex than 'common sense' would have them. Person-centred communication and care are not solely dependent on practitioners' good will and dedication to their professional role.

Health visitors and early years workers practise within organizational arrangements shaped by multiple factors and pressures. Not only do they work at the interface between primary care and local authority provision but their practice is also shaped – and often constrained – by the specific organizational arrangements of the local NHS trust, health centre, and/or GP surgery. As a consequence, the possibilities of PCC are a product of the interplay of several factors which include professional attitudes and skills, but also organizational characteristics and, at a broader level, national guidance and policy. In thinking about person-centredness in family care it is therefore important, as professionals, to be reflective about one's own practice as well as aware and informed of the context in which it takes place and what is involved in shaping that context.

Also, we need to be aware that respecting a person's choices and preferences and working towards shared decision-making, although broadly desirable, are not always straightforward in practice or in principle. This is especially so if and when these things are interpreted as handing over power or abdicating professional competence and accountability. I am thinking here of the broader argument for PCC as a shift from a 'paternalistic' approach to clinical interactions, in which the health professional makes all decisions with little consideration for the patient's perspective (or experience of care), to an approach that is meant to 'empower' patients by asking professionals to pay attention and respond to the patient's concerns, preferences and expectations of the clinical interaction (Cribb 2011). It is worth remembering here that although respecting people's choices and preferences is central to PCC, this cannot mean disregarding professional expertise, or holding parents/patients solely responsible for their health choices (and any consequences these may have) once professional advice has been offered. On the contrary, taking people's priorities seriously means engaging with their perspectives in a dialogue in which both professional advice and individual preferences are susceptible to negotiation so long as the health and wellbeing of the child are safeguarded.

Person-centred or family-centred support?

So far I have discussed essential dimensions of person-centredness in health visiting service provision but I have largely taken the idea of person-centredness as referring to parents as individuals. In this context, however, it is necessary to re-frame person-centredness to include the family as the unit around which care and support are oriented. 'Family-centred care' as a framework for paediatric nursing practice is nothing new. However, it has been examined more closely in the context of acute and hospital-based care than in that of community care (Franck and Callery 2004; Corlett and Twycross 2006; Shields *et al.*, 2006). Here I am not concerned about a terminological question – about whether, in the context of health visiting, referring to 'family-centredness' is more accurate than referring to 'person-centredness'. The distinction is largely a matter of emphasis (as family-centredness will still need to priori*tize* the wellbeing of the child and person- or even-child-centredness will need to take into account the context in which the child lives; Franck and Callery 2004) and, for this discussion, relatively unimportant. Family-centredness can be understood as reflecting the application of a person-centred approach to the relational network in which the child lives. What matters here is how we should take into account the context in which a child lives and the relationships this comprises when we offer support and advice.

Context and relationships are both very complex things to understand in enough detail to be able to tailor one's practice to respond to them effectively. Finding out whether a child's father (or second parent) lives in the family home, gathering a sense of the family's lifestyle, and learning about larger family composition may be straightforward enough through one or two home visits. But finer understanding of family dynamics may require time – which health visitors do not always have much of – and a well-developed ability to 'tune in' to parents' emotional worlds. This is particularly relevant when we consider the emphasis for health visiting practice on involving fathers. Drawing again on the interviews we did for the study, I give a few examples of the sorts of circumstances that shape the forms of 'family' support that are possible. For example, some mothers taking part in our study described their partners as 'hands-off' or taking 'more of a back seat' in the division of labour surrounding parenting tasks and responsibilities, but one father who wished to be more involved felt somewhat excluded. Other mothers sought the comfort of an exclusive relationship with the health visitor. Circumstances can vary greatly and the point I make here is that it is important to bear in mind that a person-centred approach means ensuring we pay enough attention to circumstances and cases and that we adjust our communication and practice accordingly.

For example, involving fathers at a time when couple relationships are under strain and conflict is an issue can go against developing a trusting relationship with the mother.

This was the case for Dorothy, who had found adjusting to being a mother difficult and welcomed the relationship with the health visitor as a time when she was able to offload:

> I think with it all, I felt like I wanted it to be my time for me to speak to somebody.
>
> (Dorothy, mother of one)

In the case of Dorothy's family, the health visitor did not directly involve the child's father in her conversations with Dorothy as this would have not been sensitive to her need to have a trusted person to speak to freely. Nevertheless, Dorothy also entertained the possibility that the health visitor might have had a role in mediating the communication between her and her partner:

> At times I did kind of want the health visitors to kind of explain to [my partner] how I felt. So rather than the case of when I had to explain to [my partner] how I felt, it didn't start an argument or I didn't break down in tears or whatever else.
>
> (Dorothy, mother of one)

Mother of two Hillary had a very difficult relationship with her partner and preferred one-to-one conversations with her health visitor. Hillary felt that by first checking with her whether or not her partner should be involved, her health visitor had supported her through hard times without imposing her partner's presence during home visits:

> I said I don't want him here. Because she [the health visitor] always used to ask me, 'Do you want him in the room?' And I used to say no, because he'd get in a mood if I talked about him or anything . . . . She used to say, 'Do you want him in the room? You don't have to have him in the room.' He just used to go upstairs, or he'd just go out. It helped really. I don't know, I just didn't want him in the room at that time. When I used to talk about him he just shrugged his shoulders or he'd say little comments.
>
> (Hillary, mother of two)

Some mothers described their partners as taking an observer role as opposed to becoming directly involved in consultations with the health visitors or in accessing services. Florence's comment captures this type of couple dynamic:

> He takes more of a back seat but then that's just, I talk more than he does. He's quite a quiet person. So that's just our whole dynamic is that I tend to do more talking in most experiences, because I talk too much and he doesn't talk enough . . . . I mean, I think, for us, it doesn't matter that he wasn't the most involved because it's just how our thing works. He's supportive, I do the main talking because I do the main caring and it works for us but I think the service probably, for most dads, feels like it's not as accessible as it could be but then I don't know how you could really make that different.
>
> (Florence, mother of two)

Fathers who are more inclined to be engaged in the care of their children might find the practical arrangements of home visits inconvenient or feel slightly left out by a traditional focus on the mother as the main carer. A father interviewed for our study shared his feelings of being unsupported after the birth of their first child:

> So I was getting everything second hand really. So I don't think that [my wife] didn't get good support, I don't think she didn't get good advice but I didn't get much. [. . .] I didn't feel that anybody had desperate desire to, you know, find out how I was doing and whether I was doing the right thing. They were quite sure that if they told [my wife] what to do that I would find out. Now, I did, [my wife] is very good at telling me things but if she wasn't . . .
>
> (Michael, father of two)

Being sensitive and responsive to different needs and wishes for involvement within the family requires individual attitudes and skills in practitioners but also, as already discussed, organizational structures and processes that allow for flexible and adaptive approaches to involvement. It also requires the availability of, and connection with, allied organizations and systems that can look after the needs of different members when treating the family as a unit is impossible or inappropriate (for example, when there are issues of violence or abuse, mental health concerns that require exclusive relationships with practitioners, or when a parent does not wish to be involved but would still benefit from support). These complexities highlight the extent to which PCC, far from being an unambiguous recipe for practice, is a multi-dimensional framework that can at times entail dilemmas for which there are no right or wrong answers and which can make the model problematic if not, on occasions, practically inapplicable.

Reader activity

Reflection:

> Either in your clinical practice or personal life, did you ever have to mediate between the interests and needs of different people who equally deserved your care and attention?
> Did you find that challenging in any way? How did you establish your priorities?

Summary

In this chapter I have used the example of health visiting practice and early years support to illustrate – through the accounts of parents – some dimensions of person-centred approaches to promoting the health and wellbeing of children and their families. My discussion has aimed to provide concrete examples that can be useful to practitioners but also to highlight some important complexities in applying person-centred approaches, including those relating to respecting and addressing the needs, concerns and perspectives of different members of the family.

Complexities are inherent to all healthcare practices. Exploring these complexities, remaining aware of them and reflecting upon them are key to learning and developing as a practitioner. The interview extracts above exemplify the relevance of engaging with people's experiences through their personal narratives to obtain a richer picture of what support means to different people and at different times. In healthcare research as much as practice, paying attention to parents' (and children's) experiences of care, reflecting on one's approaches to communication and practice and being aware of and involved in the organizational processes that shape services, are fundamental to the development of person-centred practitioners.

References

Berwick, D.M. (2009) What 'patient-centered' should mean: confessions of an extremist, *Health Affairs*, 28(4): 555–65.

Collins, A. (2014) *Measuring What Really Matters: Towards a Coherent Measurement System to Support Person-centred Care*. London: The Health Foundation.

Corlett, J. and Twycross, A. (2006) Negotiation of parental roles within family-centred care: a review of the research. *Journal of Clinical Nursing*, 15(10): 1308–16.

Cowley, S., Whittaker, K., Grigulis, A. *et al.* (2013) *Why Health Visiting? A Review of the Literature About Key Health Visitor Interventions, Processes and Outcomes for Children and Families*. London: King's College London.

Cowley, S., Whittaker, K., Malone, M. *et al.* (2014) Why health visiting? Examining the potential public health benefits from health visiting practice within a universal service: a narrative review of the literature, *International Journal of Nursing Studies*. DOI:10.1016/j.ijnurstu.2014.07.013

Cribb, A. (2011) *Involvement, Shared Decision-making and Medicines*. London: Royal Pharmaceutical Society.

de Silva, D. (2014) *Helping Measure Person-centred Care: A Review of Evidence about Commonly Used Approaches and Tools Used to Help Measure Person-centred Care*. London: Health Foundation.

DCSF (Department for Children, Schools and Families) (2007) *The Children's Plan: Building Brighter Futures*. London: DCSF.

DH (Department of Health) (2011) *Health Visitor Implementation Plan 2011–2015: A Call to Action*. London: Department of Health.

Donetto, S. (2012) Medical students and patient-centred clinical practice: the case for more critical work in medical schools, *British Journal of Sociology of Education*, 33(3): 431–49.

Donetto, S., Malone, M., Hughes, J. *et al.* (2013) *Health Visiting: The Voice of Service Users:– Learning from Service Users' Experiences to Inform the Development of UK Health Visiting Practice and Services*. London: King's College London.

Fisher, M. (2009) *Skill Mix in Health Visiting and Community Nursing Teams: Principles into Practice*. London: Unite the Union/The Community Practitioners' and Health Visitors' Association.

Franck, L.S. and Callery, P. (2004) Re-thinking family-centred care across the continuum of children's healthcare, *Child: Care, Health and Development*, 30(3): 265–77.

Ip, S., Chung, M., Raman, G. *et al.* (2007) *Breastfeeding and Maternal and Infant Health Outcomes in Developed Countries. Evidence Report/Technology Assessment No. 153.* Rockville, MD: Agency for Healthcare Research and Quality.

Kitson, A., Marshall, A., Bassett, K. and Zeitz, K. (2013) What are the core elements of patient-centred care? A narrative review and synthesis of the literature from health policy, medicine and nursing, *Journal of Advanced Nursing*, 69(1): 4–15.

Mead, N. and Bower, P. (2000) Patient-centredness: a conceptual framework and review of the empirical literature, *Social Science & Medicine*, 51(7): 1087–110.

NHS England (2014) *National Health Visiting Service Specification*. London: NHS England.

NHS Start 4 Life (2012) *Off to the Best Start: Important Information about Feeding your Baby*. London: Crown Copyright. Available at: www.nhs.uk/start4life/Documents/PDFs/Start4Life_Off_To_The_Best_Start_leaflet.pdf (accessed 4 November 2015).

NMC (Nursing and Midwifery Council) (2004) *Standards of Proficiency for Specialist Community Public Health Nurses*. London: NMC.

NMC (Nursing and Midwifery Council) (2015) *The Code: Professional Standards of Practice and Behaviour for Nurses and Midwives*. London: NMC.

Pugh, G. and Duffy, B. (2010) *Contemporary Issues in the Early Years*. London: Sage.

Shields, L., Pratt, J. and Hunter, J. (2006) Family centred care: a review of qualitative studies, *Journal of Clinical Nursing*, 15(10): 1317–23.

Shribman, S. and Billingham, K. (2009) *The Healthy Child Programme: Pregnancy and the First Five Years*. London: Department for Children Schools and Families.

Tiitinen, S., Homanen, R., Lindfors, P. and Ruusuvuori, J. (2013) Approaches used in investigating family support in transition to parenthood, *Health Promotion International*. DOI: doi:10.1093/heapro/das077

Chapter

5

Person-centred approaches to school age care

Andrea Cockett

Introduction

Providing care to children and their families can be both rewarding and challenging. Balancing the needs of children versus those of their parents, carers and other family members can place healthcare professionals in difficult situations and achieving a balanced approach to nursing care delivery that listens to and meets the needs of all family members requires knowledgeable and insightful nursing skill. In this chapter the aim is to outline some of the key theoretical concepts that underpin providing PCC to children and their families in order to provide the knowledge required.

These concepts will be critically analysed to provide the reader with the opportunity to explore and reflect upon how they can enhance care delivery and how our views of children and their families may hinder the delivery of truly person-centred care for this group of clients. The concepts to be explored include:

- Family-centred care
- Participation of children and its implementation into practice
- The tensions that arise between the needs of children and those of their families

This chapter focuses on children aged 4 to 13 years, as Chapter 6 will focus on the needs of adolescents and young people. Case studies will show how PCC can be facilitated and delivered in the context of caring for school age children and how nurses are essential in this process. These case studies will demonstrate how children and their families can be involved in developing both services that influence the delivery of healthcare to a specific client group and how children's voices can be heard in the development of nurse education for children's nursing. The terms 'parents' and 'family' will be used in the chapter but these terms will mean any primary carer and extended family members that are closely involved with the child.

Family Participation in Healthcare

Involving children and their families in the development and delivery of healthcare services is both an ethical and a statutory imperative. The United Nation Convention on the Rights of the Child (UNCRC) (UN 1989) sets out the importance of a child's right to participation in article 12. This states that governments have a responsibility to ensure that a child who is capable of forming his or her own views should have the right to express these freely in all matters that affect them and that this is particularly of significance in any judicial or administrative procedures that affect them (UN 1989). The United Kingdom (UK) government clearly outlines that service users should be involved in and consulted about the development, organization and delivery of healthcare services to ensure that they meet their needs in the *National Service Framework for Children, Young People and Maternity Services* (DH 2004). The UK government recently reported how progress has been made in the UK towards meeting the UNCRC articles, in particular article 12 (HM Government 2014). This progress report identified that children are able to participate in legislative activities such as the UK Youth Parliament and the Youth Select Committee, however these activities were limited to children aged 11 years and above and there are no formal government vehicles by which younger children can have their views and wishes taken into account (HM Government 2014). The limiting of activities such as these to older children will be discussed later in the chapter in relation to how society views children's ability to participate and how this affects the way in which care is delivered.

The Office of the Children's Commissioner has also identified how children and young people can be involved in strategic decisions relating to healthcare (Blades *et al.*, 2013). The report outlines that children's involvement in the development and delivery of health services is patchy and uncoordinated and often relies on individuals within organizations rather than a clear strategic plan. This haphazard approach to involvement of children and young people means that whilst children may be consulted about individual decisions that affect their own care, their ability to influence the wider configuration of services is very limited (Blades *et al.*, 2013). Children themselves identify that they would like the opportunity to have a more strategic influence but that their involvement needs to be configured so that this is possible (La Valle *et al.*, 2012). In particular they identified that they would like to:

- be istened to;
- have their recommendations acted on;
- be informed of what happens in response to their recommendations
- meet with decision makers to discuss why their recommendations haven't been implemented if this is the case.

(La Valle *et al.*, 2012)

So how do these strategic government-led initiatives affect PCC for both individual children and the healthcare professionals responsible for delivering the care? Within children's nursing as a field of nursing there are a number of theoretical concepts that have been developed and implemented to enhance the involvement of children and their families in the organization, delivery and the evaluation of the nursing care that they require. These theoretical concepts can be applied to both the delivery of individual care and also the development of healthcare at a strategic level. In order for PCC to be delivered effectively it is important that both of these aspects of care delivery are addressed. Whilst individual nurses and healthcare professionals may work with children and their families in a way which facilitates their involvement, if the overarching structures and policies do not support PCC then it will be difficult to fully provide it. This chapter will now explore these concepts and how they can help to support nursing care that is both person and family centred.

Reader activity

Think about these questions before reading the chapter and return to them again at the end.

- What are the strengths and limitations of taking a family-centred care approach to delivering nursing care?
- What key messages can be learnt about participation of children?
- What do children want from the nurses delivering care to them?
- How can we involve school age children in the decisions that affect their health and wellbeing?
- What skills, attitudes and competencies does a nurse caring for school age children and their families need to develop?

Delivering care to families and children: family-centred care and The Partnership Model

Person-centred nursing care in the context of school age children needs to be redefined as family-centred care. The use of the term family-centred care has been prevalent in children's nursing for some time and it recognizes that school age children should not be separated from their main carers when they are in receipt of healthcare interventions whatever those interventions may be (Coyne *et al.*, 2011). Family-centred care can be defined as 'a way of caring for children and their families within health services which ensures that care is planned around the whole family, not just the individual child/person and in which all the family members are recognised as care recipients' (Shields *et al.*, 2006: 1318). This concept of family-centred care arose from historical work about attachment theory and the need to minimize the effects of hospitalization on children (Coyne *et al.*, 2011). There was a recognition that families were important for the emotional and psychological wellbeing of children and that care should be constructed in such a way that the whole family was involved and was able to participate (Foster *et al.*, 2010). Family-centred care has been formally recognized as an optimal way of delivering care to children in the UK and is part of current government policy

(Coyne *et al.*, 2011). It is not however without criticism and the evidence base for its effectiveness is limited with little concrete quantitative research to demonstrate that it is a more effective care delivery mechanism than standardized care alone (Shields 2010).

Family-centred care has many different elements. The Institute for Patient and Family Centred Care (2010; see Figure 5.1) propose that it consists of the following:

Box 5.1

- **Respect and dignity.** Health care practitioners listen to and honour patient and family perspectives and choices. Patient and family knowledge, values, beliefs and cultural backgrounds are incorporated into the planning and delivery of care.
- **Information sharing.** Health care practitioners communicate and share complete and unbiased information with patients and families in ways that are affirming and useful. Patients and families receive timely, complete, and accurate information in order to effectively participate in care and decision-making.
- **Participation.** Patients and families are encouraged and supported in participating in care and decision-making at the level they choose.
- **Collaboration.** Patients and families are also included on an institution-wide basis. Health care leaders collaborate with patients and families in policy and program development, implementation, and evaluation; in health care facility design; and in professional education, as well as in the delivery of care.

The different elements identified in Box 5.1 have both micro level (individual patient care delivery) and macro level (organizational and strategic) components. For children's nurses delivering care to school age children the elements of family-centred care that apply to their work will be dependent upon their role within an organization.

Some studies have explored the perceptions that both nurses and parents have of family-centred care and the benefits and challenges of implementing family-centred care (Coyne *et al.*, 2011, Foster *et al.*, 2010; Trajkovski *et al.*, 2012; Butler *et al.*, 2013). These issues will be considered next.

Nurses' perceptions of family-centred care

Nurses' perceptions of family-centred care in developed countries have been explored by a number of researchers and these perceptions can help us to reflect upon how we deliver care to school age children in our own practice area. Nurses were asked to identify the components of family-centred care in a study by Coyne *et al.* (2011). The components identified were: family involvement in care, working in partnership with parents, negotiating care, delivering high quality care and a multidisciplinary approach to care. These are all desirable elements for quality PCC delivery, and working in partnership with both families and other healthcare professionals has been recognized in policy guidance as being pivotal to ensuring services meet clinical governance standards (Royal College of Nursing 2013). Other key elements of family-centred care that have been identified by nurses are communication, roles and relationships, meeting parental needs and resources (Foster *et al.*, 2010).

Communication with both the child and their family is key to the delivery of family-centred care. Nurses identified that appropriate communication was essential in the relationships that they developed when delivering PCC. The communication needs to focus not just on the child but the family also. Facilitating communication with parents about their child's illness, with the child themselves and also between the child and family are essential skills. This was highlighted in a study by Trajkovski *et al.* (2012) which examined neonatal nurse perceptions of family-centred care. These nurses identified that there needed to be a 'happy medium' in which the needs of the infant and the needs of the parents were met. There was also a need for nurses to not make judgements about parents' participation in their child's care as this could be affected by many different factors such as having other children, emotional distress and in the case of neonatal patients, postnatal depression (Trajkovski *et al.*, 2012). Communication with parents about their wishes and desire to participate in care were fundamental to the success of family-centred care in this context.

Box 5.2 demonstrates how family-centred care can be used in a specific clinical context: palliative care. In order to meet the needs of all family members the nurse must make decisions about how to support parents to discuss very difficult information with their child to ensure that the needs of all family members are met. It may also be necessary to support parents to discuss this information with siblings and the extended family. The skill of the nurse lies in the timing and content of these discussions with parents to ensure that their communication is timely and appropriate.

Box 5.2   Clinical context: truth telling in palliative care

In the context of palliative care truth telling is a key element of the relationship between healthcare professionals and children and their families. For some families this may mean that they need help to tell their child the truth. In these circumstances, it is the healthcare professional's role to help parents to understand the importance of telling children the truth about the disease process and the possible outcomes.

As a healthcare professional, you need to take account of:

- the context in which the family reside
- their spiritual beliefs, and
- their culture.

All of these factors must be taken into consideration when approaching what can be very difficult discussions. However, as a healthcare professional, you should ensure that your own values and beliefs do not influence the decisions that you think the family should make. Sometimes it can take a long time for families to make decisions about the right information to tell their child. For some life limited children, they may have a lengthy lifespan so families can take this time. For others, the illness is very short and the pressure to tell may be very great.

Individual families will all need to make individual decisions and whilst on the whole truth telling is seen to be good this cannot be at the cost of a breakdown in family/child or family/healthcare professional relationships.

Understanding how nurses perceive and deliver family-centred care is important as it can help practitioners to enhance the way in which they themselves deliver care. Questioning and reflecting on how we balance the needs of children versus the needs of their families can enable improved functioning for all.

Parental perceptions of family-centred care

In order for family-centred care to be successful it is important that nurses understand what parents' and families' perceptions and understanding of the concept are. Parent's perceptions of family-centred care are very similar to those of nurses however parents place differing emphasis on the components of family-centred care and what makes it successful for them (Foster *et al.*, 2010). Communication was identified as a key issue for successful implementation of family-centred care by parents but was not rated as highly as it was by nurses. Parents identified roles and relationships as being a more significant factor that affected their ability to provide effective care to their child and to have a good working relationship with professionals (Butler *et al.*, 2013). The challenges of negotiating roles within the context of care delivery is borne out by other literature relating to the care of children with complex needs and who are technology dependent (Cockett 2012). Parents identify that they struggle to balance their role as a parent with the highly nursing focused skills they have to develop in order to care for their child. Reeves *et al.* (2006) identified that when children were admitted to hospital, the parents who were perceived to be competent to care for their child at home were suddenly disenfranchized and healthcare professionals started to take control of the child's care. Because parents were used to providing their child's care they became expert at it and found it very difficult to allow others to provide the care. They also felt threatened by healthcare professionals who could be judgemental about the way parents undertook certain medical procedures. Parents also felt that there were times in hospital when staff were thin on the ground that the expectation was that they would provide all of the care for their child (Reeves *et al.*, 2006). This is supported by more general literature which identifies that family-centred care can sometimes be used as an excuse to expect parents to provide care for their child when they are in hospital (Coyne and Cowley 2007).

Negotiation was identified as a key element of family-centred care by parents (Stuart and Melling 2014). The negotiation that happens between nurses and parents is fundamental to the success of providing individualized PCC for children. Stuart and Melling (2014) found that nurses were happy to negotiate with parents about providing essential care to their child but less happy to negotiate about care that may be perceived to be 'nursing'. This focus on parents providing essential care rather than more technical care was echoed in work by Foster *et al.* (2010). With a shift to shorter hospital stays and an increase in the number

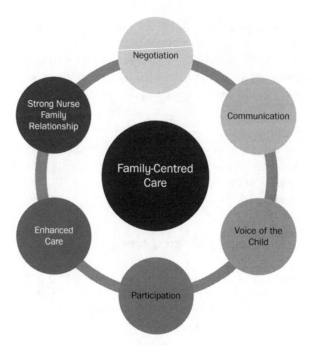

Figure 5.1 Essential elements of family-centred care

of children with ongoing and complex healthcare needs nurses need to consider what care parents can and should be participating in and delivering. Preparing parents to care for their children effectively at home is an essential element of PCC.

For family-centred care to be effective it is evident that nurses and families need to work together in partnership to achieve the best outcomes for children.

Working in partnership with children and their families

As identified previously working in partnership is a fundamental aspect of family-centred care. The theoretical model of partnership nursing is not new in children's nursing and has been adopted as a model of nursing care in many children's healthcare settings across the UK (Coyne and Cowley 2007). It arose from the recognition, like family-centred care, that children's psychological and emotional wellbeing is enhanced if their parents are able to participate in and provide care from them, particularly if they are hospitalized (Brady 2009). This recognition that care needs to be negotiated and delivered in partnership led to the development of the model from a belief that other nursing models did not meet the unique needs of children and their families (Coyne and Cowley 2007). The model identifies that 'the care of children well or sick is best carried out by their parents with varying degrees of assistance from members of a suitably qualified health care team whenever necessary' (Casey 1988: 8).

Using the partnership model of nursing in practice is not without its challenges. Parents often feel that nurses expect them to care for their child and that they are judged and found wanting if they for perfectly legitimate reasons are not able to provide that care (Shields 2010). The tension between nurses and parents has been described previously in relation to technology-dependent children particularly and parents who are experts in the care of their child often find themselves struggling to balance their roles: are they a parent or a nurse? (Cockett 2012). Children themselves identify that working in partnership is important in successful care delivery when they are hospitalized (Brady 2009). The notion of partnership is valuable but often the reality of healthcare delivery means that its implementation in practice is dependent upon factors such as the resources available, the skill of nursing staff in negotiating with parents and the skills of parents in caring for their child. Stuart and Melling (2014) found that nurses expected parents to undertake everyday tasks routinely but did not negotiate either whether this was what parents wished or to extend the care parents could provide.

Benefits and challenges of family-centred care as a model for person-centred nursing care

From the discussion above it is clear that family-centred care is a model that can be used to provide PCC for school age children. The benefits of providing nursing care in this way involve increased parental participation in decision-making relating to the care of their child, the recognition of the rights of families in relation to their child's care, enhanced care for children both physical and emotional and improved relationships between healthcare professionals and families (Foster *et al.*, 2010; Shields 2010; Coyne *et al.*, 2011). In practice factors that were identified as being important to support the delivery of family-centred care include: resources for children and their families that support parental participation in care such as adequate sleeping facilities and family rooms, financial and psychosocial support for families, improved communication between nurses and families and managerial and organizational structures that support the delivery of care in this way (Coyne *et al.*, 2011).

However as discussed above there are some challenges in providing family-centred care and an important factor to consider is where are the rights and views of the child in relation to family-centred care? If the focus is on the family as a unit supporting the child where does consideration of the child as a separate person from the family take place and how do nurses ensure the voice of the child is heard particularly if it is in conflict with those of the family? Evidence suggests that children, especially hospitalized children, are passive recipients of care and rely heavily on their parents to communicate and engage with hospital staff on their behalf (Kelly *Iet al.*, 2012). The chapter will now discuss what children's participation looks like, what theoretical influences act upon it and how nurses can encourage and develop the participation of children they care for.

Participation of children: philosophical, legal and ethical issues

What do we mean by participation?

Children's participation in the decisions that affect their lives has gained political importance both in the UK and the rest of the world in recent years. The UNCRC sets out the importance of a child's right to participation in article 12. Since the publication of the convention countries worldwide have made efforts to initiate participation with children (Wyness 2009). However participation of children was happening before the publication and adoption of the convention with Morrow (2009) identifying that the convention was not an initiator of participation but highlighted its importance by making it a political issue. In England the publication of *Every Child Matters* (DCSF 2003) identified the government's commitment to promoting children's' participation through the Change for Children programme (DfES 2004). This programme aimed to engender a culture of participation across all policy and public service areas in which children are involved. More recently the Office of the Children's Commissioner (OCC 2013) has identified a 'wheel of participation' which encourages the participation of children in three different ways in healthcare. These are involve, inform and consult. Each of these elements refers to the different contexts and ways in which children can be helped to and become true participants in decisions that affect them.

The increasing political importance of children's participation has been driven by several factors. The first of these is the recognition that children themselves are 'social actors' (Sinclair 2004). This is an acknowledgement that children, whilst being members of a family and a society, are also individuals in their own right and as such should be involved in decisions which directly affect them (Jans 2004). The second is that children are viewed as consumers of services and have a right to participate in discussion and policy formation relating to the service (Coad *et al.*, 2008). The *National Service Framework for Children, Young People and Maternity Services* (DH 2004) clearly identifies that the views of service users must be sought and acted upon both in the development and evaluation of services. The final factor is the legal pressure of documents such as the UNCRC which have enshrined the rights of children into international law (Lansdown 2001).

The term 'participation' can be defined in different ways and clarifying what is meant by the term is an important step in promoting participation of children. Sinclair (2004) highlights that participation is a multi-dimensional concept and can be open to varying degrees of interpretation by government both in the UK and abroad. Participation can be defined as active involvement in an activity (Morrow 2009) however the simplicity of this definition belies the complexity of the forces that are involved when trying to interpret and practise participation with a group such as children. Shier (2001) states that different levels of participation may be required for different activities so a flexible fluid approach is required. This is reflected in the wheel of participation from the OCC which highlights that full participation from children may need support in the form of information and guidance from adults. The activities used to promote participation are on a continuum from adult led and initiated to child led and initiated (OCC 2013). Hart *et al.* (2004) summarize children's participation as most commonly being thought of as a right and as a means of making local level development more child friendly. Whatever the model used to define participation the importance of participation cannot be underestimated in the current political climate. There is international pressure for countries to be seen to be upholding the UNCRC (DfES 2004). The benefits of participation are clearly recognized and stated by the UK government and include: better outcomes for children, families and young people, organizational benefits such as more targeted services, cost savings and happy customers and community benefits such as fresher democracies (HM Government 2014).

How do we view school age children and how does this affect their opportunities to participate?

The status of children in society has changed in recent times and children are now viewed differently by both families and society as a whole (Jans 2004). In the West children are no longer used as a means of economic income by the family and this change has meant that parents now cherish their children for emotional reasons. This has led to differences in the way families operate with a shift from a paternalistic authoritarian structure to a more democratic one (Jans 2004). This shift has also been complemented in western society with a growing body of work that examines and argues for the rights of children to be upheld (Sinclair 2004). Participation is seen as the way in which the rights of children can be realized (Lansdown 2001). This increased emphasis on the rights of the child can be in conflict with the way in which children are viewed. Children are seen as either 'at risk' or 'the risk' and their participation is hindered by a lack of trust by government in children and many adults in society (Cockburn 2005). Pascal and Bertram (2009) identify that whilst initiatives to engage in participation with children are to be applauded many English children are not listened to in their daily lives either at home or in school. This is especially true in the healthcare setting where the prevalent view of children is one of them being 'at risk' and in need of protection from both their families and professionals due to their ill health.

Children occupy different places in society (Wyness 2009). Children are either located in a 'place' which is a heavily regulated domain such as the home or school, or a 'space' which is defined as a public domain where a child can be active as a political person. A space, for example, can be an initiative that involves the child in decision-making alongside adults and where their views are given equal value to the adult participants. Participation of children in policy-making and service development requires that they are allowed access to a space that they normally may not be an active participant in. Wyness (2009) also identifies that when children are involved in projects the adults who are managing the project will often try to locate the space within a more conventional children's place. This allows the adult to control the outcome of the participation by restricting the child to a more traditional 'place' in society. Children are often constrained to what is designated the 'private' sphere of family, school and day care with the aim of protecting them from the 'public' sphere of politics (Mayall 2001). This protectionist attitude towards children stops them from developing their skills as active participants. In order to develop political skills and be able to take a full and active role in society children need exposure to political arenas.

Cockburn (2005) argues that a lack of reference to conflict in government directives on participation means that children will not develop the ability to challenge and be challenged. This infers that the participatory agenda is one of nominal participation (White 2000) rather than transformational participation that would enable the child to develop skills that would lead them to effect policy (Cockburn 2005).

Barriers to the participation of school aged children in healthcare

Barriers to children's participation can be located either within organizational structures or individuals' values and beliefs about children and their capacity. Organizations may be complex and bureaucratic and this may lead to difficulties in finding the appropriate time and space to work with children (Cavet and Sloper 2004). Internal politics may also result in reluctance to engage with children. Other organizational issues that may stop participation are the short-term nature of some projects and limited funding. Participation requires investment in time and training both of the adults involved and the children. Some projects may not have the capacity built into them to allow for the preparation required for participation to be undertaken in a meaningful manner (Cavet and Sloper 2004). Coad *et al.* (2008) identified that partnership with children implies that decision-making will be equitable. If this is not possible due to operational constraints then this needs to be clearly identified so that children do not feel their presence is tokenistic. However they argue that even young children have been shown able to make competent decisions regarding healthcare and parents' and professionals' fears may be unfounded (Coad *et al.*, 2008). In some aspects of nursing school age children such as pain management, we trust children as young as 4 to be able to self-report their pain so why can they not be seen as competent to participate on other aspects of care delivery? The tension around views of children's competence can mean that it can be very difficult for adults to relinquish control to children and allow them to be full participants. There are also sub groups within the population of children that find it even more difficult to participate due to judgements about their competence. Pascal and Bertram (2009) identified that young children in early years settings were usually not consulted and children from other minority groups such as migrant, refugee, asylum-seeking and travelling families also found it very difficult for their voice to be heard.

Participation can have a huge positive impact on the lives of children but in order for it to do this strong efforts need to be made to ensure that it is not tokenistic and part of a 'one off' process. Sinclair (2004) highlights the need to ensure that as participation of children in public decisions increases adults involved in the process learn from previous experiences and make sure that the participation is genuine. It should offer children the opportunity to make a meaningful difference to their worlds and be embedded within organizations, not seen as an 'add on' activity (Sinclair 2004). Cockburn (2005) highlights the requirement for adults to identify their own motivations for wishing children to participate and to assess their abilities to work with children in a constructive manner. The other important consideration is that the evidence has shown that children wish to participate on their own terms and allowing them to develop their own mechanisms for participation will be important in keeping children engaged in the process (Cockburn 2005).

The OCC (Blades *et al.*, 2013) identifies through its research that children hold strong views on their right to participate in decisions about their lives and the policies that affect them. Children identified that the following should be in place for them to be full and equal participants:

- Opportunity for all children to take part
- Outreach to ensure all children are aware of the opportunities to participate
- Simplicity so that children can fully understand what is required and the processes involved
- A variety of approaches and methods to ensure opportunities for participation are open to all
- Outputs and outcomes to ensure children are fed back to about the decisions that have been made

How can nurses promote participation for school age children?

Individual nurses have both a statutory and an ethical requirement to ensure that all children are given the opportunity to participate in the decisions that affect their own health and wellbeing. By facilitating participation nursing care will be person focused as the individual needs of the child will be listened to and taken account of. Sometimes this will be in conflict with the wishes or needs of the family unit as a whole and it is the role of the nurse to help the family to work through these challenging situations and to act as an advocate for the child. Communication and negotiation are key skills that the nurse requires to enable them to facilitate both participation of the child and family-centred care.

Two case studies now follow illustrating how participation and family-/person-centred care for school age children can be achieved successfully in practice.

Case study one: participation of school age children in the selection criteria for children's nursing candidates

This case study illustrates how school aged children were invited to participate in a project that elicited their views on the attributes that potential students of children's nursing should have. The project was part of the widening participation work of The Florence Nightingale Faculty of Nursing and Midwifery, King's College, London and was undertaken by the Department of Child and Adolescent Nursing. Visits to five local schools were arranged in which six focus groups were held to explore the views of children aged 8 to 13 to uncover what they thought the skills, knowledge and attributes of potential candidates should be. Parental permission was sought for involvement in the focus groups and this was managed by the schools. The format of the school visits was as follows:

- Staff were introduced to the pupils.
- Pupils were asked about their previous experience with healthcare. This was to uncover any issues that may need to be addressed sensitively in the group.
- Pupils were asked what they thought the attributes of a children's nurse should be.

Throughout the discussions the staff allowed the children and young people to lead and shape the discussion with only minimal prompting. This was to ensure the project truly reflected the views of the children and young people. As all of the staff involved were children's nurses they were all skilled at communicating with children of differing ages.

Results of the focus groups

The children and young people were very clear about the attributes they expected from potential children's nurses. In addition to the words identified in Figures 5.2 and 5.3 they also clearly articulated that they would like applicants to have:

- a knowledge and understanding of different stages of child development and the implications this has for the quality of the care that can be delivered;
- empathy and a connection with children and young people;
- respect for the rights of the child and young person and not just to consider the rights of the parents;
- the ability to listen and to know when to be quiet in a conversation;

- the ability to elicit information in a way that was reassuring without being too intrusive;
- the ability to be 'real'. The children and young people were very clear that they could identify when professionals were being fake with them.

Following these focus groups the Faculty reviewed the criteria used to score both personal statements and the group task that candidates undertook at selection to ensure that the attributes the children identified were used to select candidates both for interview and to offer a place to them.

This project received excellent feedback from the schools involved who valued the opportunity for their pupils to participate in an activity that could potentially have direct consequences for them. Many of the children who participated had engaged with local healthcare services so had direct experience of being cared for by children's nurses. They talked about their experiences of both actual engagement with nurses and other healthcare professionals and also about how images of nurses in the media and on television had influenced their views of what healthcare delivery and care that was focused on them should look like.

Case study two: developing an assessment tool for long-term ventilated children who access children's hospice services

Long-term ventilated (LTV) children are one of the fastest growing groups of technology-dependent children. Data from the LTV United Kingdom group has identified more than a 600 per cent increase in LTV children being cared for at home since 2005: 141 were identified in 1998 (Jardine *et al.*, 1999) and by 2008 this figure had risen to 933 (Wallis *et al.*, 2011). The complexity of the care they require means that it is very hard for them to access services (Noyes 2000).

At a children's hospice there was a need to offer short breaks to children using LTV but the hospice had very limited experience of providing care for this group of children. The author was employed to develop and deliver a short break service for this particular client group.

One of the challenges posed by caring for this group of children was the complexity of their care needs so the first part of the service development undertaken was to develop an assessment tool that could be used to document all of the care the children required in relation to their ventilation. In order to do this effectively families who had been referred to the hospice for short breaks were contacted to ask if they would like to be involved in the development of the assessment documentation. One family responded positively.

Tom, whose name has been changed to maintain his confidentiality (Nursing and

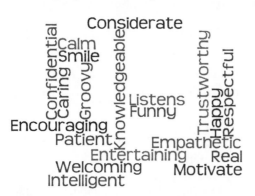

Figure 5.2 Words used to describe a 'good' children's nurse

Midwifery Council 2015) is a 4-year-old who suffers primarily from a complex form of epilepsy. Tom was born prematurely and spent a considerable amount of time in hospital prior to his discharge home. He has a tracheostomy, a gastrostomy, suffered multiple seizures and needed ventilation at night. He was discharged home to the community with a package of overnight care but no daytime care. His parents

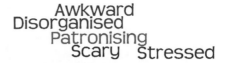

Figure 5.3 Words used to describe a 'bad' children's nurse

were very keen to help develop the documentation for the service so that Tom could start to access the hospice for short breaks. One of the challenges of working with Tom and his family was that due to the complexity of his healthcare needs his parents were reluctant to let him be cared for by staff they did not know and whose competence they had not assessed. This is a common difficulty that parents of children with very complex needs face (Kirk 2001). Tom's parents felt this burden very keenly, particularly his mother, who as a healthcare professional herself admitted that she found it very difficult to leave Tom with carers that she did not know and trust. Involving Tom's parents in the development of the documentation that would support the service was a way in which they could have some control over how the care would be delivered.

The author visited Tom and his family at home with a draft assessment tool for everyone to comment on, use and see if it met the needs of the family. The assessment tool was refined and at the suggestion of the parents, photographs of all key equipment was also included for each child so that staff could see easily how complex equipment fitted together and was used. This was invaluable as children visited the hospice from many different geographical locations so have very different equipment. The assessment tool designed in partnership with this family was later included in a national toolkit to be used by all hospices across the UK (Children's Hospice UK 2010).

Involving this particular child and family in the development of the assessment documentation had two main benefits: it helped them as an individual family to feel in control of and participants in the organization of care services that they would directly benefit from, and it helped to develop documentation that has been used to support a wide range of families across the UK. This particular example of PCC had consequences that stretched beyond the individual.

Summary

This chapter has discussed how PCC can be delivered to school age children from both a theoretical and a practical perspective. The concepts of family-centred care, partnership working and children's participation have been analysed to provide the reader with knowledge and skills about how these models of working can be used to ensure the needs of both children and their families can be met. Two case studies have been used to demonstrate how through participation of both children and their parents, services can be developed to ensure they meet their needs and not those of healthcare professionals.

In summary:

- School age children have the capacity and competence to participate in decisions that affect both their individual healthcare needs and wider strategic services.
- Participation to be successful needs to be meaningful and the adults involved need to be fully committed to it. This may require additional training for staff involved in participatory projects.
- Family-centred care is a model of nursing that can be used to provide holistic care to ensure the needs of all family members are met.
- Tension can exist between the needs of children and their families and the role of the nurse is to help families to negotiate their way through these challenging situations.
- Negotiation with both children and their families is fundamental to the success of delivering family-centred care.

Key website resources

The Institute of Patient and Family Centred Care http://www.ipfcc.org/
The National Children's Bureau http://www.ncb.org.uk/
The United Nation Convention on the Rights of the Child http://www.unicef.org.uk/UNICEFs-Work/UN-Convention/?gclid={SI:gclid}&gclid=CN6zwvXr3MECFXDHtAodpkEACg
The Office of the Children's Commissioner in England http://www.childrenscommissioner.gov.uk/

References

Blades, R., Renton, Z. and La Valle, I. (2013) *We Would Like to Make a Change: Children and Young People's Participation in Strategic Health Decision Making.* London: Office of the Children's Commissioner.

Brady, M. (2009) Hospitalised children's views of the good nurse, *Nursing Ethics*, 16(5): 543–60.

Butler, A., Copnell, B. and Willetts, G. (2013) Family centred care in the paediatric intensive care unit: an integrative review of the literature, *Journal of Clinical Nursing*, 23: 2086–100.

Casey, A. (1988) A partnership with child and family, *Senior Nurse*, 8(4): 8–9.

Cavet, J. and Sloper, P. (2004) The participation of children and young people in decisions about UK service development, *Child, Care, Health and Development*, 30(6): 613–21.

Children's Hospice UK (2010) *Tool Kit for Long Term Ventilation.* Bristol: CHUK.

Coad, J., Flay, J., Aspinall, M. *et al.* (2008) Evaluating the impact of involving young people in developing children's services in an acute hospital trust, *Journal of Clinical Nursing*, 17: 3115–22.

Cockburn, T. (2005) Children's participation in social policy: inclusion, chimera or authenticity?, *Social Policy and Society*, 4(2): 109–19.

Cockett, A. (2012) Technology dependence and children: a review of the evidence, *Nursing Children and Young People*, 24(1): 32–5.

Coyne, I. and Cowley, S. (2007) Challenging the philosophy of partnership with parents: a grounded theory study, *International Journal of Nursing Studies*, 44: 893–904.

Coyne, I., O'Neill, C., Murphy, M. *et al.* (2011) What does family centred care mean to nurses and how do they think it could be improved in practice? *Journal of Advanced Nursing*, 67(12): 2561–73.

DCSF (Department for Children, Schools and Families) (2003) *Every Child Matters*. Norwich: The Stationery Office.

DfES (Department for Education and Science) (2004) *Every Child Matters: Change for Children*. London: DfES. Available at: http://webarchive.nationalarchives.gov.uk/20130401151715/ https://www.education.gov.uk/publications/standard/publicationdetail/page1/ dfes/1081/2004 (accessed 6 November 2015).

DH (Department of Health) (2004) *National Service Framework for Children, Young People and Maternity Services*. London: DH.

Foster, M., Whitehead, L. and Maybee, P. (2010) Parents' and health professional's perceptions of family centred care for children in hospital, in developed and developing countries: a review of the literature, *International Journal of Nursing Studies*, 47: 1184–193.

Hart, J., Newman, J., Ackerman, L. and Feeney, T. (2004) *Children Changing their World: Understanding and Evaluating Children's Participation in Development*. Available at: http://www.plan-uk.org/resources/documents/28458/ (accessed 4 November 2015).

HM Government (2014) *The Fifth Periodic Report to the UN Committee on the Rights of the Child*. London: HM Government.

Institute for Patient and Family Centred Care (2010) Patient and family centred care: frequently asked questions Institute for Patient and Family Centred Care Bethesda Maryland. Available at: www.ipfcc.org/faq.html (accessed 4 November 2015).

Jans, M. (2004) Children as citizens: towards a contemporary notion of child participation, *Childhood*, 11(1): 27–44.

Jardine, E., O'Toole, M., Paton, J. and Wallis, C. (1999) Current status of long term ventilation of children in the United Kingdom: questionnaire survey, *British Medical Journal*, 318: 295–9.

Kelly, M., Jones, S., Wilson, V. and Lewis, P. (2012) How children's rights are constructed in family centred care: a review of the literature, *Journal of Child Health Care*, 16:190–205.

Kirk, S. (2001) Negotiating lay and professional roles in the care of children with complex health care needs, *Journal of Advanced Nursing*, 34(5): 593–602.

Lansdown, G. (2001) *Promoting Children's Participation in Democratic Decision Making*. Innocenti Research Centre. Available at: www.unicef-irc.org/publications/pdf/insight6. pdf (accessed 4 November 2015).

La Valle, I. Payne, L. with Gibb, J. and Jelicic, H. (2012) *Listening to Children's Views on Health: A Rapid Review of the Evidence*. London: National Children's Bureau. www.ncb. org.uk/media/723497/listening_to_children_s_views_on_health_-_final_report_july__12. pdf (accessed 4 November 2015).

Mayall, B. (2001) The sociology of childhood in relation to children's rights, *The International Journal of Children's Rights*, 8: 243–59.

Morrow, V. (2009) Children and young people's participation, in H. Montgomery and M. Kellett *Children and Young People's Worlds*. Bristol: The Policy Press.

Noyes, J. (2000) Enabling young 'ventilator-dependent' people to express their views and experiences of their care in hospital, *Journal of Advanced Nursing*, 31(5): 1206–15.

Nursing and Midwifery Council. (2015) *The Code*. London: Nursing and Midwifery Council.

OCC (Office of the Children's Commissioner) (2013) *Participation Strategy 2014–15*. London: OCC. Available at: www.childrenscommissioner.gov.uk/sites/default/files/publications/Research%20Strategy%20May%202014.pdf (accessed 6 November 2015).

Pascal, C. and Bertram, T. (2009) Listening to young citizens: the struggle to make a real participatory paradigm in research with young children, *European Early Childhood Education Research Journal*, 17(2): 249–62.

Reeves, E., Timmons, S. and Dampier, S. (2006) Parents' experiences of negotiating care for their technology-dependent child., *Journal of Child Health Care*, 10(3): 228–39.

Royal College of Nursing (2013) *Developing an Effective Clinical Governance Framework for Acute Children's Services*. London: RCN.

Shields, L. (2010) Questioning family-centred care, *Journal of Clinical Nursing*, 19: 2629–38.

Shields, L., Pratt, J. and Hunter, J. (2006) Family centred care: a review of qualitative studies, *Journal of Clinical Nursing*, 15: 1317–23.

Shier, H. (2001) Pathways to participation: openings, opportunities and obligations, *Children and Society*, 15(2): 107–17.

Sinclair, R. (2004) Participation in practice: making it meaningful, effective and sustainable, *Children and Society*, 18: 106–18.

Stuart, M. and Melling, S. (2014) Understanding nurses and parents' perceptions of family centred care,*Children and Young People's Nursing*, 26(7): 16–20.

Trajkovski, S., Schmeid, V., Vickers, M. and Jackson, D. (2012) Neonatal nurses' perspectives of family centred care: a qualitative study, *Journal of Clinical Nursing*, 21: 2477–87.

UN (United Nations) (1989) *Convention on the Rights of the Child*, UN General Assembly, Document A/RES/44/25. Geneva: United Nations.

Wallis, C., Paton, J., Beaton, S. and Jardine, E. (2011) Children on long term ventilatory support: 10 years of progress, *Archives of Diseases of Childhood*, 96(11): 998–1002.

White, S. (2000) Depoliticising development: the uses and abuses of participation, in D. Eade (ed.) *Development, NGOSs and Civil Society*. Oxford: Oxfam.

Wyness, M. (2009) Adult's involvement in children's participation: juggling children's places and spaces, *Children and Society*, 23: 395–406.

Further reading

Carter, C. and Brown, K. (2014) Service user input in pre-registration children's nursing education, *Children and Young People's Nursing*, 26(4): 28–31.

Elf, M., Rystedt, H., Lundin, J. and Krevbers, B. (2012) Young carers as co designers of a web based support system – the views of two publics, *Informatics for Health and Social Care*, 37(4): 203–16.

John, T., Hope, T., Savulescu, J. *et al.* (2008) Children's consent and paediatric research: is it appropriate for healthy children to be the decision makers in clinical research? *Archives of Diseases of Childhood*, 93: 379–83.

Lambert, V. and Keogh, D. (2014a) Health literacy and its importance for effective communication Part 1, *Nursing Children and Young People*, 26(3): 31–7.

Lambert, V. and Keogh, D. (2014b) Health literacy and its importance for effective communication Part 2, *Nursing Children and Young People*, 26(4): 32–6. Maconochie, H. and McNeill, F. (2010) User involvement: children's participation in a parent-baby group, *Community Practitioner*, 83(8): 17–20.

Price, B. (2010) Techniques to use when consulting families about child health services, *Paediatric Nursing*, 22(5): 26–33.

Rhodes, C.A. (2013) Service user involvement in pre-registration children's nursing education: the impact and influence on practice: a case study, *Issues in Comprehensive Pediatric Nursing*, 326(4): 291–308.

Shields, L., Zhou, H., Pratt, J. *et al.* (2012) Family Centred Care for hospitalised children age 0 to 12, *Cochrane Database of Systematic Reviews*.

Summers, K. (2013) Children's nurse duration – what is important to service users? *British Journal of Nursing*, 22(13): 747–50.

White, S. (2000) Depoliticising development: the uses and abuses of participation, in D. Eade (ed.) *Development, NGOs, and Civil Society*. Oxford: Oxfam.

Whiting, M. (2014a) Children with disability and complex health needs: the impact on family life, *Children and Young People's Nursing*, 26(3): 26–30.

Whiting, M. (2014b) Support requirements of parents caring for a child with disability and complex health needs, *Children and Young People's Nursing*, 26(4): 24–7.

Adolescent participation in care: listening to young people

Joan Walters

Introduction

Reader activity

Reflect on any experiences you have had caring for an adolescent and their families and write down a few positive and negative points that you feel were significant.

What do these experiences tell you about the healthcare needs of adolescents?

Adolescence can be described as a transition period between childhood and adulthood. It can be a stressful developmental period filled with major changes in physical maturity and sexuality, cognitive processes (ways of thinking and thought content), emotional feelings and relationships with others (Coleman and Hagell, 2007). Addressing the healthcare needs of this age group requires not only addressing identified health concerns, but also considering the complicated interactions of developmental changes on healthcare needs, the effectiveness of treatment, health education and health promotion (Viner 2005; Coleman *et al.*, 2007; Curran *et al.*, 2013).

Since the late 1980s research in both developed and developing countries has drawn attention to the barriers young people face in accessing health services. This research has resulted in a growing recognition that young people require services that are sensitive to their needs and a vision has developed of how health services can be made more youth friendly. The World Health Organization (WHO) criteria (2002) are the template which nations are now utilizing to assess and design their services. In England and Wales this has led to the Department of Health (DH 2011a) policy document the *You're Welcome – Quality Criteria for Young People Friendly Health Services* (YWQC).

The YWQC policy's stated aim is that 'All young people are entitled to receive appropriate health care wherever they access it' (DH 2011a: 7). It is directed at commissioners at Primary Care Trusts (PCTs) and local authorities (LAs). It lays out principles to help health services 'to get it right and become young person friendly'.

These criteria require a knowledgeable and skilled healthcare workforce. This does not always mean the ability to give direct care but to use referral processes appropriately, have a good knowledge of existing local resources and the ability to work across agencies. Therefore, it could be argued that healthcare staff across all agencies require ongoing training to care for adolescents at both pre- and post-registration level (DH 2011b).

It is relevant to ask: why focus on the health of adolescents? However the evidence we have has shown us that many of the behavioural patterns acquired during adolescence – for example, gender relations, sexual conduct, the use of tobacco, alcohol and other drugs, eating habits, and dealing with conflicts and risks – will last a lifetime (DH 2004). These patterns of behaviour will also affect the health and wellbeing of future children. However, we can also see adolescence as a gateway that provides opportunities to prevent the onset of health-damaging behaviours and their future repercussions (Coleman *et al.*, 2007; Umeh 2009).

This chapter will include the following:

- Defining adolescence
- An overview of adolescent development
- Morbidity and mortality data with a focus on chronic illnesses
- Defining adolescent participation in healthcare
- Case studies to highlight key aspects of the adolescent as a service user (the examples look at transition and outpatient services).

Defining Adolescence

Reader activity

Think about your key memories of what it was like to be an adolescent.

What do these tell you about being an adolescent?

Around one in six persons in the world is an adolescent: that is 1.2 billion people aged 10 to 19. About 85 per cent live in developing countries and the remainder live in the industrialized world (WHO 2014). In the UK there are 7.4 million 10–19-year-olds currently living in the UK, accounting for 12 per cent of the population.

The DH (2005) uses the term 'young people.' as adopted by The United Nations General Assembly adopted during the International Year of Youth in 1985 and which has been generally used by United Nations agencies and other partners. Adolescents, young people and youth are defined as 'young people' through differentiation and an amalgamation of terms:

- 'Adolescence' covers ages 10 to 19 years
- 'Youth' covers ages 15 to 24 years
- 'Young people' covers ages 10 to 24 years

The term 'young people' is increasingly being seen as useful in terms of healthcare delivery because increasing knowledge shows that the brain continues to mature into a least the mid-20s, particularly in the areas of judgement, reasoning and impulse control (Giedd *et al.*, 1999). With this comes a general acknowledgement that although young people share many characteristics with adults, their health-related adolescent problems and needs are different in a number of significant respects. Therefore, although in most parts of the world at the end of adolescence young people are accorded many rights and responsibilities, we may be right to question the young person consistently being able to make safe decisions without the appropriate support in place (Giedd *et al.*, 1999; Tylee *et al.*, 2007).

Adolescent development

The emphasis during adolescence tends to be on the physiological changes known as puberty. However, at the same time that these physiological changes are occurring so are many cognitive, social and emotional changes. Some of the changes outlined in Table 6.1 may not occur to the same degree in certain social groups owing to certain expected cultural norm; nevertheless a western understanding of adolescence includes all or some of these changes (Coleman *et al.*, 2007; Roche *et al.*, 2007). These can be broken down into three key phases known as early adolescence, middle adolescence and late adolescence.

Having considered the definition of adolescence and its development, we will now move on to the health context of this age group and will start with the health data on mortality.

Morbidity and Mortality overview

Reader activity

Have a look at the admissions to the clinical areas over a three-month period.

Is there a difference in reason for admission in the under 10s from the over 10s?

After infancy, late adolescence is the second riskiest time for death under the age of 19 years (see Figure 6.1). The considerable recent improvements seen in mortality for 0–4-year-olds have not been matched in adolescents and death rates among 15–19-year-olds are now higher than in the 1–4-year-olds (Wolfe *et al.*, 2014).

Table 6.1 Key milestones in adolescent development

Phase	Key changes
Early adolescence (10–13 years)	• Significant physical/sexual maturation. Intense concern with body image • Beginnings of abstract thought but still some concrete thinking • As young people enter adolescence they begin to redefine their relationship with their parents. They become increasingly resistant to complying with family rules and attempt to redefine boundaries. There is often increased negotiation and conflict over parental control and their capacity to make decisions • Feeling attracted to others begins
Middle adolescence (14–16 years)	• Continuing physical/sexual changes. Less concern with body image • Continual growth of capacity to think abstractly • There is a strong drive to conform to a peer group that may ultimately influence and define the way the young person dresses and how they speak and provides them with a moral code relating to what behaviours are and are not permissible • Initially there is little tolerance of difference and increasing rejection of those outside the selected peer group, which may have a unique way of dressing, a preferred style of music, etc. Each group may be disparaging of, or in active conflict with, other groups • Increase in sexual interest • There is a strong identification with mixed gender peer groups to affirm self-image and help develop a social and behavioural code
Late adolescence (17–19 years)	• Most physical/sexual changes complete. Greater acceptance of physical appearance • Capacity to think abstractly is in place • Communication can be almost as hard for the parents as it is for the young person who may swing in and out of a more adult communication style when circumstances dictate • There is a move away from a reliance on the peer group as individual and potentially intimate relationships become increasingly important • Biological and social changes enable more efficient processing of behaviours and situations and result in a more reliable calculation of potential consequences • As young people move through late adolescence, there tends to be the development of greater tolerance of difference and a move away from the 'tribe mentality' that exemplified the middle adolescent period • Serious intimate relationships begin to develop

There are relatively few deaths due to illnesses in adolescents, and instead many young people die prematurely due to other causes such as accidents and risky behaviour see Fig. 6.1 (WHO 2014). This is due to the rise of 'social' causes of mortality, including road traffic injuries, other injuries (e.g. self-harm) and suicide, which have replaced communicable diseases as the most common causes of death in adolescents. Also, there is a record rise in suicides in young men (Viner and Booy 2005).

Health problems among adolescents seem to be increasing. Morbidity in young people is commonly caused by chronic illness and mental health problems, with the risk of long-term

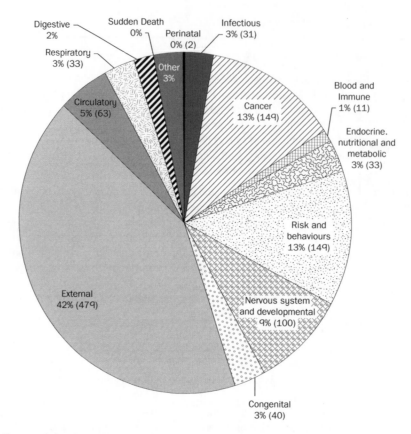

Figure 6.1 Cause of death among 15–19-year-olds in the UK
Source: WHO (2014).

adverse consequences. However, this partly also reflects a rise in the proportions of black and other minority ethnic groups in the adolescent population. Ethnic diversity is greater in young people than in the general UK population, and minority ethnicity is linked to poor health outcomes in adolescence, such as suicide, teenage pregnancy, sexually transmitted infections and mental disorders; the most plausible link is through socio-economic disadvantage (Hagel *et al.*, 2013; Wolfe *et al.*, 2014).

When morbidity is considered across all socio-economic and ethnic groups the key issues that can be identified are as follows (summarized from Hagel *et al.*, 2013):

- 16–24-year-olds were the most likely group to binge drink.
- England has the worst record for teenage pregnancies in Europe – the teenage birth rates are twice as high as Germany, three times as high as France and six times as high as the Netherlands.
- Young adults are most at risk of being diagnosed with a sexually transmitted infection – 50 per cent of all new diagnoses.
- For people aged 15–24, suicide is the second largest cause of death after road traffic accidents.

- One in every five young women, age 16–24 years, has some form of eating disorder.
- 85 per cent of children with chronic illness survive to adult life.

Chronic Illness in Adolescence

Reader activity

Think about what it is like to be an adolescent and have an ongoing health problem.

How involved would you want to be in managing your care?

It is predicted that by 2020, worldwide, 623 million children younger than 5, and 1.2 billion children aged 5 to 14 will have some kind of significant chronic disease. The incidence and prevalence of chronic conditions is rising in most developed and developing countries and will constitute the main cause of death by 2020 (WHO 2014).

There are several reasons for this growth in adolescents with chronic illness and key amongst these are:

- Advances in medical science and technology – new diagnostic testing, medical procedures and pharmaceuticals – are being used to treat acute illnesses and maintain a level of health and functioning that results in increased numbers of people living with chronic conditions.
- We are also screening and diagnosing chronic conditions with greater frequency and success. Earlier detection means people can live with chronic conditions that used to grow to acute care stages before diagnosis.

Defining Chronic illness

The term chronic illness is part of a collection of terms that are commonly used interchangeably and include chronic disease, chronic condition, lifelong disease/condition, long-term disease/condition and non-communicable disease/condition (DH 2005). Chronic illnesses can be grouped as follows:

- sudden onset conditions, for example acquired brain injury or spinal cord injury, followed by a partial recovery
- intermittent and unpredictable conditions, for example epilepsy, sickle cell disease, asthma
- progressive conditions, for example muscular dystrophy, cystic fibrosis, where progressive deterioration in function leads to increasing dependence on help and care from others.
- stable conditions, but with changing needs due to development or ageing, for example cerebral palsy.
  (Modified from the National Service Framework for Long-term Conditions DH 2005)

Psychological and Social Impact of Having a Chronic Illness

Reader activity

How may having a health problem make you feel about yourself and respond to your treatment?

Michaud *et al.* (2007) argue that while any chronic condition can potentially affect these developmental processes, the reverse is also true; that is, both physiological change and psychosocial adjustments can have an impact on chronic conditions. For example, certain chronic illnesses such as diabetes and sickle cell disease are known to have long-term neuropsychological effects in adolescence; as a result of the disease process (hypoglycaemia in diabetes and cerebrovascular accidents in sickle cell disorders) rather than representing a generic chronic illness effect. Chronic illness may also delay growth, puberty and the maturation of other biological systems through the lack of nutrients caused by malabsorption as seen in cystic fibrosis and other gastrointestinal disorders, as well as through competition for nutrients from chronic inflammation and infection (Michaud *et al.*, 2007).

With the described physiological disturbances it is probably not surprising that the adolescent with a serious medical illness is at risk of developing associated emotional problems (Judson 2004; Sawyer *et al.*, 2007); unlike a child with a temporary sickness such as the flu, the child with a chronic illness must cope with knowing that the disease is here to stay and may even get worse (Judson 2004). Child and adolescent psychiatrists point out that almost all of these children initially refuse to believe they are ill and later feel guilt and anger (Michaud *et al.*, 2007).

The demands of managing a chronic illness and the restrictions on lifestyle inherent in many disabling conditions increase dependence on the family, and carers, at a time when this should be decreasing (Michaud *et al.*, 2007). At the same time, young people may also become dissociated from their peer group, particularly in those with taxing medical conditions and those that mark them out as very different, which may escalate their risk-taking behaviour (La Greca 1990). The lack of acceptance of potential future consequences also has an impact on the management of a chronic illness. Peer pressure can also strongly influence a young person's ability to manage their condition (La Greca 1990).

Adolescents' evolving capacities and participation in healthcare

Reader activity

Think about a time when you were not involved in a decision that directly affected you. How did you feel?

How did you react?

Adolescent competence

Adolescence is notable for a shift in the relationship from parent–child to adult–adult. However, this period of transition can be quite complex. Successful transition to adult independence requires young people to be psychologically, emotionally and financially independent. These can occur at different times, for example some young people see themselves as 'adult' but are still living at home and do not have a job (Coleman *et al.*, 2007; Roche *et al.*, 2007). This is the stage when young people may begin to withdraw from family social gatherings and spend increasing amounts of time alone, in their bedrooms, on the computer or watching TV (Curran *et al.*, 2013).

Abstract thinking is essential in order to question identity, as well as imagine multiple possible selves, which is at the core of the adolescent search for identity. When working with an adolescent, health practitioners should recognize they are working with someone who is developing the capacity to assess situations as well as being someone who may be working on their personal identity, thereby developing notions to describe their goals, interests, values, religious beliefs, political belief, gender, sexual identity, ethnic identity, and so on. It is the brain development during this period often called maturity that allows development particularly in the areas of judgement, reasoning and impulse control (Giedd *et al.*, 1999).

Viner (2005) argues that the management of confidentiality and consent issues are central to the management and examination of young people, who are potentially underage. Services which are not considered to be confidential are less likely to be used by young people. Full confidentiality, including keeping confidentiality from parents, should be assured unless the young person is found to be at risk to themselves, for example through suicide or abuse, or reveals plans to harm another (Fortin 2009).

Adolescent Interests and Rights

As identified by Cockett in Chapter 5 of this volume, the child's best interests are a primary consideration and practitioners are balancing the rights of the young person between protection and autonomy. Health practitioners need to work with young people with an understanding of the following:

- All children are entitled to be involved in decisions that affect them – but the extent to which they exercise control over decision-making will be determined by their capacities.
- Parental responsibilities exist in order to enable the child to exercise his/her rights.
- Parental rights only extend for so long as the child is unable to exercise those rights for her or himself.
- There is a need to balance respect for the child's evolving capacities while also promoting their best interests.

(Lansdown 2005; Fortin 2009)

Adolescent Participation

In line with other areas of health policy, direct feedback from young patients and adolescents attending our services is increasingly being sought (e.g. via patient surveys) and where possible used to shape service provision and planning. This process enables adolescents to define their needs themselves. UNICEF (2001) declared that the participation rights of adolescents require a strategic approach that uses a developmental approach, taking account of the context of adolescent lives. They define adolescent participation 'as adolescents partaking in and influencing processes, decisions and activities' (2001: 1). In youth work Sapin (2013) argues that providing opportunities for young people to have a voice can have a positive impact on the ways in which decisions are made including improving existing services and processes or making demands for new services to address their particular needs.

However participation as a concept must be explored as it is concerned with power and control, where the young person's experience can range from passive recipient to active decision-makers. In 1992 Hart created a ladder of participation for children which professionals working with young people have adapted (see Figure 6.2). Hart argued that having clear identification of roles and communication can protect against false expectations. Acceptable levels of participation do not expect young people to be 'managers' in control at all times, but young people need to know where they stand.

Assessing Adolescent Participation

The Department of Health (2011a) YWQC recommends several ways in which an organization can assess the participation of adolescents in the service. This includes them being routinely consulted in relation to current services and relevant new developments; including

RUNG 8 - **Youth initiated shared decisions with adults**: Youth-led activities, in which decision-making is shared between youth and adults working as equal partners

RUNG 7 - **Youth initiated and directed**: Youth-led activities with little input from adults

RUNG 6 - **Adult initiated shared decisions with youth:** Adult-led activities, in which decision-making is shared with youth

RUNG 5 - **Consulted and informed:** Adult-led activities, in which youth are consulted and informed about how their input will be used and the outcomes of adult decisions

RUNG 4 - **Assigned, but informed:** Adult-led activities, in which youth understand purpose, decision-making process and have a role

RUNG 3 - **Tokenism:** Adult-led activities, in which youth may be consulted with minimal opportunities for feedback

RUNG 2 - **Decoration:** Adult-led activities, in which youth understand purpose, but have no input in how they are planned

RUNG 1 - **Manipulation:** Adult-led activities, in which youth do as directed without understanding of the purpose for the activities

Figure 6.2 Youth participation ladder
Adapted from Hart (1992) and UNICEF (2001).

them in patient satisfaction surveys; having processes are in place to ensure that young people's views are included in governance service design and development; encouraging them to give their opinions of the service offered and whether it met their needs and that these are reviewed and acted on as appropriate. Building on from this the CQC is developing an approach to involving children and young people in its inspection activity. This will include using children and young people as 'experts by experience' to support its inspectors when they inspect registered providers. It is also developing information about CQC in a child and young person friendly format to help them understand more about CQC and what to expect in providers that are registered with CQC. CQC has run a number of workshops with children and young people to progress this work (DH 2013).

Barriers to Adolescent Participation

However, there can be several barriers to valuing adolescents as health service users which can lead to a young person facing discrimination, mainly based around perceptions of 'youth'. In Western cultures adolescents can be seen as socially significant and psychologically complex (Hehily 2007). Some of the more common bases for discrimination are, age (amount of experience), gender, obsession with sexual activity, emotional volatility, use of common language, modes of dress, social interests, where they live and past history of trouble (UNICEF 2001; Curran *et al.*, 2013). Alongside, this communication can be almost as hard for the parents and adult figures such as teachers, health workers, as it is for the young person who may swing in and out of a more adult communication style when circumstances dictate (WHO 2002; Viner 2005). This can lead to the adolescent being seen as 'other'.

Case Studies

Reader activity

Think about the first time you went onto a hospital ward or attended a GP appointment on your own.

How did you feel?
What made you feel safe and able to function effectively?

Box 6.1 Case study 1: Transition to adult services

Alex (pseudonym) is an 18-year-old young man with sickle cell disease, a hereditary long-term condition of the blood which can require emergency hospital admissions to hospital as well as regular hospital appointments. He attends King's College Hospital,

London. When interviewed on his views on the service, Alex described his first encounter with adult services at the age of 16 to me:

'I was always tall for my age. I was at school when the pains started coming on. So I rang my mum and told her I was taking myself to the Emergency Department (ED). When I signed in at reception the lady sent me to an area I had never been to before (the adult section of ED) where I waited and waited and waited. When the doctor came he asked me did I really need painkillers or was I after drugs or bunking off school. They did give me painkillers eventually and then when it got no better sent me to a new ward, with grown-ups. I hadn't been there before. I asked why I could not go to my usual ward (the children's ward) and they said that I was now an adult. It was horrible. Nobody knew me and they would not let my mum in to see me as they had a strict visiting policy. It was the first time that my mum was not there to speak for me. It was even harder for my mates to come and see me. It was so bad that next time I felt ill I hung on as I was scared of where they would send me.'

Alex's experience of moving from child to adult service could be described as a transfer (see Box 6.1). The process was not planned: it was abrupt, focused only on his physical wellbeing, and Alex's views and desires were not asked for. His 'participation' in his care management was limited. Alex's reaction to his experience illustrates Max-Neef's (1991) contention that if the young people's needs to participate are not satisfied it can interfere with other aspects of their lives. Alex felt distrustful, disempowered and alienated from the service set up to meet his health needs. Applying Hart's (1992) ladder it is clear that Alex was at rung one; he felt manipulated in that he was directed but had no understanding of why the organization chose to organize his care in a particular way.

Models of Adolescent Transition

Ideally, the support of adolescents with a long-term condition moving from child to adult services should be managed under a process known as 'transition'. It is a 'process that addresses the medical, psychosocial and educational/vocational needs of adolescents and young adults with chronic physical and medical conditions as they move from child-centred to adult-oriented healthcare systems' (DH 2006: 14). It can be understood as a guided, educational, therapeutic process, rather than an administrative event (DH 2004). Young people such as Alex with additional, and sometimes complex, needs such as mental health problems or physical difficulties or disabilities may find it more difficult to make these transitions successfully and they and their families may require additional support. However, as Alex's case illustrates these young people often have experiences of poor support during their transition to adulthood.

In Alex's case it could be argued that participation for transitioning to adult services started too late. The RCN (2013) suggests that that responsibility for decision-making should occur gradually with key milestones marked out. In their key document *Adolescent Transition Care* they give examples of how to consider the adolescent's emerging capacity to be partners in their care by using the three stages of adolescent development to break down the transition process into early, middle and late transition stage. The RCN (2013) transition framework allows for the fact that adolescents are undergoing changes far broader than just their clinical needs.

Practitioners need to be aware that they may have to contend with low parental, young person and professional expectations; lack of self-advocacy skills and lack of opportunity to develop and practise these skills; differing views of independence and success and a lack of knowledge of existing career and vocational education services (Michaud *et al.*, 2007). The responsibility for ensuring effective transition does not stop at the point of transfer of the young person to a different consultant. Joint multi-disciplinary working is essential and longer consultation times are required for adolescents working through transition than in children's or adult clinics. Experiences such as Alex's were the driver for the creation of a nurse specialist post in transition for sickle cell and thalassaemia working across both paediatric and adult services. This arose from emerging evidence that well organized transition protocols and programmes do have measurable benefits for young people and their parents, that is changes in morbidity and mortality, through:

- parents and carers feeling more confident in 'letting go'
- improved follow-up
- better disease control and
- improved documentation of transitional issues.

(Michaud *et al.*, 2007; RCPE 2008)

Adolescent Adherence to Treatment

There is much research to say that the involvement of patients in adolescent care increases adherence with treatment (Haynes *et al.*, 1979). In children and adolescents with long-term health disorders most of this work has been done with those with diabetes, cystic fibrosis, sickle cell disease and solid organ transplant, the consistent messages being that children and adolescents knowing the purpose of their treatment increases the likelihood of their cooperation. Knowing their treatment plan helped children and adolescents appreciate the logic and the intentions underlying painful, frightening procedures (Michaud *et al.*, 2007). For the health practitioner there arises a tension between the 'liberationist' and 'caretaking' or protectionist view of childhood. The staff have a strong desire to believe in the capabilities of the child but also wish to protect them from the consequences of their actions. As discussed earlier staff will often find it challenging giving up control to the adolescent as it can be difficult to understand where they sit with their evolving capacities and yet are legally being seen as minor in law (see Box 6.2).

Reader activity

- How might you gain access to adolescent service users' experience data?
- What skills, attitudes and competencies does a nurse caring for an adolescent and their family need to develop?

Box 6.2   Case study 2: Clinical services

The Variety Children's Unit at King's College Hospital, London wished to explore if the existing Outpatients services for adolescents with cystic fibrosis or sickle cell disease was meeting their needs and if not were there any ways in which the services could adapt to meet any additional needs.

Prior to this posters were put up and letters were sent out to adolescents above 11 years (34) and their parents/carers (37) inviting them to take part. It was made clear that if they chose not to complete the questionnaire that it would not affect their treatment in any way. Two surveys, one directed at the adolescent and one directed at parents/carers, were given out during outpatient appointments. The questions included the following:

- What is the appropriate environment for managing adolescent health needs?
- Which health personnel should be involved?
- At what time should clinics be held?
- Do you feel you have any control over your illness?
- Are you asked about/involved in making decisions concerning treatment?
- How much responsibility do you take for your condition?
- Who gives you your treatment at home?
- Has anyone talked to you about Adult Services?
- At what age should transfer occur?
- At what age do you think young people should leave children's services?
- At what age should preparation for transfer begin?

There was also the opportunity to answer some open questions at the end of each section.

The questionnaires used several traditional rating scales to detect beliefs and attitude. Reaction was evaluated by self-completed questions as they are a low cost and quick way to gather data and make the least demand on the time of the participants. In keeping with this, the questionnaires were distributed and collected as part of the Outpatients appointment. Also to minimize the disadvantages of this method, that is, low response rates, the questions (apart from the open questions at the end of each section) were in a check box form that could be coded more easily.

In designing the survey it is necessary to understand why slightly different forms were given to the adolescents and their parents/carer. When utilizing health services parents/carers can go from being experts in caring for their child at home to someone who has to share the care of their sick child with healthcare 'experts'. As observed by Darbyshire (1994) it is the parents/carers who have to enter the domain and discourse of the childcare 'experts'. Their ideas of control and ownership of the child diminished but the project wished to acknowledge the family unit as service user each with their unique perspectives.

There was concern that if only one survey was given that the young person might be overly influenced by the parent's attitudes and beliefs as they work through the balance of independence and interdependence. There may be a tension between the young person trying to please the researcher and trying to please their parent/carer (Dashiff *et al.*, 2009). Table 6.2 illustrates some of these tensions.

Table 6.2 Differentiating adolescent needs from their parents in the transition process

Young person	Parent/carer	General comments
Transfer preferred between 15 and 19 years	Transfer preferred between 18 and 21 years	For the young people it was dependent on what age they left school. Particularly if they had jobs it felt uncomfortable being seen in children's services Parents/carers felt young people were not adults until 18 years of age and if still at college or university they were still highly dependent
Begin preparation between 11 and 14 years	Begin preparation between 16 and 18 years	Many of the young people felt that they were highly knowledgeable already about their care and would like more control (65%) Many parents/carers felt that the young person did not fully understand their condition, required a lot of prompting and needed to be free of responsibility (70%)
Most young people (85%) wanted some time to talk to healthcare professionals on their own	Most parents/carers (70%) were uncomfortable with the young person having some time to talk to healthcare professionals on their own	The young people did not necessarily want all of the appointment on their own but felt some time should be given to discuss personal issues on their own Many parents felt that that there was no need for separate discussion as their child told them everything and that their child would have to have any decision run by them
Most young people preferred clinic appointments and other treatments to be during school hours	Most parents/carers preferred clinic appointments and other treatments not to be during school hours	Parents worried about clinic and treatment times affecting their child's education, whereas more than 70% of young people liked that idea of missing school and wanted evenings and weekends to spend at home or out with their friends

The open text box obtained some other useful information from the adolescents about the setup of our services:

- Expect variable involvement in decision-making and participation in care
- Children's outpatients departments (COPDs) cater predominantly for younger children – would like to spend time with other patients similar in age
- COPDs lack age-appropriate material
- COPDs can be noisy, with no separate quiet area that can be used – did not like to be in with younger children
- COPDs have rigid seating arrangements
- If treatment had to be in the evening or weekend they would like time spent with young people of a similar age and to have health promotion sessions delivered.

The information collected has led to certain service changes such as including the following:

- Some time is offered during clinic appointments for the young person to speak to a health professional at the time of their transition.
- In specialities where there were sufficient numbers of adolescents the clinics are set up by age to assist socializing with peers.
- Treatments and investigations such as transfusions and health checks are set up either as a weekend club with peers (transfusion for sickle cell patients) or organized by age and gender (annual health checks for cystic fibrosis and liver patients).
- Where clinics are age graded, health information is laid out appropriate to their age; this includes videos and leaflets as well as the young people being allocated a designated spot in the department where possible if it is mixed clinic.
- Nurse specialists begin assessing young people from the ages of 10–11 years as to their readiness to begin preparing for transition.

In order to achieve some of these changes the various specialities have held workshops with the young people and parents/carers (some jointly and some separately). This is to enable the service to work with them on the changes requested but also to assist them in understanding the changes occurring in adolescence and the need for the increasing involvement of the young person in their own care and the help available for them on this journey. The process can be described as the 'adult initiating shared decisions with youth' type in that the adults led the activities, in which decision-making was shared with youth.

Summary

We know that fortunately, adolescents are receptive to new ideas; they are keen to make the most of their growing capacity for making decisions. Their curiosity and interest are a tremendous opening to foster personal responsibility for health (Hagel *et al.*, 2013). Furthermore, engaging in positive and constructive activities provides occasions to forge relationships with adults and peers as well as to acquire behaviours that are crucial to health (Coleman *et al.*, 2007). Their differing forms of communication can give the impression that the adolescent cannot assess a situation and be future orientated. As with adults, when assessing adolescent comprehension it is important to see them as individuals and consider the following:

- Explore the adolescent's ability to paraphrase.
- Explore whether the adolescent is able to compare alternatives, or to express thoughts on possible consequences on what they have been told.
- Explore whether the adolescent applies the information to their own case.

Learning from adolescent service users' experience of healthcare services: what do adolescents, parents and carers want from nurses?

Adolescents require the support of their family, carers and peers but also healthcare practitioners who are able to:

- provide information appropriate for the adolescent's maturational stage (to be future orientated and able to assess risk accurately requires cognitive and social maturity);
- take into account underlying psychological and social factors;
- tailor the treatment to the patient's individual process and stage (emotional development);
- communicate information in a straightforward way, trust the adolescent;
- recognize levels of participation;
- ask for proposals from the patient;
- tailor the doses of the medication to the patient's physiological status (puberty/growth);
- adapt the therapy to the adolescent's lifestyle. (We know that the duration of the treatment has an equivocal effect on compliance; to the point that adherence to treatment decreases with time).

Useful websites

WHO (Adolescent Health) – http://www.who.int/maternal_child_adolescent/topics/adolescence/second-decade/en/

UNICET child and adolescent participation guide – http://www.unicef.org/adolescence/index_38074.html

References

Coleman, J. and Hagell, A. (eds) (2007) *Adolescence, Risk and Resilience: Against the Odds.* London: Wiley.

Coleman, J., Hendry L.B. and Kloep, M. (eds) (2007) *Adolescence and Health.* London: Wiley.

Curran, S., Harrison, R. and Mackinnon, D. (2013) *Working with Young People*, 2nd edn. London: Sage with The Open University.

Darbyshire, P. (1994) *Living With a Sick Child in Hospital: The Experiences of Parents and Nurses.* London: Chapman and Hall.

Dashiff, C., Vance, D., Abdullatif, H. and Wallander, J. (2009) Parenting, autonomy and self-care in adolescents with Type 1 Diabetes, *Child Health Care and Development,* 35(1): 79–88.

DH (Department of Health) (2004) *National Service Framework for Children, Young People and Maternity Services.* London: Department of Health.

DH (2005) *The National Service Framework for Long-term Conditions.* London: DH.

DH (2006) *Transition: Getting it Right for Young People.* London: DH.

DH (2011a) *You're Welcome – Quality Criteria for Young People Friendly Health Services.* London: DH.

DH (2011b) *Self-review Tool for Quality Criteria for Young People Friendly Health Services.* London: DH Children and Young People.

DH (2013) *Improving Children and Young People's Health Outcomes: A System Wide Response.* London: Department of Health.

Fortin, J. (2009) *Children's Rights and the Developing Law*, 3rd edn. Cambridge: Cambridge University Press.

Giedd, J., Blumenthal, J., Jeffries, N. *et al.* (1999) Brain development during childhood and adolescence: a longitudinal MRI study, *Nature Neuroscience,* 2(10): 861–3.

Hagell, A., Coleman, J. and Brooks, F. (2013) *Key Data on Adolescence 2013: The Latest Information and Statistics about Young People Today.* London: Association for Young People's Health.

Hart, R. (1992) *Children's Participation: The Theory and Practice of Involving Young Citizens in Community Development and Environmental Care.* London: Earthcare.

Haynes, R.B., Taylor, D.W. and Sackett, D. (eds) (1979) *Compliance in Health Care.* Baltimore, MD: Johns Hopkins University Press.

Hehily, M.J. (ed.) (2007) *Understanding Youth: Perspectives, Identities and Practices.* London: The Open University/Sage Publications Ltd. Judson, L. (2004) Global childhood chronic illness, *Nursing Administration Quarterly,* 28(1): 60–6.

Judson, L. (2004) Global childhood chronic illness. *Nursing Administration Quaterly* 28(1): 60–66.

La Greca, A.M. (1990) Issues in adherence with pediatric regimens, *Journal of Pediatric Psychology,* 15(4): 423–36.

Lansdown, G. (2005) *The Evolving Capacities of the Child.* Florence, Italy: Save the Children/UNICEF.

Max-Neef, A. (1991) *Human Scale Development: Conception, Application and Further Reflections.* New York: Apex Press.

Michaud, P.A., Suris, J.C. and Viner, R. (2007) *The Adolescent with a Chronic Condition.* Geneva: WHO.

Roche, J., Tucker, S., Flynn, R. and Thomson, R. (eds) (2007) *Youth in Society: Contemporary Theory, Policy and Practice.* London: Sage.

Royal College of Nursing (RCN) (2013) *Adolescent Transition Care,* 2nd edn. London: Royal College of Nursing.

Royal College of Physicians of Edinburgh (RCPE) Transition Steering Group (2008) Think Transition: Developing the Essential Link Between Paediatric and Adult Care. Available at: www.cen.scot.nhs.uk/files/16o-think-transition-edinburgh.pdf (accessed 4 November 2015).

Sapin, K. (2013) *Essential Skills for Youth Work Practice,* 2nd edn. London: Sage.

Sawyer, S.M., Drew, S., Yeo, M.S. and Britto, M.T. (2007) Adolescents with a chronic condition: challenges living, challenges treating, *Lancet,* 36: 1481–9.

Tylee, A., Haller, D.M., Graham, T. *et al.* (2007) Youth-friendly primary-care services: how are we doing and what more needs to be done? *The Lancet* 369 (9572): 1565–73.

Umeh, K. (2009) *Understanding Adolescent Health Behaviour: A Decision Making Perspective.* New York: Cambridge University Press.

UNICEF (2001) *The Participation Rights of Adolescents: A Strategic Approach.* New York: WHO.

Viner, R. (ed.) (2005) *ABC of Adolescence.* London: Blackwell.

Viner, R. and Booy, R. (2005) ABC of adolescence: epidemiology of health and illness, *British Medical Journal,* 330: 411–14.

WHO (2002) *Adolescent Friendly Services.* Geneva: WHO.

WHO (2014) *Health for the World's Adolescents: A Second Chance in the Second Decade.* Geneva: WHO.

Wolfe, I., MacFarlane, A., Donkin, A. *et al.* (2014) Why children die: deaths in infants, children and young people in the UK. London: Royal College of Paediatrics and Child Health; National Children's Bureau and British Association for Child and Adolescent Public Health.

PERSON-CENTRED APPROACHES FOR ACUTE AND LONG-TERM CONDITIONS IN ADULTS

Person-centred approaches to adult critical care

Suzanne Bench

Introduction

More than 110,000 people are admitted to a Critical Care Unit (CCU) annually in the UK (NICE 2009). Experiencing a critical illness has been described as *'an unexpected, life-threatening and traumatic event'* (Löf *et al.*, 2008: 108) and a time during which patients and their families face major challenging and often life-changing experiences (Tembo *et al.*, 2012).

To optimize the service provided to these patients and their families, patient-focused healthcare provision is widely advocated (DH 2004, 2005, 2013). To achieve this, active engagement with service users is required (Coulter and Ellis 2006; INVOLVE 2012, Morrow *et al.*, 2012). These are people who have had previous experience of being in a CCU, either as a patient or as a visitor, visitors being family members (relatives), but who may also be significant others, caregivers or friends. This chapter uses the narratives of three former critically ill patients and two relatives to illuminate the key issues faced during the illness and recovery trajectory, and to identify the patient/family-centred care priorities which arise from these experiences. All those involved have agreed to waive their anonymity, thus all names and details are real.

For the purpose of this chapter, critical care is defined according to the Department of Health (DH 2000) classifications from the UK, focusing on patients requiring either level 2 (high dependency) or level 3 (intensive) care.

Reader activity

Reflect on the points below before and after reading the rest of this chapter:

- Think about the first time you went onto a hospital ward or into a CCU. How did you feel? Next think of how critically unwell people and their families may experience this, and write down a few points that you feel are significant.
- What do you think patients need from healthcare staff to optimize their recovery from critical illness?
- What national and international initiatives currently exist, which address the physical, psychological and social needs of patients who have had a critical illness, and their families?
- What competencies (knowledge, attitude and skills) does a nurse caring for a critically ill person and their family need to develop?
- What key messages can be learnt from critical care service users' experiences?
- How can you access critical care service users' experience data?

Case examples of critical illness

The following individuals will be referred to throughout the chapter to illuminate the lived experience of various aspects of adult critical care.

Peter (see Fig. 7.1) had a serious cycling accident on 24 April 2003, during which he sustained 'a brain haemorrhage, a broken rib that punctured my left lung, a fractured vertebra in my neck and two broken vertebrae in my back'. Peter recalls that he and a friend were training 'to make sure we were in peak condition and ready to tackle the Freeraid Classic; a forty mile Alpine bike ride'. Peter was airlifted by helicopter to hospital, where he spent 22 days in an Intensive Care Unit (ICU).

Dawn (see Fig. 7.2) suffered a postpartum haemorrhage following the birth of her son in 1998. Dawn was transferred to an ICU, where she developed acute respiratory distress syndrome (ARDS). Dawn was later referred

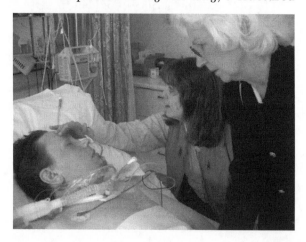

Figure 7.1 Peter and his family: in the ICU, April 2003

to a trauma psychologist 'who I saw for 7 years for chronic and enduring PTSD'.

Bill, aged 52, was admitted to hospital on 18 December 2010 with 'what I thought was a chest infection'. . Bill spent a total of 103 days in hospital, 88 of which were in an ICU, where he was ventilated for 19 days. Bill was diagnosed with severe sepsis, ARDS and multiple organ failure and continues to suffer with 'post ARDS pulmonary fibrosis'.

Shirley, Bill's wife, was 49 years old at the time of his illness. She spent most days at the hospital but also recalls, 'I had to deal with many other things happen-

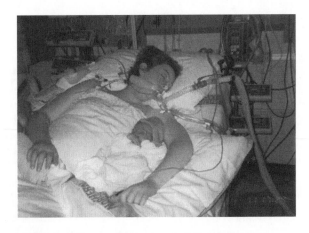

Figure 7.2 Dawn and her son in ICU (1998)

ing at the same time. The possibility of losing my job . . . my dad had a massive heart attack and died'. She says 'We had many scares and a lot of visits where nothing seemed to change'.

Colin's wife Andrea became critically ill on 13ʰ December 2003, after falling through 'a hole in our bedroom floor'. Andrea sustained severe damage to her lungs and 'two unstable crush fractures in her spine'. Andrea was transferred to a hospital two hours away, where she spent 15 days in an ICU. During this time, Colin stayed at the hospital and his children travelled to visit every day. On 29 December 2003, Andrea was transferred back to the ICU in her local hospital, where she stayed for another two weeks. Over ten years later Colin reflects that 'It has been a very long and slow road to recovery with many ups and lots of downs and has changed our lives completely.'

Further details of these and other patients' and relatives' experiences can be found on the ICUsteps website: www.icusteps.org.

Admission to Intensive Care

Many patients remember little about their admission to an ICU. The last thing that Peter remembers is 'being at a Placebo gig at Brixton Academy the night before'. Bill also says, 'I barely remember the 10 minute journey to the hospital .. . . I was taken into A&E . . . then taken straight to ITU, something I have no memory of.'

Many patients are sedated on or soon after their arrival into ICU. This, in addition to the poor cerebral oxygenation associated with critical illness, may account for the lack of recall during this period. Even though they were unable to fully grasp what was happening, some of the eight patients interviewed by Löf *et al.* (2008) at three and 12 months after hospital discharge did, however, describe experiencing fear and dread, and feeling that they were gravely ill and could die. Löf *et al.* (2008) also found that those patients who were conscious on admission had extensive unpleasant emotions, a finding supported by the earlier work of Perrins *et al.* (1998), who adds that patients admitted as emergencies (such as in the case of Peter, Bill and Dawn) may have more unpleasant memories than patients admitted electively.

In contrast to the limited memories of ICU admission that many patients have, relatives remember the event in great detail. Colin's story exemplifies this. He says:

> December 13 2003 will be etched in my life forever . . . I shot out of bed and to my horror I saw . . . my wife, Andrea, lying sprawled on the lounge floor . . . all covered in dust and grit saying she was having difficulty in breathing. . . . Waiting for assessment was unbearable . . . [the doctor] told us that the next 48 hours were very crucial. . . . He also said that if we believed in god then we should pray that night. . . . after the doctor left I just broke down and cried, I think I cried nearly all night.'

Shirley also clearly remembers the day of Bill's admission to ICU. She recalls:

> The morning of 18 December 2010 – weather was bad and our road very icy so could not get to work . . . at 7ish I was alarmed that his breathing was so fast and he looked a funny colour and I found it difficult to wake him. I first tried to call the emergency doctor but could not get through so called an ambulance, it was while I was on the phone and they asked me what colour were his lips I noticed they were blue!!!!. . . they took Bill into A&E and within five minutes . . . said that they were taking him straight to ITU.

Shirley and Colin's narratives highlight the significant emotional distress that relatives experience before and during a patient's admission to an ICU: traumatic events which are seldom or never forgotten by those who experience them (Löf *et al.*, 2008). Verhaeghe *et al.* (2005) point out that admission to an ICU can generate strong emotions including shock, denial, anger, despair, guilt and fear for the loss of the family member. Most people have never been into the highly technical world of an ICU, an environment which can be intimidating and alien (Brysiewicz andBhengu 2010). Qualitative data from Brysiewicz andBhengu's (2010) study of nine ICU nurses suggest that families need additional attention from staff at this time as the admission is often unexpected, and the family may be facing the possibility that their loved one may die. Jamerson *et al.* (1996) further describe the admission to ICU as a phase characterized by uncertainty, stress and confusion for relatives as they wait to gain access to the ICU and to obtain information about the patient's diagnosis and the prognosis. Furthermore relatives' perception of time changes, and they become unaware of their own needs (Verhaeghe *et al.*, 2005).

Being in the ICU

Patients report variable memories of their time in the ICU (Zetterlund *et al.*, 2012; Cutler *et al.*, 2013), often aided by information given to them by staff, friends and family. Bill describes his first memory when waking from sedation: 'I heard a radio playing, on the news they said that Gary Moore the former Thin Lizzie guitarist had died of a heart attack aged 56.' He goes on to say, 'I remember trying to talk but no words came out.' Approximately 15 to 33 per cent of patients have no recollection of being in the ICU (Samuelson *et al.*, 2006; Rattray *et al.*, 2010). For example, Peter says, 'To my perception, I went to bed one night and when I woke up nearly three weeks were missing and my life had been turned on its head.' The findings of a literature review of 26 studies by Stein-Parbury and McKinley (2000) suggest, however, that many patients do remember this period, sometimes in vivid detail.

Memories, nightmares, hallucinations and delirium

Although some recollections of time in the ICU are positive and associated with a perceived sense of safety and security promoted by nurses, memories are often related to more negative experiences, such as problems with sleeping, pain and anxiety (Granja *et al.*, 2005; Rattray *et al.*, 2010). The experience of delusional memories and nightmares is also persistently reported in the literature (Adamson *et al.*, 2004; Granja *et al.*, 2005; Löf *et al.*, 2008; Rattray *et al.*, 2010; Tembo *et al.*, 2012), and is associated with higher levels of anxiety, depression, Post-Traumatic Stress Disorder (PTSD) and other cognitive impairments (Davydow *et al.*, 2008; Kiekkas *et al.*, 2010; Desai *et al.*, 2011; Nouwen *et al.*, 2012).

Both Bill and Dawn describe experiencing harrowing dreams and hallucinations whilst in the ICU. Bill reflects:

> that time for me had just been full of strange nightmares, believing I was dead . . . had done a deal with the grim reaper to get back, then the hallucinations started, I saw the grim reaper was walking around the ward looking at everyone then taking someone away, a nurse then said don't worry he'll be back for you, it was a terrifying time.

Dawn expresses that waking from sedation was 'the worst type of nightmare' and describes 'people constantly trying to kill me, bury me alive, keeping the people who I knew could save me away from me'. She further recalls 'in fear and frustration physically lashing out at staff' and says, 'I was in ultimate survival mode . . . made worse by the fact I was tied to a bed (by the machines keeping me alive) and unable to escape.' Peter also says, 'the slightest inconsistency drew my attention, convincing me that this reality that I now found myself in was no more real than any other dream'.

Many of these experiences can be attributed to the presence of delirium, a state 'character-ized by disturbed consciousness, cognitive function *or* perception, which has an acute onset and fluctuating course' (NICE 2010: 4). Finding out later that she probably experienced delirium, Dawn says, 'has never managed to even slightly shift the absolute terror of this experience'.

The impact of hallucinations and delirium on visitors is illustrated by Colin who recalls that when Andrea came off sedation, 'she began to have hallucinations, which to me was very frightening . . . she would not stop pushing one foot against the metal side of the bed and was very restless. We now know she thought she was kicking over a metal flower stand.' Shirley further recalls, 'I found it so distressing to watch the man (Bill) I knew and loved turning violent.'

Physical care

Patients in ICU are frequently dependent on nursing staff for all of their care needs (Lykkegaard and Delmar 2013), including toileting, personal hygiene and mobilizing. In a multi-centre Portuguese study conducted by Granja *et al.* (2005) the physical factors reported to cause patients (*n* = 464) most stress included tracheal tube aspiration (81 per cent), nose tubes (75 per cent), pain (64 per cent), immobilization in bed (64 per cent) and general discomfort (58 per cent).

A prominent memory for Dawn was 'being cleaned and my personal hygiene needs being taken care of'. She says, 'I had always imagined the thought of someone having to sort my toileting messes up would be unbearable. It's a testament to the staff that I never once felt dirty or as if I had lost my dignity.' Dawn recalls, 'They treated me with such compassion and respect. The only time I ever felt I lost my dignity . . . the hoist had to be used . . . . The indignity of people seeing me being winched out of bed like a stranded whale to be dumped hunched in a chair with no ability to even sit myself comfortably was awful. It filled me with absolute dread every day.'

Dependence and control

Because of their physical dependence, patients often perceive a lack of control whilst in ICU, a feeling expressed by Dawn who says, 'the feeling of helplessness is so easy to contact with'. The distress associated with being critically ill in the highly technological environment of ICU and the evocative and powerful sense of loss of control that this can produce has been reported by many authors (Almerud et al., 2007; Tembo et al., 2012; Lykkegaard and Delmar 2013). Patient's bodies are invaded with numerous lines and tubes containing infusions of sedation and other drugs, and they are attached to equipment that monitors their every move. One former ICU patient describes this as 'my chest locked to the bed with wires and straps' and 'an invisible force pinning my body down' (Wake and Kitchener 2013: 1). Kelly (2013) further describes a patient whose hands are wrapped in gauze 'so she won't pull things' (Kelly 2013: 7). These experiences are made worse by the frequently experienced fragmented delusional memories and paranoia often described (White 2013).

Dawn says, 'I was so scared . . . I remember the nurse connecting me to CPAP (sic) and telling me to relax when I began to panic'. She goes on to say, 'I never imagined feeling safe enough to sleep again.' Dawn's narrative also illustrates the key role that the staff played in alleviating this fear. She says, 'I built some amazing relationships with the staff . . . they made me feel safe. They were honest when I needed it most. . . . One amazing member of staff eventually worked out I needed to know what was happening and turned all the monitors to face me and explained what all the numbers meant. From this moment forward I felt safer . . . I might not have liked what was being done, but I understood why .'

Communication

Patients in ICU experience frequent communication challenges (Almerud et al., 2007; Tembo et al., 2012). Being sedated and ventilated makes it very difficult to verbalize feelings and wishes. Dawn says, 'One of the hardest things as I became more aware was being unable to communicate my fear.' Colin further explains, 'Watching her (Andrea) try to communicate while she was coming out of sedation was difficult . . . . I used to hold writing paper up and let her try and write but she had no strength to form the letters.' This inability to verbally communicate can add to the sense of disempowerment felt by patients as they are unable to tell staff what they need, or explain how they are feeling (White 2013).

The importance of family

Friends and family members are also affected by a patient's critical illness (Holden et al., 2002; Verhaeghe et al., 2005; Wartella et al., 2009). Patients report that close relatives and friends give them a feeling of being in contact with something real and increase their feelings of safety and security (Bench and Day 2010). Dawn recalls, 'Throughout my sedation she (her mum) had felt like my anchor to life.' Some relatives also help with the physical care of their loved one (Mitchell and Chaboyer 2010). Colin describes helping care for his wife Andrea whilst she was in ICU and the value of this for him. He says, 'The nurses started to let me help with the suction from her mouth when she coughed up mucus, give her water on her lips from a sponge and wipe her brow when she was clammy . . . they started to call me Nurse Colin which was nice as I felt I contributed to her recovery.'

Having a loved one in ICU can have a huge impact on a relative's wellbeing (Hughes *et al.*, 2005), with mean anxiety levels during this period reported as 45.41 (SD = 15.27) (Bailey *et al.*, 2010). Relatives (*n* = 7) of critically ill patients interviewed in a study by Blom *et al.* (2013) felt, however, that being allowed to participate in care helped them feel secure and as if they were safeguarding the patient's needs. These relatives saw themselves as an important link to the patient's personality, identity and ordinary life, preventing them from becoming dehumanized (Blom *et al.*, 2013). The need to participate in care and the extent of that participation does, however, vary from person to person (Blom *et al.*, 2013). It is also important to consider the potential wishes of the patient, who at this point, is unlikely to have the capacity required for informed consent.

Discharge from ICU

A meta-synthesis of qualitative studies (Bench and Day 2010) identifies a complex array of physical and psychological symptoms experienced at the point of critical care discharge, with commonly reported physical symptoms including impaired mobility, pain, loss of appetite and difficulties with sleeping, swallowing and eating: problems compounded by overwhelming feelings of weakness and fatigue (Bench and Day 2010). Bill recalls: 'The first time I was got out of bed and sat in a chair it felt like I was sitting on broken glass it was so painful.'

Many patients and their relatives find the discharge from ICU to either a level 2 (HDU) area or a general ward a particularly difficult period, and a time during which they and the healthcare staff feel most concerned over the patient's safety (Bench and Day 2010; Bench *et al.*, 2011). Dawn recalls: 'From the moment the words HDU were uttered constant fear raged through my entire being. This place (ICU) and the people who had "held me captive and tortured me" was also the safest place in the world.'

Patients frequently cite feelings of fear, isolation, vulnerability and dependence at this point (Bench and Day 2010; Bench *et al.*, 2011). Dawn says, 'Leaving them (ICU) behind was extremely difficult . . . I was still being tube fed, catheterized and no amount of lorazepam or tamazepam (sic) would lead to sleep.' Bill also recalls: 'I was moved to HDU on 27 February still with my tracheotomy. . . . I was totally unprepared for life on a general ward. . . . I was put in a side room I felt totally abandoned . . . I then found myself moved into a ward bay which was the worst time spent in hospital. . . . I was glad the day came that I finally left.' Dawn's story supports that these are common experiences. She explains that on arrival to the ward 'I was introduced briefly to a nurse . . . she told me to push the buzzer (still attached to the wall behind me) if I needed anything and left. Thirty minutes later food was placed on the table at the end of the bed and ninety minutes after that I was 'told off' for not eating it . . . I could not move to sitting by myself, I could not reach my buzzer and I had no voice. . . . I felt totally abandoned, paralysed and dependent. . . . I spent a week in this room and was scared of dying for every single minute of it because I was left for hours without any contact.' These narratives are supported by the research literature. The majority of participants in a study by Field *et al.* (2008) felt, for example, that they had not received appropriate levels of care on the ward, a view endorsed by other authors (e.g. Russell 2000; Gardner *et al.*, 2005).

During the ICU-ward relocation period, many patients and relatives report feelings of anxiety, fear and abandonment, symptoms associated with 'relocation/transfer anxiety' (Leith 1998). This is not, however, true for everyone. Bench and Day's (2010) meta-synthesis reports data suggests that some patients associate the move to a general ward with recovery and are excited about having technical equipment removed and being able to look forward; highlighting the very personal and individual nature of critical illness and recovery.

In-hospital follow up and rehabilitation

Patients' experiences of in-hospital critical illness follow up vary widely. Some patients like Dawn describe receiving visits from ICU staff: 'A nurse from ICU came back to my ward and explained to the staff how ill I had been . . . and that I would probably need supporting with the basic care needs.' In contrast, others report little or no follow up support whilst on the ward (Bench and Day 2010; Bench *et al.*, 2011).

Expectations of progress

A person's recall and subjective interpretation of the CCU experience may relate to their emotional outcome (Rattray and Hull 2008; Kiekkas *et al.*, 2010; Nouwen *et al.*, 2012). Peter says, 'I had no real perception of how seriously injured I'd been. . . . I still fully expected to be going on my mountain biking holiday in a few months' time.' He goes on to say, 'as time went on I became increasingly convinced that there was a conspiracy to keep me in that place.' Talking about his attempt to leave the hospital, he says, 'The idea of a man escaping hospital in his pyjamas with a zimmer frame may seem almost comical as it is bewildering and pathetic, but in the state of mind that I was in . . . it was the only conceivable course of action.'

Dawn also describes the unrealistic expectations of others and the impact that this can have. At the point of discharge to the ward, she says, 'They were happy with my progress. By this they meant I had been weaned from a ventilator, I could move from the bed to a chair and walk five steps with considerable assistance and I could whisper a couple of words if I pressed my tracheostomy wound site.' She goes on to say, 'The hardest thing though was the people around me were overjoyed that I had survived and because they had seen me at my worst and could see me now they believed I was better.'

Life after hospital

Seventy-five per cent of patients with a critical illness survive beyond hospital discharge (NICE 2009). The narratives shared by former patients and relatives highlight, however, the significant physical, emotional and social challenges faced after leaving hospital. Bill remembers, 'On the journey home I became so emotional, in tears all the way. Finally the realization of what I had been through took its toll, I had no idea how the next few months would turn into my darkest days.' Dawn's experience was no easier and she says, 'What I soon realized was despite the awfulness of my hospital stay actually that was the easy bit and I was only just starting to recover.'

International research publications report a wide array of physical, emotional and social consequences of critical illness. Research studies support that patients can suffer significant fatigue, cognitive impairment and symptoms of PTSD and that, after hospital discharge, there can be long-standing consequences, which impact on all aspects of quality of life (physical, psychological, social), both for the patient and their family (Desai *et al.*, 2011; Davidson *et al.*, 2012; Griffiths *et al.*, 2013). Some of the longer-term physical, emotional and social consequences of critical illness experienced by Bill, Shirley and Dawn are described in Table 7.1.

Despite the wide range of physical and psycho-social problems identified, the availability of support services aimed at addressing patients' and relatives' needs after discharge from hospital remains inconsistent. Although Dawn describes 'amazing support from my GP', she also explains that 'when I asked for additional support there was nothing available' and was told 'what I was experiencing was normal'. Part of this problem may be attributed to insufficient communication between primary and secondary care providers. In a longitudinal interview study exploring patients' and their families' (*n* = 24) views about their critical illness recovery in Scotland, conducted one to twelve months after hospital discharge, patients perceived that GPs had little understanding of their needs (Ramsay *et al.*, 2012). A study of

Table 7.1 The longer-term consequences of critical illness

Physical consequences	'Finding it hard to do anything as I had lost so much muscle and weight' (Bill)
	'I could not believe how hard it was (getting to the toilet)' (Dawn).
	'They expected me to be able to do things which were not yet physically possible for me . . . every little thing felt like climbing a mountain' (Dawn)
	'Everything was hard . . . I didn't have the strength to hold him (the baby) by myself or change his nappy . . . I was dependent and I did not like it' (Dawn)
Emotional consequences	'I felt I had become a burden on them (family) and didn't want to live in constant pain and just wanted it all to end, it was just an endless nightmare' (Bill)
	'I was beginning to think that life just isn't worth living any more. I had lost all energy to fight and on more than one occasion on my drive to work I thought about crashing the car and ending it all' (Shirley)
	Dawn describes experiencing ongoing problems with sleeping, nightmares, flash backs and symptoms of PTSD 16 years after her critical illness.
Social consequences	'I found life so difficult having to sell my van and equipment, watching my business I had built up over 20 years disappear' (Bill)
	'Our life had changed completely. . . . We were both struggling to accept this' (Shirley)
	'My family had to return to work and a series of well-meaning friends/ acquaintances volunteered or were paid to look after me, my son or both' (Dawn)

UK ICU discharge communication practice by Wong and Wickham (2013) also reported that only 22 (36.7 per cent) of the ICUs they surveyed sent a discharge letter to the patient's GP, with significant variation in the type of information given.

Life after critical illness

Bill explains: 'It was several month (sic) later when I finally found the strength to read the diary my wife had kept of my time in ICU. It made me realize how lucky I was to survive and what a traumatic time they must have all gone

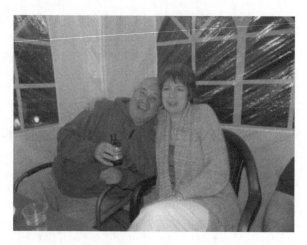

Figure 7.3 Bill and Shirley, June 2011

through, something none of us will ever forget.' Three years after his critical illness Bill writes, 'Thanks to my very special family I'm beginning to enjoy life again, with our first grandchild born in May 2013 it makes life even more worth surviving for.' Bill's wife Shirley, further comments that 'life is worth looking forward to again' (see Fig. 7.3).

The experience of critical illness often makes people re-evaluate their life, a point supported by Dawn who says, 'I now view each and every day (no matter what it holds) as something precious and to be celebrated.'

The experience can, however, have a significant impact on quality of life. Six months after hospital discharge, of the 464 patients who reported fatigue in the study by Granja *et al.* (2005), 65 per cent were unable to return to their previous level of activity/employment. Work by Davidson *et al*, (2012) and Griffiths *et al.* (2013) further highlights the significant socio-economic burden of critical illness on both the patient and their family.

Many patients feel the need to give something back to the community after their critical illness experience and research data suggest that interaction with former patients is helpful for recovery (Deacon 2012). Bill's narrative supports this view. He says:

> The turning point for me came when I was asked at a follow-up clinic if I would speak to a patient in ICU who was having a tough time. . . . I now put my experience of being an ICU patient to good use, doing presentations to healthcare professionals raising awareness of the trauma ICU patients and their relatives can go through, I also run a local support group, it's my way of giving something back for the second chance of life.'

Since his critical illness, Peter (see Fig. 7.5) has also been active in advocating support for patients and relatives. He has served as a patient representative on two National Institute of Clinical Excellence guidelines (NICE 2007, 2009) and is currently Chief Executive of ICUsteps, the intensive care patient support charity he co-founded. Peter led on the production of a patients' and relatives' guide to intensive care, now used by 50 per cent of ICUs around the UK. Peter is also working as a website and web-user interface developer.

Dawn's narrative helps explain why many former patients choose to volunteer in an area that can be so traumatic and painful for them. She says, 'It's because for a brief period of time I feel I belong and the people around me understand' (see Fig. 7.4).

Learning from service users' experience of critical illness: what do patients and relatives want from nurses and what services currently exist to support the critical care service users' needs?

Care, competence and compassion

Just as in all other areas of healthcare, patients and their families want to feel safe and to be treated with compassion, and should be able to expect this from all nurses and other health-care staff (DH 2012; Francis 2013). The narra-

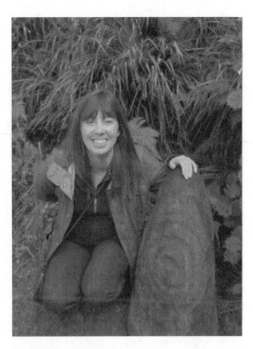

Figure 7.4 Dawn in her garden, 2014

tives described in this chapter highlight that, for patients and relatives, perceptions of safety are closely related to trust in the nursing staff. This in turn requires staff to have the knowledge, skills and attitudes needed to build these relationships. Staff working with patients experiencing or recovering from a critical illness should acquire specific competencies, national guidelines for which are now available for both nursing and medicine (GMC 2011; CC3Na 2012). Similarly, patients should expect to be cared for in an environment which meets the minimum requirements for critical care laid out by the Core Standards Working Party of the Joint Professional Standards Committee (2013).

Local and national evidence-based protocols, guidelines and assessment tools can aid nurses and other healthcare professionals to provide safe, optimum care to their patients. Examples of these are available for many different care pathways and processes including assessment and management of pain (Gélinas *et al.*, 2006), sedation (Sessler *et al.*, 2002), delirium (NICE 2010), ventilator weaning (Blackwood *et al.*, 2011), rehabilitation (NICE 2009) and many others.

Longer-term or specialist patient groups (such as the older person) may have complex needs that require additional skills and attention,

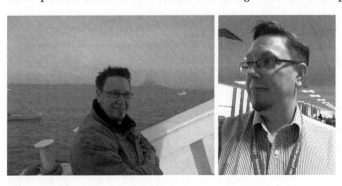

Figure 7.5 Peter: 2013/2014

over an extended period of time in the ICU. In such cases, multi-professional case conferences and referral to other services such as long-term weaning centres, pain teams and occupational therapists may be particularly important to optimize recovery (NICE 2009). In addition, a fifth of patients do not survive their ICU admission (Higginson *et al.*, 2013). The provision of good end of life care is therefore also a priority, and can be enhanced by collaborative working with specialist palliative care professionals (Higginson *et al.*, 2013).

Preparation for discharge to the ward

Preparing a patient for ICU discharge should include the gradual withdrawal of observation and monitoring, encouragement of self-care interventions, such as personal hygiene and toileting, and effective collaboration and communication with the patient, family and staff from relevant departments (NICE 2009). Findings of an observational study of critical care nurses (n = 218) by Watts *et al.* (2006) also highlight the importance of having an identified person to coordinate the discharge process. Discharge liaison nurses (Chaboyer *et al.*, 2007; St-Louis and Brault 2011) can optimize discharge by undertaking pre-transfer assessments, coordinating transfer and communicating between departments, to help the patients, families and ward staff feel prepared and well supported during the transition period.

Avoiding the discharge of patients from a CCU at night time (22:00–07.00hrs) or at weekends is also recommended (NICE 2007, 2009). These discharge times are associated with greater risks to patient safety and can lead to increased CCU readmission rates and a longer hospital length of stay (Campbell *et al.*, 2008; Hanane *et al.*, 2008). NICE (2009) recommendations (see Box 7.1) and data from Wong and Wickham (2013) and Lin *et al.* (2013) further stress the importance of a good inter-departmental handover.

Box 7.1   Recommended CCU discharge/handover information

- The structure and process of the rehabilitation care pathway.
- Differences between critical care and ward-based care; how to adjust to this and ways to cope.
- The transfer of clinical responsibility to different medical and nursing teams.
- Potential short and/or long-term physical and non-physical problems e.g. sleeping problems and hallucinations.

NICE (2009)

Effective support after discharge

An increasing awareness of the difficulties faced by critical care patients and their relatives during and after discharge from a CCU has led to a range of service improvements in the UK over the last 10 to 15 years (Endacott *et al.*, 2009). Critical care outreach services formally commenced in the UK in 2000, following a recommendation from the Department of Health for England (DH 2000). Outreach teams are commonly nurse led and usually involve a multi-professional group of staff including nurses, doctors and allied health professionals (for example, physiotherapists). Critical care outreach teams provide practical advice, education and support for ward staff to help them prevent, recognize and manage deteriorating patients (NICE 2007). Some hospitals have also developed models which involve the patient and their family in recognizing and responding to signs of patient deterioration on the ward (Odell *et al.*, 2010).

A Cochrane review by McGaughey *et al.* (2007) concluded that it is currently unclear whether such services reduce either ICU admission or hospital mortality and to date, the DH in England has avoided fully recommending their introduction (NICE 2007, 2009). The findings of an integrative review and meta-synthesis of the literature ($n = 20$) by Endacott *et al.* (2009) however, indicate that outreach services do have a beneficial impact on mortality, re-admission to ICU, discharge delays and the rate of adverse events.

Multi-professional phase specific rehabilitation programmes, commenced prior to discharge to the ward, are strongly recommended to optimize both physical and emotional recovery after critical illness (NICE 2009). Since publication of the NICE (2009) critical care rehabilitation guidelines, a variety of interventions have been developed and/or evaluated across Europe and in the US (Cuthbertson *et al.*, 2009; Jackson *et al.*, 2012; Ramsay *et al.*, 2012; Samuelson and Corrigan 2009; Walsh *et al.*, 2012). In some hospitals, specialist counselling services for critical care patients have also been introduced to help reduce patients' psychological distress (Jones and Griffiths 2007; Jones *et al.*, 2008).

Follow-up services after hospital discharge

Patients report finding the first few months after hospital discharge the most difficult period of their recovery (Prinjha *et al.*, 2009); yet the narratives included in this chapter support other research data highlighting that access to critical care follow-up services after hospital discharge remains inconsistent (Prinjha *et al.*, 2009), with clinics often funded and resourced by the acute hospital CCU. Interview data from 34 former ICU patients (Prinjha *et al.*, 2009) identifies the key perceived benefits of attending a follow-up clinic to be continuity of care and the opportunity for referral; receipt of information; the provision of expert reassurance; and the chance to give feedback to ICU staff. Additional work is, however, required in this area to further develop the role of primary care services in supporting critical illness rehabilitation.

The provision of effective information

Effective information delivery can facilitate psychological wellbeing, improve perceptions of coping, empowerment and control (Bench and Day 2010; Bench *et al.*, 2011; Bench *et al.*, 2012; Bench *et al.*, 2014) and optimize critical illness recovery (NICE 2007, 2009). Sharing health information in a way that meets individual needs enables patients to feel involved and to maintain a sense of control throughout their critical illness, even when they may be unable or unwilling to make decisions for themselves (Bench *et al.*, 2014).

National organizations, such as the Intensive Care Society (ICS) and charities such as ICUsteps have produced commercially designed information resources (ICUsteps 2010; ICS 2011) many of which provide details about the ICU environment, staff and processes.

A number of published papers also describe the development of booklets or leaflets, which include information for both patients and their relatives about discharge from ICU and on-going recovery (for example, Paul *et al.*, 2004; Mitchell and Courtney 2005; Bench *et al.*, 2014,). Applications for portable devices with internet access (such as the Apple iPhone and iPad©) are also under development for use within the ICU (Hayden and Pinto 2012). ICUsteps, for example, have produced an iPhone application which provides information for both critical care patients and their relatives. In addition, a number of websites are currently available (Healthtalkonline; ICAN-UK; ICUsteps) or under development (Ramsey 2013), which detail service users' experiences of critical illness and include information about the rehabilitation process with links to support forums and other resources.

Verbal and written communication provided throughout the critical illness trajectory underpins the delivery of compassionate care (DH 2012) and Bench (2014) suggests that effective information comprises three distinct, but overlapping elements: (1) information that helps an individual make sense of their critical illness experience and recognize the progress they have made; (2) information that is personalized to the needs of the individual; (3) information provided within a supportive context of care.

Help to make sense of the experience

Filling in memory gaps and helping patients understand what happened to them has been identified as an important part of the recovery process for the critically ill patient (NICE 2009). One way of doing this is to complete diaries for patients who are in an ICU, an intervention which Bill received. Diary entries, written by staff and visitors, contain information about the ICU stay, details of the patient's illness, treatment and progress (Egerod and Bagger 2010). They can also include photographs, which provide information to the patient about what they looked like and cues as to how ill they were. The use of diaries has been shown to improve psychological wellbeing post CCU discharge (Knowles and Tarrier 2009; Jones *et al.*, 2010) and to enhance feelings of control and safety (Forsberg *et al.*, 2011). Similar interventions, aimed at enhancing understanding, have also been developed. For example, Bench *et al.* (2014) describe the development and evaluation of a personalized patient discharge summary, a short 'lay' account of events, written by critical care nurses and given to the patient when they are discharged from the CCU. Significantly, however, Bench *et al.* (2014) point out the importance of healthcare staff who can facilitate patients' use of such 'sense-making' interventions.

Relatives

The narratives detailed in this chapter clearly highlight the impact of critical illness on family members. Research data suggest, however, that family members consider their own material needs least important and that they give absolute priority to everything that concerns the patient (Verhaeghe *et al.*, 2005).

A review of 26 research studies by Verhaeghe *et al.* (2005) emphasizes the need for relatives to be given accurate and comprehensible information, with regular opportunities to speak to a doctor about the patient's condition and prognosis, and nurses to explain to them about the care, the unit, the equipment and what they can do for the patient. Family members also place great importance on being called at home if the condition of the patient changes. Verhaeghe *et al.* (2005) further identify the importance of being able to feel hope and having reassurance. Relatives may also need help with financial or family problems.

Proximity to the patient and being able to see them regularly is crucial; yet many ICUs in the UK (BACCN 2012) and internationally (Liu *et al.*, 2013) still restrict visiting to some degree. Verhaeghe *et al.*'s (2005) review highlights the importance of flexible visiting hours, a view supported by ICU nurses, doctors and physiotherapists (da Silva Ramos *et al.*, 2013). It is worthy of note, however, that open visiting can have an impact on patient care due to an increased number of interruptions, and that nurses need the time and skills to effectively communicate with and support visitors (da Silva Ramos *et al.*, 2013).

A position statement by the British Association of Critical Care Nurse (BACCN) summarizes the relative benefits of visitors to the ICU, both for the patient and the nursing staff (BACCN 2012) and makes recommendations for minimum standards of care, both for the patient and their relatives (see Box 7.2).

Box 7.2   Standards on visiting in adult critical care units in the United Kingdom

Patients should expect:

- To have their privacy, dignity and cultural beliefs recognized
- Confidentiality
- The choice of whether or not to have visitors
- The choice to decide who they want to visit including children and other loved ones
- The choice of care assisted by their relatives
- A critical care team who recognize the importance and value of visiting.

Relatives should expect:

- A comfortable and accessible waiting room with bathroom facilities nearby
- Access to overnight accommodation in the vicinity of the ICU
- Easy access to food and drink
- A telephone nearby
- Access to relevant information
- A separate area for private discussions with healthcare professionals
- Involvement in patient care as the patient would wish
- Not have to wait for long periods of time in the waiting room without regular updates
- Access to interpretation facilities if needed

BACCN (2012)

Summary

Using the narratives of former patients and relatives, this chapter has explored the service user experience of critical illness. Patients and their families suffer significant physical, emotional and social challenges during and after an admission to a CCU. Nurses, as part of the wider healthcare team, have a pivotal role to play in minimizing the complications of critical illness and optimizing recovery.

Key website resources

EPIC website: Engaging with Patients to understand and improve recovery after Intensive Care (EPIC): a patient and family focused website for use following critical illness (Currently under development by research team in Edinburgh: Ramsay P 2014).

Health talk online: www.healthtalkonline.org/Intensive_care/

ICU steps website: www.icusteps.org

References

Adamson, H., Murgo, M., Boyle, M. *et al.* (2004) Memories of intensive care and experiences of survivors of critical illness: an interview study. *Intensive & Critical Care Nursing*, 20(5): 257–63.

Almerud, S., Alapack, R., Fridlund, B. and Ekebergh, M. (2007) Of vigilance and invisibility: being a patient in technological intense environments, *Nursing in Critical Care*, 12(3): 151–8.

Bailey, J., Sabbagh, M., Loiselle, C. *et al.* (2010) Supporting families in the ICU: a descriptive correlational study of informational support, anxiety, and satisfaction with care, *Intensive & Critical Care Nursing*, 26(2): 114–22.

Bench, S. (2014) Self-regulation and coping during early critical illness recovery: the contribution of critical care discharge information. Unpublished Phd thesis.

Bench, S. and Day, T. (2010) The user experience of critical care discharge: a meta-synthesis of qualitative research, *International Journal of Nursing Studies*, 47(4): 487–99.

Bench, S., Day, T. and Griffiths, P. (2011) Involving users in the development of effective critical care discharge information: a focus group study with patients, relatives and health care staff, *American Journal of Critical Care*, 20(6): 443–52.

Bench, S., Day, T. and Griffiths, P. (2012) Developing user centred critical care discharge information to support early critical illness rehabilitation using the medical research council's complex interventions framework, *Intensive & Critical Care Nursing*, 28(2): 123–31.

Bench, S., Heelas, K., White, C. and Griffiths, P. (2014) Providing critical care patients with a personalised discharge summary: a questionnaire survey and retrospective analysis exploring feasibility and effectiveness, *Intensive & Critical Care Nursing*, 30(2): 69–76.

Blackwood, B., Alderdice, F., Burns, K. *et al.* (2011) Use of weaning protocols for reducing duration of mechanical ventilation in critically ill adult patients: Cochrane systematic review and meta-analysis, *British Medical JournalI*, 342: c7237.

Blom, H., Gustavsson, C. and Sundler, J. (2013) Participation and support in intensive care as experienced by close relatives of patients: a phenomenological study, *Intensive & Critical Care Nursing*, 29(1): 1–8.

BACCN (British Association of Critical Care Nurses) (2012) *Position Statement on Visiting in Adult Critical Care Units in the United Kingdom.* Available at: www.baccn.org.uk/about/downloads/BACCNVisiting.pdf (accessed 4 November 2015).

Brysiewicz, P. and Bhengu, B. (2010) The experiences of nurses in providing psychosocial support to families of critically ill trauma patients in intensive care units: a study in the Durban metropolitan area, *Southern African Journal of Critical Care*, 26(2): 42–51.

Campbell, A., Cook, J., Adey, G. and Cuthbertson, B. (2008) Predicting death and readmission after intensive care discharge, *British Journal of Anaesthesia*, 100(5): 656–62.

Chaboyer, W., Thalib, L., Alcorn, K. and Foster, M. (2007) The effect of an ICU liaison nurse on patients and family's anxiety prior to transfer to the ward: an intervention study. *Intensive & Critical Care Nursing*, 23(6): 362–9.

Core Standards Working Party of the Joint Professional Standards Committee (2013) *Core Standards for Intensive Care Units (edition 1).* Available at: www.ficm.ac.uk/sites/default/files/Core%20Standards%20for%20ICUs%20Ed.1%20%282013%29.pdf (accessed 4 November 2015).

Coulter, A. and Ellis, J. (2006) *Patient Focused Interventions: A Review of the Evidence.* London: The Health Foundation.

Critical Care Network-National Nurse Leads (CC3Na) (2012) *National Competency Framework for Adult Critical Care Nurses.* Available at: www.cc3n.org.uk/competency-framework/4577977310 (accessed 4 November 2015).

Cuthbertson, B., Rattray, J. and Campbell, M. (2009) The PRACTICAL study of nurse led, intensive care follow up programmes for improving long term outcomes from critical illness: a pragmatic randomised controlled trial, *British Medical Journal*, 339(b3723). DOI: http://dx.doi.org/10.1136/bmj.b3723.

Cutler, L., Hayter, M. and Ryan, T. (2013) A critical review and synthesis of qualitative research on patient experiences of critical illness, *Intensive & Critical Care Nursing*, 29(3): 147–57.

da Silva Ramos, F., Fumis, R., Azevedo, L. and Schettino, G. (2013) Perceptions of an open visitation policy by intensive care unit workers, *Annals of Intensive Care*, 3: 34.

Davidson, J., Jones, C. and Bienvenue, J. (2012) Family response to critical illness: post intensive care syndrome-family, *Critical Care Medicine*, 40(2): 618–24.

Davydow, D., Gifford, J., Desai, S. *et al.* (2008) Posttraumatic stress disorder in general intensive care unit survivors: a systematic review, *General Hospital Psychiatry*, 30(5): 421–34.

Deacon, K. (2012) Re-building life after ICU: a qualitative study of the patients' perspective, *Intensive & Critical Care Nursing*, 28(2): 114–22.

Desai, S., Law, T. and Needham, D. (2011) Long-term complications of critical care, *Critical Care Medicine*, 39(2): 371–9.

DH (Department of Health) (2000) *Comprehensive Critical Care; a review of adult critical care services.* London: DH.

DH (2004) *Making Partnership Work for Patients, Carers and Service users: a strategic agreement between the Department of Health, the NHS and the voluntary and community sector.* Available at: http://webarchive.nationalarchives.gov.uk/+/www.dh.gov.uk/en/Publicationsandstatistics/Publications/PublicationsPolicyAndGuidance/DH_4089515 (accessed 4 November 2015).

DH (2005) *Self Care: A Real Choice. Self Care Support: A Practical Option.* London: DH.

DH (2012) *Compassion in Practice: Nursing, Midwifery and Care Staff: Our Vision and Strategy.* London: DH.

DH (2013) *The NHS Constitution: the NHS Belongs to Us All.* London: DH.

Egerod, I. and Bagger, C. (2010) Patients' experiences of intensive care diaries: a focus group study, *Intensive & Critical Care Nursing*, 26(5): 278–87.

Endacott, R., Eliott, S. and Chaboyer, W. (2009) The scope and impact of intensive care liaison and outreach services: an integrative review and meta-synthesis, *Journal of Clinical Nursing*, 18(23): 3225–36.

Field, K., Prinjha, S. and Rowan, K. (2008) 'One patient amongst many': a qualitative analysis of intensive care unit patients' experiences of transferring to the general ward, *Critical Care*, 12: R21.

Forsberg, A., Lindgren, E. and Engström, Å. (2011) Being transferred from an intensive care unit to a ward: searching for the known in the unknown, *International Journal of Nursing Practice*, 17(2): 110–16.

Francis, R. (2013) *Report of the Mid Staffordshire NHS Foundation Trust, Public Inquiry: Executive Summary.* London: HMSO.

Gardner, G., Elliott, D. and Gill, J. (2005) Patient experiences following cardiothoracic surgery: an interview study, *European Journal of Cardiovascular Nursing*, 4(3): 242–50.

Gélinas, C., Fillion, L., Puntillo, K. *et al.* (2006) Validation of the critical-care pain observation tool in adult patients, *American Journal of Critical Care*, 15(4): 420–7.

General Medical Council (GMC) (2011) *Intensive Care Medicine 1. Approved Specialty Curriculum and Associated Assessment System 2011 – ICM Single.* Available at: www.gmc-uk.org/education/intensive_care_medicine.asp (accessed 4 November 2015).

Granja, C., Lopes, A., Moreira, S. *et al.*, for the JMIP Study Group (2005) Patients' recollections of experiences in the intensive care unit may affect their quality of life, *Critical Care*, 9(2): R96–109.

Griffiths, J., Hatch, R., Bishop, J. *et al.* (2013) An exploration of social and economic outcome and associated health-related quality of life after critical illness in general intensive care unit survivors: a 12 month follow up study, *Critical Care*, 17(3): R100.

Hanane, T., Keegan, M., Seferian, E. *et al.* (2008) The association between night time transfer from the intensive care unit and patient outcome, *Critical Care Medicine*, 36(8): 2232–7.

Hayden, P. and Pinto, N. (2012) *AssIsT'U: an innovative application for the Apple IPad® to improve communication and rehabilitation on the intensive care unit.* Poster presentation. Intensive Care Society State of the Art Meeting, EXCEL, 10–12 December, London.

Higginson, I., Koffman, J., Hopkins, P. *et al.* (2013) Development and evaluation of the feasibility and effects on staff, patients, and families of a new tool, the Psychosocial Assessment and Communication Evaluation (PACE), to improve communication and palliative care in intensive care and during clinical uncertainty, *BMC Medicine*, 11: 213.

Holden, J., Harrison, L. and Johnson, M. (2002) Families, nurses and intensive care patients: a review of the literature, *Journal of Clinical Nursing*, 11(2): 140–8.

Hughes, F., Bryan, K. and Robbins, I. (2005) Relatives' experiences of critical care, *Nursing in Critical Care*, 10(1): 23–30.

ICUsteps (2010) *Intensive Care: A Guide for Patients and Relatives.* Available at: www. icusteps.org (accessed 4 November 2015).

Intensive Care Society (ICS) (2011) *Discharge from Intensive Care: Information for Patients and Relatives.* Available at: www.ics.ac.uk (accessed 4 November 2015).

INVOLVE (2012) *Briefing Notes for Researchers: Public Involvement in NHS, Public Health and Social Care Research.* Available at: www.invo.org.uk/wp-content/uploads/2012/04/ INVOLVEBriefingNotesApr2012.pdf (accessed 4 November 2015).

Jackson, J., Ely, E., Wesley, M. *et al.* (2012) Cognitive and physical rehabilitation of intensive care unit survivors: results of the RETURN randomized controlled pilot investigation, *Critical Care Medicine*, 40(4): 1088–97.

Jamerson, P., Scheibmeir, M., Bott, M. *et al.* (1996) Experiences in the ICU: The experiences of families with a relative in the intensive care unit, *Heart and Lung: Journal of Acute and Critical Care*, 25: 467–74.

Jones, C. and Griffiths, R. (2007) Patient and caregiver counselling after the intensive care unit: what are the needs and how should they be met? *Current Opinion in Critical Care*, 13(5): 503–7.

Jones, C., Bäckman, C., Capuzzo, M. *et al.*, for the RACHEL group (2010) Intensive care diaries reduce new onset post-traumatic stress disorder following critical illness: a randomised controlled trial, *Critical Care*, 14(5): R168.

Jones, C., Hall, S. and Jackson, S. (2008) Benchmarking a nurse-led ICU counselling initiative, *Nursing Times*, 104(38): 32–4.

Kelly, J. (2013) *Where Night is Day: The World of the ICU.* London: Cornell University Press.

Kiekkas, P., Theodorakopoulou, G., Spyratos, F. and Baltopoulos, G. (2010) Psychological distress and delusional memories after critical care: a literature review, *International Nursing Review*, 57(3): 288–96.

Knowles, R. and Tarrier, N. (2009) Evaluation of the effect of prospective patient diaries on emotional well-being in intensive care unit survivors: a randomized controlled trial, *Critical Care Medicine*, 37(1): 184–91.

Leith, B. (1998) Transfer anxiety in critical care patients and their family members, *Critical Care Nurse*, 18(4): 24–32.

Lin, F., Chaboyer, W., Wallis, M. and Miller, A. (2013) Factors contributing to the process of intensive care patient discharge: an ethnographic study informed by activity theory, *International Journal of Nursing Studies*, 50(8): 1054–66.

Liu, V., Read, J., Scruth, E. and Cheng, E. (2013) Visitation policies and practices in US ICUs, *Critical Care*, 17:R71.

Löf, L., Berggren, L. and Ahlström, G. (2008) ICU patients' recall of emotional reactions in the trajectory from falling critically ill to hospital discharge: follow-ups after 3 and 12 months, *Intensive & Critical Care Nursing*, 24: 108–21.

Lykkegaard, K. and Delmar, C. (2013) A threat to the understanding of oneself: intensive care patients' experiences of dependency, *International Journal of Qualitative Studies of Health & Well-being*, 8: 10.3402/qhw.v8i0.20934. DOI: 10.3402/qhw.v8i0.20934.

McGaughey, J., Alderdice, F., Fowler, R. *et al.* (2007) *Outreach and Early Warning Systems (EWS) for the Prevention of Intensive Care Admission and Death of Critically Ill Adult Patients on General Hospital Wards, Cochrane Database of Systematic Reviews 2007*, Issue 3. Art. No.: CD005529. DOI: 10.1002/14651858.CD005529.pub2.

Mitchell, M. and Chaboyer, W. (2010) Family Centred Care – a way to connect patients, families and nurses in critical care: a qualitative study using telephone interviews, *Intensive & Critical Care Nursing*, 26(3): 154–60.

Mitchell, M. and Courtney, M. (2005) Improving transfer from the intensive care unit: the development, implementation and evaluation of a brochure based on Knowles' adult learning theory, *International Journal of Nursing Practice*, 11(6): 257–68.

Morrow, E., Boaz, A., Brearley, S. and Ross, F. (2012) *Handbook of Service User Involvement in Nursing and Healthcare Research*. Chichester: Wiley-Blackwell.

NICE (National Institute for Health and Clinical Excellence) (2007) *Acutely Ill Patients in Hospital: Recognition of and Response to Acute Illness in Adults in Hospital*. NICE clinical guideline 50. Developed by the Centre for Clinical Practice at NICE. Available at: www.nice.org.uk/guidance/cg50/evidence (accessed 4 November 2015).

NICE (2009) *Rehabilitation after Critical Illness*. NICE clinical guideline 83. Developed by the Centre for Clinical Practice at NICE. Available at: www.nice.org.uk/guidance/cg83/evidence (accessed 4 November 2015).

NICE (2010) *Delirium: Diagnosis, Prevention and Management*. Clinical Guideline 103. Commissioned by the National Institute for Health and Clinical Excellence. Available at: www.nice.org.uk/guidance/cg103/evidence (accessed 4 November 2015).

Nouwen, M., Klijn, F., van den Broek, B. and Slooter, A. (2012) Emotional consequences of intensive care unit delirium and delusional memories after intensive care unit admission: a systematic review, *Journal of Critical Care*, 27(2): 199–211.

Odell, M., Gerber, K. and Gager, M. (2010) Call 4 concern: patient and relative activated critical care outreach, *British Journal of Nursing*, 19(22): 1390–5.

Paul, F., Hendry, C. and Cabrelli, L. (2004) Meeting patient and relatives' information needs upon transfer from an intensive care unit: the development and evaluation of an information booklet, *Journal of Clinical Nursing*, 13(3): 396–405.

Perrins, J., King, N. and Collins, J. (1998) Assessment of long-term psychological well-being following intensive care, *Intensive & Critical Care Nursing*, 14: 108–16.

Prinjha, S., Field, K. and Rowan, K. (2009) What patients think about ICU follow-up services: a qualitative study, *Critical Care*, 13(2): R46. DOI:10.1186/cc7769.

Ramsay, P. (2013) Engaging with Patients to understand and improve recovery after Intensive Care (EPIC): a patient and family focused website for use following critical illness. Oral presentation. Whats new in ICU? Edinburgh Critical Care Research Group, 6th annual meeting, Royal Infirmary of Edinburgh, 26 June 2013.

Ramsay, P., Huby, G., Rattray, J., Salisbury, L., Walsh, T. and Kean, S. (2012) A longitudinal qualitative exploration of healthcare and informal support needs among survivors of critical illness: the RELINQUISH protocol, *British Medical Journal Open*, 2(4), e001507. DOI:10.1136/bmjopen-2012-001507.

Rattray, J. and Hull, A. (2008) Emotional outcome after intensive care: literature review, *Journal of Advanced Nursing*, 64(1): 2–13.

Rattray, J., Crocker, C., Jones, M. and Connaghan, J. (2010) Patients' perceptions of and emotional outcome after intensive care: results from a multicentre study, *Nursing in Critical Care*, 15(2): 86–93.

Russell, S. (2000) Continuity of care after discharge from ICU, *Professional Nurse*, 15(8): 497–500.

Samuelson, K. and Corrigan, I. (2009) A nurse-led intensive care after-care programme-development, experiences and preliminary evaluation, *Nursing in Critical Care*, 14(5): 254–63.

Samuleson, K., Lundberg, D. and Fridlund, B. (2006) Memory in relation to depth of sedation in adult mechanically ventilated intensive care unit patients, *Intensive Care Medicine*, 32(5): 660–7.

Sessler, C., Gosnell, M., Brophy, G. *et al.* (2002) The Richmond Agitation-Sedation Scale: validity and reliability in adult intensive care unit patients, *American Journal of Respiratory Critical Care Medicine*, 166(10): 1338–44.

St-Louis, L. and Brault, D. (2011) A clinical nurse specialist intervention to facilitate safe transfer from ICU, *Clinical Nurse Specialist*, 25(6): 321–6.

Stein-Parbury, J. and McKinley, S. (2000) Patients' experiences of being in an intensive care unit: a select literature review, *American Journal of Critical Care*, 9(1): 20–7.

Tembo, A., Parker, V. and Higgins, I. (2012) Being in limbo: the experience of critical illness in intensive care and beyond, *Open Journal of Nursing*, 2(3): 270–6.

Verhaeghe, S., Defloor, T., Van Zurren, F. *et al.* (2005) The needs and experiences of family members of adult patients in an intensive care unit: a review of the literature, *Journal of Clinical Nursing*, 14(4): 501–9.

Wake, S. and Kitchener, D. (2013) Post-traumatic stress disorder after intensive care, *British Medical Journal*, 346(f3232). DOI: 10.1136/bmj.f3232.

Walsh, T., Salisbury, L., Ramsay, P. *et al.* (2012) A randomised controlled trial evaluating a rehabilitation complex intervention for patients following intensive care discharge: the RECOVER study, *British Medical Journal Open*, 2:e001475. DOI:10.1136/bmjopen-2012-001475

Wartella, J., Auerbach, S. and Ward, K. (2009) Emotional distress, coping and adjustment in family members of neuroscience intensive care patients, *Journal of Psychosomatic Research*, 66: 503–9.

Watts, R., Pierson, J. and Gardner, H. (2006) Co-ordination of the discharge planning process in critical care, *Journal of Clinical Nursing*, 16(1): 194–202.

White, C. (2013) Intensive care and rehabilitation- a patient's perspective, *Journal of the Intensive Care Society*, 14(4): 299–333.

Wong, D. and Wickham, A. (2013) A survey of intensive care unit discharge communication practices in the UK, *Journal of the Intensive Care Society*, 14(4): 330–3.

Zetterlund, P., Plos, K., Bergbom, I. and Ringdal, M. (2012) Memories from intensive care unit persist for several years – a – longitudinal prospective multi-centre study, *Intensive & Critical Care Nursing*, 28(3): 159–67.

Person-centred approaches to diabetes

Annie Holme and Jakki Berry

Introduction

This chapter explores the provision of PCC for people with Diabetes Mellitus. People with diabetes are expected to have a much greater involvement in the daily management of their condition than those with other long-term conditions. Healthcare professionals and patients in this field have led the way in developing ways of working together effectively. In this chapter, three different person-centred approaches that can be taken by nurses and other health professionals working with people with diabetes are reviewed along with potential outcomes for health and wellbeing. The views and experiences of people with diabetes illustrate the discussion throughout. Pseudonyms are used to preserve confidentiality.

Diabetes Mellitus is a global health problem with 347 million people worldwide living with the condition (WHO 2015). In the UK there are 3.2 million people who are known to have diabetes plus an estimated 630,000 who have diabetes but are not yet diagnosed (Diabetes UK 2014). Current spending on diabetes accounts for about 10 per cent of the NHS budget (Diabetes UK 2012). Diabetes is a long-term condition that needs to be managed and monitored well to prevent a range of serious and potentially life-threatening consequences for health. Optimal management of diabetes is often complex, varies from individual to individual and changes over time.

'Diabetes Mellitus is a chronic complex metabolic disorder characterised by a high level of blood glucose and caused by defects in insulin secretion and/or action' (NICE 2011). There are two main types of diabetes, classified as type 1 and type 2. Type 1 diabetes is usually caused by an autoimmune process that destroys the pancreatic islet cells (American Diabetes Association 2014). Whilst it can affect all age groups it is often diagnosed in childhood or young adulthood. Type 2 is associated with insulin resistance and/or insulin insufficiency and results from a complex interaction between the environment and genetics (Lyssenko and Laakso 2013). Those more at risk of type 2 diabetes include older people, the overweight or obese, those of South Asian, Chinese, African-Caribbean and black African descent (NICE 2012), and those with a family history of diabetes or previous gestational diabetes (Lyssenko and Laakso 2013).

Diabetes has a profound effect on the lives of people with the condition and those around them from the moment of diagnosis onwards. Both type 1 and type 2 diabetes lead to a rise in blood glucose levels. Insulin is the treatment for type 1 diabetes and is injected subcutaneously with an insulin syringe, pen device or continuous subcutaneous insulin infusion (CSII or insulin pump). There are a range of therapies for type 2 diabetes including dietary modification, exercise, oral hypoglycaemic agents, injectable non-insulin treatments and insulin. Treatment regimens can be complex for both types of diabetes. Blood glucose levels are significant determinants of Initial and ongoing treatment decisions.

Different clinical indicators are used to assess how well diabetes is being managed. Capillary blood testing with a glucometer gives an immediate reading of the blood glucose level. People who have been diagnosed with diabetes may need to monitor their blood glucose levels up to 10 times a day and adjust their treatment accordingly. The frequency of testing depends on a range of factors including type of diabetes, treatment and lifestyle.

Glycated haemoglobin (HbA1c) provides a measure of the amount of blood glucose in red blood cells and indicates average blood glucose levels over the previous three months. This test is used to show how well diabetes is being managed over a period of time, also known as glycaemic control. Glucose levels below or above the target range can lead to acute complications of diabetes such as hypoglycaemia or problems related to hyperglycaemia such as diabetic ketoacidosis. Long-term poor glycaemic control can lead to chronic complications of diabetes due to blood vessel and nerve damage including retinopathy, neuropathy and nephropathy.

Reader activity

Think about people you have met with diabetes either as patients or friends or family.

What activities do they need to undertake every day to manage their diabetes?
How might this impact on their day-to-day life and plans for the future?
How could you take this into consideration when caring for someone with diabetes?

Person-centred approaches in diabetes

The description of diabetes in the previous section and reflection on the daily lives of people with diabetes demonstrates how important monitoring and maintaining glycaemic control is for short- and long-term health outcomes. To live independent lives and achieve good levels of glycaemic control people with diabetes need to understand their condition and be competent and confident in performing the technical, clinical tasks needed to monitor and manage their blood glucose levels effectively. Most people learn and perform these skills for themselves but in some cases it may be the role of a carer.

From the activity above you probably identified some of these tasks as part of the daily life of people with diabetes: measuring blood glucose, injecting with insulin, taking oral medication, diet management and preventing and managing hypoglycaemia. To learn and undertake these skills requires more active participation by patients in their healthcare than for many other conditions. It has been estimated that people with a long-term condition such as diabetes spend on average three hours of every year with a health professional and 8,757 hours managing their condition alone (Wallace *et al.*, 2012). This highlights both the need for self-management skills on the part of the person with diabetes and the importance of the time spent with a professional to enable and facilitate these skills. As a consequence person-centred approaches have been recognized as key to effective diabetes care for many years.

Janice and Susan have both been living with type 2 diabetes for many years. We asked them for their views on how they work with health professionals to manage their condition. In Box 8.1 they explain what PCC means to them.

Box 8.1

'Person-centred care means rather than care being the same for everyone and you as the patient fitting in with a care facility being your only option, you can decide where and how the care you require is provided. It is arranged around you.' (Janice, person with diabetes)

'To me person-centred care is where the person with diabetes is at the centre. The person with diabetes is empowered by working with healthcare professionals to be able to make decisions about their condition through education, and . . . the goals made between the person with diabetes and the healthcare professionals need to be patient focused and ideally patient driven. Healthcare professionals may help individuals to identify their goals' (Susan, person with diabetes)

The centrality of the person with diabetes in treatment decisions and care planning is recognized in government policies, guidelines and guidelines. For example in England, Standard 3 of the National Service Framework for Diabetes (DH 2001) enshrines the need for a service that encourages partnership in decision-making and care planning:

All children, young people and adults with diabetes will receive a service which encourages partnership in decision-making, supports them in managing their diabetes and helps them to adopt and maintain a healthy lifestyle. This will be reflected in an agreed and shared care plan in an appropriate format and language. Where appropriate, parents and carers should be fully engaged in this process.

(DH 2001: 5)

The different person-centred approaches used with people with diabetes can be grouped into the following categories:

- Individualized care planning
- Shared decision-making
- Support with self-management.

Individualized care planning

As we have seen diabetes is a complex condition. Health professionals need to consider not only the major differences between type 1 and type 2 diabetes, but also the potential impacts of age, co-morbidities, disability, life changes such as pregnancy and individual physiological responses to treatment.

Reader activity

Ahmed is a 52-year-old computer programmer and has recently been diagnosed with type 2 diabetes. He is overweight with a Body Mass Index (BMI) of 32.5 and has border-line hypertension. He has no other health problems. He lives with his wife, four children and extended family.

Mary is an 83-year-old retired teacher. She was diagnosed with type 2 diabetes 16 years ago. She has raised cholesterol and has had two Transient Ischaemic Attacks (TIAs) in the last three years. She has osteoarthritis in both knees, which affects her mobility. Recently Mary has become increasing forgetful and at times gets confused about where she is. She lives alone.

Identify short- and long-term goals for Ahmed and Mary's diabetes care.

Type 2 diabetes is frequently diagnosed in people aged between 40 and 60 years old. The aim of treatment is to reduce contributory factors such as obesity and maintain good glycaemic control to prevent the long-term health consequences. The core component of treatment is dietary modification. Dietary advice needs to consider social and cultural norms for individual patients.

The physiological changes associated with ageing can affect an individual's capability in managing their condition and their response to treatment. Waterman (2012) and Da Costa (2014) both express concern that the emphasis on achieving HbA1c target levels may compromise the safety of some old, frail patients with co-morbidities such as declining renal function and dementia. The risk of hypoglycaemia may increase while the benefits of glycaemic control are reduced. Quality of life issues such as the freedom to eat and drink for enjoyment may also become more important than rigorous glycaemic control as part of end of life care. However, diabetes care for an older person who is functionally and cognitively able should be the same as for someone younger (Waterman 2012). A person-centred approach ensures that factors such as age do not determine the care given but are considered as part of an individualizedand holistic assessment and care planning process.

In planning the care for both Ahmed and Mary, treatment with medication but also dietary and other lifestyle interventions are important to limit the short- and long-term negative consequences of their diabetes. How these goals are to be achieved would be different for each of them taking in to consideration their individual capabilities, preferences and social circumstances.

Reflection on the day-to-day impact of diabetes-related activities undertaken in Activity 8.1 may have highlighted other factors such as employment, education, housing, family and lifestyle that also need to be considered in planning the care of an individual with diabetes. Taking into consideration simple and practical aspects of daily life is important, such as whom in the household buys and cooks food, as their cooperation and understanding may be needed to bring about the necessary dietary changes.

The role of nurses in individualized care planning

Nurses play a key role in helping patients monitor and manage their diabetes from diagnosis onwards. Hospital- and community based Diabetes Nurse Specialists and Practice Nurses may be the principal and ongoing contact for patients. In-depth knowledge and understanding of their patients facilitates care planning which meets the different needs of individual patients (Stenner *et al.*, 2011). The following quotes indicate the importance to people with diabetes of getting good advice and support.

> Having access to healthcare professionals has been key, whether that's by email, phone or face to face appointment as I think that has built up my confidence and understanding and allows me to get on with life with the knowledge that if I have a problem or think I need to change something, I have support available.
>
> (Susan, person with diabetes)

> What matters most to me is being confident I am being given the best advice and having access to health professionals with knowledge of diabetes care.
>
> (Janice, person with diabetes)

A hospital admission poses a challenge for both people with diabetes and for the nurses caring for them. The physiological effects of illness, trauma and surgery will affect blood glucose levels and treatment. People may find they are temporarily no longer able to manage their diabetes independently. They are often cared for by a team of health professionals who do not know them and may not have expertise in managing diabetes.

> I think where patient centred approach with diabetes sometimes fails is when people are in-patients and ward staff have a lack of understanding of the condition.
>
> (Susan, person with diabetes)

The need to take a person-centred approach in care planning is essential for safe and effective care. Assessment should include exploring how the patient normally monitors and manages their diabetes, how effective this is and what their priorities are. Care planning should be aimed at returning a patient to their previous level of independence as soon as they are able or taking the opportunity to improve their management through involvement of a hospital or community-based diabetes team. Taking an individualized approach and knowing when to refer to others means that PCC for people with diabetes can be provided by nurses without specialist knowledge of diabetes in a range of settings.

Shared decision-making

Ahmad *et al.* (2014) view shared decision-making as an important person-centred activity as it is enabling, allowing people to develop their own capabilities to manage their condition and improves patient satisfaction with their care. Central to shared decision-making is the belief that both clinicians and patients have expertise; the knowledge and experience they bring to decisions are different but equally important (Coulter and Collins 2011). People with diabetes have knowledge of their own individual experience of the disease and its impact on their lives (see Fig. 8.1).

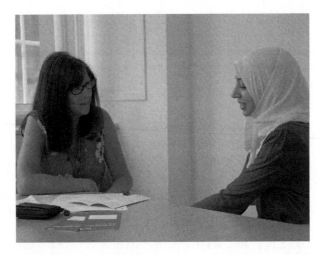

Figure 8.1 A Diabetes Clinical Nurse Specialist and a person with diabetes review ongoing management of the condition

They know their own social and economic circumstances; and also importantly their own values and attitudes in relation to health, illness and risk as well as their preferences in relation to management and treatments. This expertise can be used alongside the health professional's evidence-based clinical knowledge, to help people with diabetes to make the best decisions about treatment, self-management or lifestyle changes.

All patients with diabetes in the UK are offered an annual review of their condition with a doctor or nurse. This provides an opportunity to review their health, their glycaemic control and to screen for the micro and macro vascular long-term consequences of diabetes. The Year of Care (YOC) Programme aims to actively involve people with long-term conditions in the management of their care through personalized care planning and shared decision-making. The pilot studies for this programme were carried out with people with diabetes and were successful in transforming this annual review into an interaction based on an holistic and partnership approach that increased the satisfaction of both people with diabetes and the health professionals with the care provided (Year of Care 2011): 'Before, things seemed to get forced on you . . . Whereas this way I prefer to discuss it myself . . . there's more of a choice now, it's my choice rather than someone else's choice, that's why I like it' (Person with diabetes, reporting on their experience of the YOC approach to care planning; Year of Care 2011: 2).

Reader activity

Reflect on interactions between people with diabetes and health professionals you have observed.

- Can you think of examples where there was shared decision-making?

- What were the characteristics of the interactions that facilitated shared decision-making?
- Where did these interactions take place?

The role of nurses in shared decision-making

You may have noticed that the health professionals in the interactions you identified as exemplars of shared decision-making listened carefully to the person with diabetes, acknowledged and utilized their knowledge and understanding of their condition, shared information, agreed agendas, offered choices and negotiated and agreed goals and actions.

Many of these interactions may have taken place in a primary care setting or at home. Practice nurses and other community nurses are often responsible for ongoing management including the annual review and therefore play a key role in enabling and empowering people with diabetes to be involved in decision-making about their care.

Coulter and Collins (2011) acknowledge that sharing decision-making with patients may be challenging and requires good communication skills. They propose that the health professional needs to be 'curious, supportive, non-judgemental' and to present unbiased evidence about benefits and risks (p. 25). They suggest following the simple model of 'ask-tell-ask' when sharing complex information (see Box 8.2).

Box 8.2   Example of using ask-tell-ask model

Sue is 60 and has poorly controlled type 2 diabetes. You notice that she is eating sweets that have been left by a family member. She tells you that she has eaten them all her life, that eating a few sweets does not make her feel unwell and that she does not really understand why the nurses are telling her she must not eat them.

Ask her if it is alright if you tell her why the nurses are concerned about her eating sweets. If Sue agrees this is alright, reassure (**tell**) her that many people with diabetes feel the same and find it hard to understand why eating certain foods is a problem for their health. Then explain (**tell**) why her body can no longer deal with sugary foods and the possible consequences of a raised blood sugar level for her health in the long term. **Ask** if Sue has any questions, needs anything explaining again and what this information means to her.

Decision aids can also be very useful tools in helping people make the right decisions for them. Several have been designed with the aim of improving glycaemic control in diabetes, an example can be found on the NHS England Shared Decision making web pages http://sdm.rightcare.nhs.uk/pda/diabetes-improving-control/.

Support with self-management

At the beginning of this chapter the knowledge and skills that people with diabetes need to independently monitor and manage their condition effectively on a daily basis were identified.

A person-centred approach is essential to optimize an individual's ability to self-manage their diabetes. The engagement with and ability to self-manage care is often referred to as patient activation (Wallace *et al.*, 2012). Individualized care planning and shared decision-making are fundamental to the process of maximizing activation and are also central to a range of initiatives introduced to help people manage their diabetes successfully (see Fig. 8.2).

One approach that was first introduced in the UK in 2002 is the Expert Patient Programme (DH 2002). As the title suggests the underlying premise for this programme is that people with long-term conditions are often more knowledgeable about their dis-

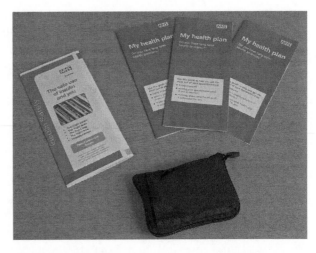

Figure 8.2 Examples of documents used to help people with diabetes manage their health and a patient glucometer used to monitor blood glucose levels

ease and the impact on them as individuals than the health professionals caring for them and should therefore take the lead in managing their health. The programme offers people courses that help them with issues such as healthy eating and communicating with family and health professionals. More information can be found on the NHS Choices website http://www. nhs.uk/NHSEngland/AboutNHSservices/doctors/Pages/expert-patients-programme.aspx.

Co-creating Health is a more recent programme that aims to integrate self-management approaches into routine healthcare for people with long-term conditions including diabetes. It comprises self-management training for patients, knowledge, skills and attitude education for health professionals and service improvements so health systems and processes support people in managing their conditions. Early evaluation demonstrated that participation in the programme increased both the activation and quality of life of people with diabetes (Wallace *et al.*, 2012). More information can be found at the Health Foundation website http://www. health.org.uk/publications/co-creating-health-evaluation-phase-1/

Structured education programmes are offered to many people with diabetes to help them develop the knowledge and skills they need to manage their condition effectively. Dose Adjustment for Normal Eating (DAFNE) is a course that provides people with type 1 diabetes with skills to accurately judge the amount of carbohydrates in each meal and adjust their dose of insulin accordingly. This leads to better glycaemic control and a more flexible approach to eating which allows diabetes to fit around the person's lifestyle and can therefore improve their quality of life (Lawton and Rankin 2010).

> I found going to the DAFNE course changed my diabetic control dramatically and has made it so much easier to live with. It fits in with my lifestyle and has given me so much more freedom to do whatever I want to do. It's still hard work to keep good control and I find carbohydrate measurement can still be a bit hit and miss but compared to the other very regimented methods it's so much easier.
>
> (Janice, person with diabetes)

The DESMOND programme includes modules, toolkits and pathways for people who are at risk of or who have type 2 diabetes. The structured education component is usually provided as a group session(s) with the aim of encouraging participants to identify their own risk factors and develop their own goals for lifestyle changes to improve their health (Khunti et al., 2012).

Both DAFNE and DESMOND are provided by health professionals who have undergone the specialist training needed. The importance of structured education programmes to enable self-management of diabetes is reflected in national guidelines issued by organizations such as NICE in the UK, for example the Quality Standard on Diabetes in Adults http://www.nice. org.uk/guidance/qs6

Despite the importance of self-management for effective diabetes control some people struggle to develop the motivation and skills needed to be successful in this. Motivational interviewing has been identified as an intervention that can help people improve their self-management skills and glycaemic control (Deakin et al., 2005; Greaves et al., 2010; Chen et al., 2012).

Motivational interviewing uses a person-centred counselling approach to encourage people to develop their own motivation to change rather than having it imposed by someone else. Ambivalence towards and barriers to change are explored, possible solutions identified and action plans made. The need for the client to be ready for change is core to the approach and resistance to change is viewed as an indication of the client's lack of readiness rather than as a problem (Greaves et al., 2010).

The role of nurses in supporting self-management

All the interventions above require specialist training which is often undertaken by nurses particularly those who work with diabetic patients. It is important for all nurses to be aware of the existence of these and similar schemes. Patients who have experienced structured education are likely to be more confident and effective in their diabetes self-management and therefore will be able to contribute significantly to or lead care planning in relation to their condition.

Challenges in providing PCC

There are many reasons why a person with diabetes might find it hard to manage their condition independently and effectively. There are also many challenges for health professionals in enabling and facilitating their patients to achieve the knowledge, skills and confidence to achieve optimal self-management.

Reader activity

List factors that might make it difficult for a person with diabetes to manage their condition safely and effectively.

What are the challenges for health professionals in providing PCC to people with diabetes?

Barriers to effective self-management

You may have identified barriers to effective self-management that are intrinsic to the person with diabetes and include age, co-morbidities including mental health problems such as anxiety and depression, poor cognitive function and physical disabilities, as well as individual physiological responses to insulin therapy and other medication. Health beliefs and values can influence understanding of diabetes and its causes and treatments. People may also have expectations about the roles of health professionals and patients in managing diabetes that run counter to the fundamental principles of shared decision-making and self-management.

Some of these barriers can be overcome by treating concurrent conditions such as depression and anxiety. Approaches such as motivational interviewing may help people perceive self-management of their condition more positively and change their behaviour accordingly. Other intrinsic factors such as disability may require a more flexible approach in finding the best solution on an individualized basis.

Individual social and economic circumstances such as poverty, poor housing, irregular working hours and the need to care for others can all have a significant impact on a person's ability to self-manage their diabetes (Weaver *et al.*, 2014). An integrated approach with social care providers is needed to address these broader issues. This requires individual health professionals to have knowledge of the range of services available but also systems that enable partnership working so care can be personalized and coordinated (Ahmad *et al.*, 2014).

Taking a person-centred approach means that the aim of care is not to impose self-management on a person with diabetes but to work with their preferences, including those for participation in shared decision-making and agree on outcomes that are realistic and important for that individual at that time (Ahmad *et al.*, 2014). For this to happen effectively healthcare professionals have to be committed to individualized care planning and the principles of shared decision-making.

Challenges for health professionals

When reviewing the challenges faced by health professionals in providing PCC for people with diabetes you may have identified lack of knowledge, skills and time as key factors. The need for a greater focus on providing health professionals with the knowledge and skills they need has been identified (Brown 2005; Willis Commission 2012). As already discussed many of the person-centred interventions that have been evaluated as effective in diabetes self-management such as motivational interviewing require specialist training.

Individualized care planning and shared decision-making should be achievable for all nurses working with patients with diabetes. Time pressures and habitual ways of working may present challenges for some health professionals in some settings. Nurses and other clinicians may be used to making decisions for patients particularly in acute settings and may feel uneasy about relinquishing some of the responsibility or feel that they do not have the time available to facilitate the process.

Healthcare systems

Effective PCC is also dependent on the healthcare systems in which service provision is embedded. People with diabetes may receive care in a range of settings including acute, mental health and primary care and in hospitals, clinics, health centres and their own homes. Consistency in information shared and approach taken is essential (Ahmad *et al.*, 2014). The extent to which this integration is achieved can be very variable depending on the individuals, teams and organizations involved. Exemplars of effective PCC initiatives such as the Co-creating health programme described previously that work to improve the capability of health systems to support person-centred approaches demonstrate how important these factors can be to patient experience and effective management of conditions like diabetes.

Another challenge can be ensuring the right services are available to meet the different needs that people with diabetes experience at different stages of their lives. For example, women with diabetes will need more specialist services during pregnancy and birth. As discussed earlier physiological changes associated with ageing, other illness and changing personal priorities and preferences mean that people will need varied levels and types of support at different times. At some points in their lives people may prefer to access a more generic service offered locally in the community rather than specialist hospital-based provision but this may change as priorities and needs alter. Providing choice is core to PCC and requires flexibility in service provision where possible. Health professionals who take an individualized approach can help a person with diabetes achieve the personalized care they need from the varied and complex health and social care services provided: 'I have changed back to getting my care from the diabetic clinic at the hospital because the hospital was more knowledgeable about DAFNE and treatment of type 1 diabetes' (Janice, person with diabetes).

NICE have produced Diabetes Pathways to help ensure that commissioning for and provision of diabetic health services are consistent in quality and approach (NICE 2014). The NICE Quality Standard (2011) states that 'an integrated approach to provision of services is fundamental to the delivery of high quality care to people with diabetes'.

There are clearly many potential challenges to providing PCC. Yet, it can be seen that adhering to the core tenets of individualized care planning and shared decision-making in every interaction with people with diabetes will ensure that they are listened to, that their knowledge and experience are acknowledged and utilized and that their priorities and preferences are central to care decisions. Understanding of the whole health system in which the person receives their treatment can facilitate a more consistent and integrated approach.

Summary

This chapter has shown that diabetes is a complex, dynamic and potentially life-threatening disease that requires constant and lifelong monitoring and treatment. Effective management of blood glucose levels can prevent the long-term consequence of diabetes. People with diabetes have to play an active role in monitoring and treating their condition on a daily basis throughout their lives. They are supported in this role by a range of health professionals, with nurses playing a key role.

Evidence shows that a person-centred approach can optimize effective self-management by people with diabetes. Individualized care planning and shared decision-making are fundamental to this approach. People are viewed as individuals within their own social, economic and cultural context. Their priorities and preferences are respected, including their wishes around participating in decision-making and self-management. Their knowledge, experience and priorities shape care decisions.

There are a range of person-centred programmes and initiatives available that can enable and help people in becoming more effective and independent in managing their diabetes. There are also a growing number of strategies aimed at enhancing the capability of health systems to provide person-centred and integrated care to people with long-term conditions including diabetes. Individual nurses and other health professionals with their knowledge of individual patients and the services available can help people with diabetes get the flexible and personalized care they need to live successfully with their condition.

References

Ahmad, N., Ellins, J., Krelle, H. and Lawrie, M. (2014) *Person-centred Care: From Ideas to Action.* London: The Health Foundation.

American Diabetes Association (2014) Diagnosis and classification of Diabetes Mellitus, *Diabetes Care (Supp)*, January 37(1): 81–90.

Brown, F. (2005) Nurse consultations: a person-centred approach, *Diabetes and Primary Care (Supp)*, 7(2): 86–8.

Chen, S.M., Creedy, D., Lin, H.S. and Wollin, J. (2012) Effects of motivational interviewing intervention on self management, psychological and glycemic outcomes in type 2 diabetes: a randomized controlled trial, *International Journal of Nursing Studies*, 49: 637–44.

Coulter, A. and Collins, A. (2011) *Making Shared Decision Making a Reality: No Decision About Me Without Me.* London: The King's Fund.

Da Costa, S. (2014) Care of the older person with diabetes: when the target misses the person, *Journal of Diabetes Nursing*, 18(4): 144.

Deakin, T., McShane, C., Cade, J. and Williams, R. (2005) *Group Based Training for Self-management Strategies in People with Type 2 Diabetes Mellitus (Review).* Cochrane Database of Systematic Reviews 2005, Issue 2. Art. No.: CD003417.

DH (Department of Health) (2001) *National Service Framework for Diabetes.* London: The Stationery Office.

DH (2002) *The Expert Patient: A New Approach to Chronic Disease Management for the 21st Century.* London: The Stationery Office.

Diabetes UK (2012) *State of the Nation 2012 England.* Available at: www.diabetes.org.uk/documents/reports/state-of-the-nation-2012.pdf (accessed 5 November 2015).

Diabetes UK (2014) *What is Diabetes*? Available at: www.diabetes.org.uk/Guide-to-diabetes/What-is-diabetes/ (accessed 5 November 2015).

Greaves, C., Sheppard, K. and Evans, P. (2010) Motivational interviewing for lifestyle change, *Diabetes and Primary Care* (Supp), 12(3): 178–82.

Khunti, K., Gray, L., Skinner, T. *et al.* (2012) Effectiveness of a diabetes education and self management programme (DESMOND) for people with newly diagnosed type 2 diabetes mellitus: three year follow-up of a cluster randomised controlled trial in primary care, *British Medical Journal*, 344: e2333.

Lawton, J. and Rankin, D. (2010) How do structured education programmes work? An ethnographic investigation of the dose adjustment for normal eating (DAFNE) programme for type 1 diabetes patients in the UK, *Social Science & Medicine*, 71: 486–93.

Lyssenko, V. and Laakso, M. (2013) Genetic screening for the risk of type 2 diabetes. Worthless or valuable? *Diabetes Care*, 6 Supplement 2: 120–6.

NICE (2011) Diabetes in Adults Quality Standard. Available at: www.nice.org.uk/guidance/qs6 (accessed 5 November 2015).

NICE (2012) *Preventing Type 2 Diabetes: Risk Identification and Interventions for Individuals at High Risk. NICE Public Health Guidance 38.* Available at: www.nice.org.uk/guidance/ph38 (accessed 5 November 2015).

NICE (2014) NICE pathways: Diabetes overview. Available at: http://pathways.nice.org.uk/pathways/diabetes (accessed 5 November 2015).

Stenner, K.L., Courtenay, M. and Carey, N. (2011) Consultations between nurse prescribers and patients with diabetes in primary care: a qualitative study of patient views, *International Journal of Nursing Studies*, 48: 37–46.

Wallace, L.M., Turner, A., Kosmala-Anderson, J. *et al.* (2012) *Evidence: Co-creating Health: Evaluation of the First Phase.* London: The Health Foundation.

Waterman, B.J. (2012) A person-centred approach to determining target HbA1c for older people with diabetes, *Diabetes and Primary Care*, 14(1): 22–33.

Weaver, R.R., Lemonde, M., Payman, N. and Goodman, W.M. (2014) Health capabilities and diabetes self-management: the impact of economic, social and cultural resources, *Social Science & Medicine*, 102: 58–68.

WHO (2015) *Diabetes Fact Sheet No 312.* Available at: www.who.int/features/factfiles/diabetes/en (accessed 6 November 2015).

The Willis Commission (2012) *Quality with Compassion: The Future of Nursing Education. Report of the Willis Commission on Nursing Education.* London: The Willis Commission.

Year of Care (2011) *Year of Care: Report of Findings from the Pilot Programme.* Available at: www.diabetes.org.uk/upload/Professionals/Year%20of%20Care/YOC_Report.pdf (accessed 5 November 2015).

Person-centred approaches to Rheumatoid Arthritis

Julie Bliss and Nicola Wilson

LEARNING OUTCOMES

- To explore the impact of living with Rheumatoid Arthritis
- To consider the importance of a holistic approach to care
- To understand the contribution of inter-professional working
- To examine who are the important partners in care

Introduction

Rheumatoid Arthritis (RA) affects approximately 400,000 people in the UK with around 12,000 new cases per year (NICE 2013). An inflammatory disease, mainly of the synovial joints, RA covers a continuum of joint problems from minor aches to total immobility (Daker-White *et al.*, 2014). Living with RA impacts upon the quality of life of both the individual and their family. NICE (2013) identified the impact of RA on individuals, their families and society which is without doubt immense, and this includes: the personal impact for the individual living with RA and their family, indirect costs to the economy as a consequence of reduced productivity and direct costs to the NHS and associated healthcare services. The cost of RA is estimated at £3.8 to £4.75 billion per year, including indirect costs and work-related disability (NICE 2013). However it is important that healthcare professionals focus on the individual with RA, the impact the condition has on the individual and quality of life and their interactions with their family and social network. The RA guidelines (NICE 2013) provide best practice advice and state clearly that the care and treatment of people living with RA must take into account the preferences and needs of individuals. Furthermore people living with RA must be empowered to make informed choices about their healthcare and work in partnership with healthcare professionals. This chapter utilizes a case study to explore the variety of factors which impact on the lives of one individual and their family living with RA.

Reader activity

Consider people you have met who are living with RA: this could be as patients, family or friends.

How does the RA impact upon their daily living?
Consider if it has required any changes in their life or plans for the future.

The first activity has been an opportunity to spend some time thinking about people that you have met with RA and the impact that RA has had on their lives. In this chapter one individual, Nicola, shares her experiences of living with RA to illustrate the importance of PCC.

Living with RA

Nicola

I am 47 years old and live in a small village. I am married and have a daughter who is 15 years old. We live in a bungalow with our small dog which I take for a walk every day. I work two mornings a week in the local post office and sometimes provide holiday cover. I enjoy reading, knitting, arts and crafts and gardening. My husband has built raised beds in the garden and we have just heard that the development of the village allotments will be completed next spring. I am excited about sharing an allotment with a friend (her son will do the digging!). I was first diagnosed as having RA when I was 19 years old.

Generally developing in late or middle age, RA affects more women than men (Daker-White *et al.*, 2014). The incidence of RA is at its peak in men and women over 70 years of age although the disease can be developed across the age range (NICE 2013). It is possible that the people that you considered in Activity 9.1 were older, but RA is not a disease of middle and older age and can affect anyone. From Activity 9.1 you may have identified a number of ways in which RA impacts upon individuals, for example reduced mobility, fatigue and the unpredictable nature of the disease with episodes or remission and flare up. In the case of Nicola, she is able to work two mornings a week and continues to enjoy gardening by the use of raised beds. Nicola and her family have adopted a lifestyle that means that the RA is not central to their lives but part of their lives. This reflects the findings of Headland (2006) who analysed individual narratives of people living with arthritis. In one narrative a male respondent who had been living with arthritis for twenty years reported that he had been able 'to place arthritis in (his) life' (Headland 2006: 108). In order to provide PCC it is imperative that nurses and other healthcare professionals are able to engage holistically with the individual and not focus on the disease.

Nicola enjoys gardening and has been able to continue with this as a result of the raised beds in the garden and going forward by sharing an allotment and therefore the work. Loeppenthin *et al.* (2014) identified that for people who have RA physical activity can be viewed as a resource which supports staying healthy whilst not surrendering to disability and provides a meaningful structure to life. It is important as healthcare professionals not to assume that people living with RA are unable to undertake physical activity; for example it is possible to continue to participate in triathlon at an international level (Jackson 2011).

A holistic approach to care

Nicola's medical history

My RA is quite well managed now as a result of changes in the medication over the last decade. Initially it took a long time to get a diagnosis and during that time I was in hospital on bed rest. I started having weekly injections ten years ago and they have been a real turning point in managing my symptoms. Over the years I have had a number of joint replacements, the first was a right hip replacement before my daughter was born. I have also had a left hip replacement, a left shoulder replacement and a right knee replacement. My consultant has identified that I need a left knee replacement, but I am reluctant to have this done, he has told me to phone his secretary when I am ready for the knee replacement. As we are writing this chapter I am recovering from day surgery to my foot. I have had toes two, three and four on my right foot straightened and pins inserted. I have also had a bony nodule removed from the large toe.

NICE (2013) identify a need for a specialist opinion if the individual has had the start of symptoms and has attended the GP for medical advice. In Nicola's case, some 28 years ago, the diagnosis took several months after she first saw her GP. More recently Headland (2006) identified that for younger people living with RA the initial diagnosis took several months. A delay in diagnosis could impact on the ongoing trajectory of the disease and quality of life for the individual. It is important that healthcare professionals consider RA as a possible diagnosis regardless of age of the individual presenting with symptoms.

A combination of disease-modifying anti-rheumatic drugs (DMARDs) is the first line treatment (NICE 2013) and the development in DMARDs has had a positive impact on Nicola's quality of life.

Reader activity

Note that Nicola has experienced a number of joint replacements in the past and is currently reluctant to have a left knee replacement.

Take some time to consider what factors may be making her reluctant.

Previous experience of healthcare inevitably impacts upon the individual's ongoing interaction with health professionals. You may have considered that Nicola's previous experience of surgery may have made her more reluctant to undergo further surgery. You may have identified that she has had day surgery recently and it may be that she is concerned about being an inpatient.

Nicola's surgery

I have already listed the number of joint replacements that I have had. They have taken place over the last twenty years and it is clear that people are discharged home earlier post operatively and staff are increasingly busy. In the past when I had a synovectomy I was not given the physiotherapy I required and it was much more difficult to recover. During my shoulder replacement my arm was broken; this was only picked up when I complained of pain in my arm following the surgery. I am nervous about having the second knee replacement and have been putting it off. I want the healthcare team caring for me when I have my next knee replacement to recognize that the treatment, for example physiotherapy, is different for someone with RA compared to Osteoarthritis.

Reader activity

Take some time to reflect on Nicola's comments regarding her experiences of surgery and identify the key points for consideration by healthcare professionals.

You may have picked up on Nicola's anxiety regarding her humerus being broken during surgery and her statement that following a knee replacement it is important that the care provided reflects the needs of the individual and not just the operation that has taken place. Nicola is a person, not 'the shoulder replacement in bed three'.

When taking into consideration the nature of the surgery required to replace a shoulder joint and impact of the RA it is perhaps not surprising the humerus was broken. Hayward (1975) identified a relationship between anxiety and pain. The fractured humerus was a complication of the shoulder replacement which should have been picked up during surgery rather than when Nicola complained of pain. It may also have helped to reduce anxiety if the fact that it was a possibility had been raised prior to the surgery by the healthcare team involved. An understanding of what is happening, and perhaps more importantly what to expect, during an episode of healthcare reduces anxiety and pain. Person-centred care requires that healthcare professionals consider the person as a partner in care and provide the information to facilitate informed consent. Surgical informed consent requires an exchange of information between competent doctor and a patient resulting in the patient giving consent. However a recent review of the literature identified that surgeons are not given education and training to develop competence required for surgical informed consent (Leclercq *et al.*, 2010).

With regards to joint replacement surgery, in this case the knee, it is important to consider the cause of the surgery. Since the pathophysiology of RA and osteoarthritis are different the care post operatively is also different. This is of particular importance for exercise post operatively and illustrates the importance of providing PCC at all points of the patient's journey.

It is evident that Nicola's consultant has listened to her concerns and has given her a choice regarding when she will have her left knee replacement. By working in partnership with Nicola he is promoting choice and ensuring that Nicola is in control of her own health and wellbeing. The Five Year Forward View (NHS England 2014) sets out steps to empower patients, keeping them at the centre of care. This includes providing information and supporting people to make informed choices regarding their condition, treatment and avoiding complication. The use of patient decision aids can be helpful for shared decision-making, where the 'patient' and healthcare professional discuss the options and make a decision together. The NHS Right Care Shared Decision Making programme is part of the Quality Improvement Productivity and Prevention (QIPP) Right Care programme and includes a patient decision aid for people living with RA (Right Care NHS 2014). The information is provided in a format that people without healthcare expertise can understand and utilize to make an informed choice.

Nicola has undergone a considerable amount of surgery as a result of her RA. However her quality of life has been enhanced since she commenced on injections as a result of the medication on managing the symptoms of her RA.

Nicola's medication

My regular medication is as follows; I inject Etanercept 50 mg weekly, in addition I take Meloxicam 15 mg, Lansoprazole 15 mg and Folic acid 5 mg daily and Methotrexate 15 mg once a week. Currently I am also taking Zinc 25 mg daily as my Zinc levels are very low. I have to have regular blood tests whilst I am having the injections as it affects my immune system. If I get an infection I have to stop the injections. I set the alarm on my phone to remind me to take the injections, sometimes I put off having the injection because although I know they make a difference they do sting. Sometimes when Healthcare at Home phone about my injections they ask if I have been taking them weekly.

Managing regular injections in the home requires an infrastructure in place to support the process. In this case Nicola receives her injections and the equipment from an independent healthcare provider; in addition the independent healthcare provider has a helpline that Nicola can contact if she has any queries regarding her injections. This supplements the support received from the rheumatology specialist nurse. The NAO (2009) identified that 59 per cent of the 1400 people surveyed felt that it would be helpful to have a named person to turn to if they experienced a flare up. The RA guidelines (NICE 2013) set out the importance of access to the multi-disciplinary team for people living with RA, in particular a named member of the team responsible for coordinating care. This is often the specialist nurse who may be better placed to develop an ongoing relationship with the person and discuss treatment options. It is important to note that one of the key benefits of multi-disciplinary team working is the pooling of knowledge and skills.

The monthly blood tests are done at the local community hospital. It is important that medication is taken at the correct intervals, in the case of the Etanercept (a type of biologic drug known as anti-tumour necrosis factor) weekly, in order to maintain the therapeutic levels within the blood stream. It is interesting to note that although Nicola has clearly stated that the injections have made a difference to her quality of life she remains reluctant on occasions to do the injection because of the stinging, this could be described as non-adherence. If healthcare delivery is to be person centred it is important that episodes of non-adherence are not regarded as 'the patient's problem' (NICE 2009: 3). Medication adherence has been described as the extent to which the patient actions reflect the actions agreed at the time of prescribing the medication (NICE 2009). The prescribing pyramid sets out the stages required for effective prescribing; these include discussing the options with the patient, and may result in decision not to prescribe medication (National Prescribing Centre 1999). In this case Nicola has articulated her rationale for not always taking the medication on time; she has made an informed choice.

The contribution of inter-professional working

Nicola's medication management and surgery

When I have surgery I have to stop the injections three weeks prior to surgery. My recent foot surgery was cancelled twice due to staff shortages. I appreciate the challenge of delivering healthcare but for me not knowing if and when the surgery would happen was difficult. I choose not to restart my injections and although the surgery was done a month after it was originally scheduled by that time I was really struggling with my arthritis. I contacted the rheumatology nurse and asked for a steroid injection to calm the symptoms of my arthritis. I will be able to restart my injections once I have a clear blood test.

The podiatrist is a key member of the multi-disciplinary team for assessment and period review of the needs of an individual with RA (NICE 2013). The current configuration of healthcare services means that this may result in working across organizations. The NAO (2009) identified that only 12 per cent of primary care trusts were providing RA care in the primary care setting, despite the strategy for long-term conditions set out to promote a patient-centered approach in primary care. In Nicola's case the delay to the surgery was a result of the need to work across two healthcare providers to ensure patient safety and quality at a time when the local clinical commissioning group (CCG) was in the process of commissioning the service. It is without doubt important that services are commissioned to deliver safe quality care but it is equally important the user of the healthcare service remains central. Cowley *et al.* (2002) undertook research using a multiple case study design to examine multi-disciplinary working across three organizations in four different areas. The research found that where the patient was at the centre of the multi-disciplinary team inter-professional working and working across organizations was more effective as everyone involved was focused on delivering PCC.

Reader activity

Taking into consideration the information that you have available regarding Nicola and her family, take some time to consider who may have been involved in her care since she was diagnosed with RA.

You may have identified a range of healthcare professionals, for example it is evident from what Nicola has already said that she has received care from a rheumatology consultant, an orthopaedic surgeon, podiatrist, medical secretary, an independent healthcare provider, physiotherapists and a range of nurses, for example the rheumatology specialist nurse, out-patient nurses and surgical nurses. You may also have identified the GP, midwife and health visitor.

Nicola: more than a person with arthritis

When my husband and I got married we talked to my consultant about having a family. We needed to think about the medication I was taking at the time and how it could impact on a pregnancy. I was admitted to the maternity unit with a urinary tract infection when I was eight months pregnant, I was given a steroid injection in case the baby was born early. The most helpful thing during that time was being shown the labour suite and having an opportunity to try out the stirrups. I had already had my first hip replacement and was still able to have a normal vaginal delivery. When my daughter and I went home it became clear that as a family we would need to move from our two-bedroom Victorian cottage with steep stairs. Before we moved the local authority arranged for a home help to visit when my husband was at work to carry my daughter down the stairs in the morning or upstairs in the evening. This was something that we had to pay for but it made a big difference to me as I was able to care for my daughter with the additional support. The health visitor was able to direct us to the Children's Centre for support, she also told us that if she had known about my RA before my daughter was born she would have been able to refer us to a specialist team who could have offered advice and equipment for managing as a young mother with RA. We moved to our current bungalow before my daughter was one year old.

The opportunity to see the labour suite before going into labour clearly reduced Nicola's anxiety (Hayward 1975). In this text Nicola identifies the importance of the local authority input and the home help during the period before they moved to their bungalow. The move to a bungalow is another example of how Nicola and her family have adapted their lifestyle to accommodate the RA whilst ensuring that it does not dominate their lives. Daker-White *et al.* (2014) undertook a meta-ethnography of qualitative studies focusing on the experience of living with RA. One of the themes identified in their work was re-defining normal life and included identifying new ways to live with the disease. It is important that healthcare professionals empower the individual and their families to master the condition and identify new ways of living. You may not have considered the local authority and the services that they can provide in activity (p.159), however it is important to consider all services which have the potential to impact upon individuals' quality of life. For Nicola in this case the home help was provided by the local authority, it is also important to consider providers across the health economy for example the third sector and independent healthcare providers when involved in PCC.

It would appear that Nicola was not referred to the health visitor during the antenatal period; this meant that Nicola and her husband were unaware of the specialist team that could have provided information and support regarding equipment for a young mother with RA. This oversight was not a deliberate act on behalf of the GP or midwife but it may be that Nicola's RA was not considered during her pregnancy which gives rise to the question 'was it person centred?' An alternative explanation may be that the GP and midwife were unaware of the specialist team. The unintended consequence, regardless of the reason, was that Nicola and her husband did not gain access to the service and perhaps more importantly the advice available. Access to multi-disciplinary team is central to the management of RA (NICE 2013). Nicola's daughter was born some 15 years ago; however inadvertent gatekeeping remains a concern.

The current primary healthcare-based system in the UK requires the generalist to refer to specialist services and to act as a care coordinator and potentially a gatekeeper. Garrido *et al.* (2011) undertook a systematic literature review to explore the effects of gatekeeping in healthcare and identified that there did appear to be a lower uptake of services and lower expenditure. It is of interest to note that they identified that the impact of gatekeeping on patient-related outcomes was explored less and the results were inconclusive. To ensure PCC, it is imperative that healthcare professionals involved in working in partnership with patients, whatever their condition and circumstances, are aware of the available services and refer to other services that may have specialist expertise from which individuals would benefit.

Partners in care

Whilst PCC is key to delivering effective health and social care which meets individual need it is important to consider the family as a whole. In England 5.4 million people are providing unpaid care, which includes over 166,000 young carers aged 5–17 (Office for National Statistics 2012). The Carers Strategy (DH 2014) sets out a number of priority areas, the first of which is identification and recognition. People with caring responsibilities may not consider themselves to be carers; in a similar way to gatekeeping this may result in not being able to access appropriate services.

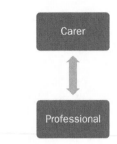

Figure 9.1 The Triangle of Care Worthington *et al.* (2013: 6).

Carers possess knowledge and experience of the individual for whom they provide care and as such should be involved as equal partners in care planning. The triangle of care was originally developed by carers and staff in the mental health setting; it sets out six standards including staff being carer aware and the need for a carer introduction to the service (Worthington *et al.*, 2013). Although initially developed for mental healthcare the triangle of care, where the dialogue is two way between all interested parties, can be used in all areas of health and social care – see Figure 9.1.

In Activity 9.4 you may have identified Nicola's family as being involved in her care. In reality her husband and daughter do not consider themselves to be carers as the support they offer is part of being a family unit. However PCC does need to take the family and unpaid care into consideration to ensure that personalized support is available to ensure that the carers and those that they support are able to engage in family and community life.

Experiences of the health service

I find that I don't see the GP very much; when I do because of the large practice I find I am explaining my medication and history to the GP. The practice nurse knows me by name and I feel that there is continuity. I have a good relationship with the outpatient nurses who have been there for me, for example holding my hand when I have had steroid injections. My experience of being an inpatient is mixed; one charge nurse asked me about my concerns prior to surgery and made sure that the staff addressed my concerns about being sick after surgery. As an inpatient it is important that I am valued as an individual and given information about what is happening. Much of my time as an inpatient has been on orthopaedic wards, it is quite hard to look around a ward and see older people with more severe arthritis and think that will that be me in twenty years' time?

In the case of the charge nurse who asked Nicola about her anxieties prior to her surgery he focused on Nicola as a person and was clearly providing PCC. The NHS values set out in the NHS Constitution (NHS England 2013) provide a framework for PCC, – see Figure 9.2.

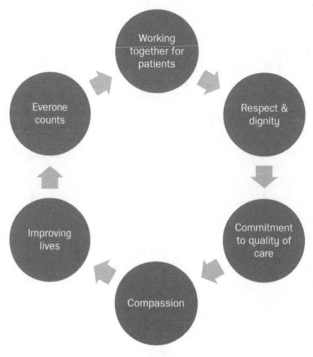

Figure 9.2 NHS Values
NHS England (2013).

Reader activity

Take some time to reflect on Nicola's comment: 'it is quite hard to look around a ward and see older people with more severe arthritis and think that will that be me in twenty years' time?'.

Nicola's concern about seeing people older people with severe arthritis is very real and potentially a difficult topic to explore. In some ways Nicola's own health trajectory provides an answer to this concern. Since she commenced on the Etanercept her symptoms have been managed much better. The advances in treatment means that Nicola's care trajectory will be different to that of people who have had arthritis for longer and whose disease trajectory progressed further before the advances in treatment. It is important that the psychological needs of people living with a long-term condition are considered as part of PCC. Coventry *et al.* (2011) undertook a number of in-depth interviews with healthcare professionals, service users and carers along with focus groups to examine the diagnosis and management of depression in people living with diabetes or coronary heart disease. The research found that depression was considered normal for people living with a long-term condition and as a consequence comprehensive assessment and treatment was often neglected. Whilst the work by Coventry *et al.* (2011) focused on depression it is possible that findings could be extrapolated to other psychological aspects of living with a long-term condition.

Reader activity

Taking into consideration what you know now about Nicola reflect on her health and wellbeing.

What do you think Nicola considers to be important?

Having reflected on what you have read about Nicola and her health and wellbeing read Nicola's thoughts in the box below. Patient-centred care should focus on the experiences and needs of the individual.

The importance of being me

I use a number of aids to help me with my daily living, for example I have a knicker stick and a sock putter on (helping hands); these make life easier. We have a traditional kettle as I can't lift a jug kettle, the height of chairs is important and when my husband redecorated the bungalow he put all the sockets at hip height. Like the raised beds for gardening, these are all things that enable me to live independently and maintain my dignity. I am a person who happens to have arthritis; I am not an arthritis sufferer.

In your reflection for Activity 9.5 you may have identified that independence and dignity are central to Nicola's health and wellbeing. Perhaps the most important statement is that she 'happens to have arthritis'. For many people living with a long-term condition the long-term condition is something that is part of them but does not define who they are. In order to work in partnership with individuals and provide PCC it is crucial that focus is the individual and their family and not the condition they happen to have. By utilizing one case study this chapter has provided an opportunity to explore these issues from the perspective of the individual around who the care is centred.

Acknowledgment

The authors would like to acknowledge the support of Dr Carole Jackson who read the initial drafts.

References

Coventry, P., Hays, R., Dickens, C. *et al.* (2011) Talking about depression: a qualitative study of barriers to managing depression in people with long term conditions in primary care, *BMC Family Practice*, 12:10. DOI:10.1186/1471-2296-12-10.

Cowley, S., Bliss, J., Mathew, A. and McVey, G. (2002) Effective interagency and interprofessional working: facilitators and barriers, *International Journal of Palliative Nursing*, 8(1): 30–9.

Daker-White, G., Donovan, J. and Campbell, R. (2014) Redefined by illness: a meta-ethnography of qualitative studies on the experience of rheumatoid arthritis, *Disability and Rehabilitation*, 36(13): 1061–71.

DH (Department of Health) (2014) *Carers Strategy: Second National Action Plan 2014–2016.* London: Department of Health.

Garrido, M., Zentner, A. and Busse, R. (2011) The effects of gatekeeping: a systematic review of the literature, *Scandinavian Journal of Primary Health Care*, 29: 28–38.

Hayward, J. (1975) *Information: A Prescription Against Pain.* London: Royal College of Nursing.

Headland, M. (2006) Using a website containing patient narratives to understanding people's experiences of living with arthritis, *Journal of Orthopaedic Nursing*, 10: 106–12.

Jackson, C. (2011) Competing with Arthritis. Arthritis Care. Available at: www.arthritis-care.org.uk/@2496/Onlinecommunity/Reallives/CompetingwitharthritisCaroleJackson (accessed 5 November 2015).

Leclercq, W., Keulers, B., Scheltinga, M. *et al.* (2010) A review of surgical informed consent: past, present and future. A quest to help patients make better decisions, *World Journal of Surgery*, 34: 1406–15.

NAO (National Audit Office) (2009) *Services for People with Rheumatoid Arthritis.* London: The Stationery Office.

National Prescribing Centre (1999) Signposts for prescribing nurses: general principles of good prescribing, *Prescribing Nures Bulletin*. Available at http://homepage.ntlworld.com/john-campbell/Nurse%20Prescribing/signpostsvol1no1%2520.pdf (accessed 26 October 2015).

NHS England (2013) *The NHS Constitution.* London: Department of Health.

NHS England (2014) *Five Year Forward.* London: NHS England.

NICE (National Institute for Health and Care Excellence) (2009) *Medicines Adherence: Involving Patients in Decisions about Prescribed Medicines and Supporting Adherence. NICE clinical guideline 76.* Manchester: National Insitute for Health and Care Excellence.

NICE (2013) *Rheumatoid Arthritis: The Management of Rheumatoid Arthritis in Adults NICE Clinical Guideline 79.* Manchester: National Institutue for Health and Care Excellence.

Office for National Statistics (2012) *2011 Census: Key Statistics for England and Wales, March 2011.* London: ONS.

Right Care NHS (2014) Shared decision making. Available at: http://sdm.rightcare.nhs.uk/pda/rheumatoid-arthritis/ (accessed 5 November 2015).

Worthington, A., Rooney, P., Hannan, R. and Martin, K. (2013) *The Triangle of Care. Carers Included: A Guide to Best Practice in Mental Health Care in Scotland.* London: The Carers Trust.

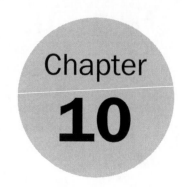

Chapter

10

Optimizing medicine management

Promoting person-centred care

Angela Parry

Introduction

A prescribed medicine is the most common clinical intervention provided in the NHS, and covers all sectors and ages of care: primary, secondary, public and community health. Medicine management involves inter-professional working, commonly involving doctors, pharmacists and nurses working with the service user to ensure that the five rights of medicine safety are upheld[1] and that medicines are prescribed, dispensed and administered safely and effectively.

This chapter explores the provision of PCC for adults who need to take prescribed medicines on a regular basis in order to manage and/or maintain their health condition. Many of the principles that will be discussed can be applied to other modes of prescription, for example one off medicines prescribed or administered in the community, walk-in centre or hospital setting. The chapter will also consider challenges in providing high quality care for this important aspect of health management. In addition, the experience of service users who need to take medicines both when going about their everyday life, as well as when they become inpatients, will be explored, together with the role of health professionals in promoting person-centred medicine management. Words from two service users will be used to inform some of the key points raised.

---

[1] Right patient, right medicine, right time, right route, right amount (DH 2004).

LEARNING OUTCOMES

This chapter will provide you with the opportunity to:

- Appreciate the range, type and delivery mode of medications that service users may have to take
- Consider the impact, both positive and negative, that prescribed medications may have on the daily life of a service user
- Explore the role of the nurse in promoting person-centred medication management

The scope of the issue

After staffing costs, medicines comprise the second highest area of spending in the NHS. Whilst exact data on the number of medicines prescribed nationally is difficult to obtain, it is known that most medicine prescriptions originate in the community, through attendance for diagnosis or maintenance of a health condition at GP/nurse practitioner consultations. The number of medications prescribed has increased threefold since 2009, with 886 million prescription items issued in England in 2009, equating to the 17.1 items being the average number of prescriptions per head of the UK population (Prescribing Support Unit 2010). The net cost of these prescription items was £8,539 million, roughly 15 per cent of all NHS costs (Duerdin *et al.*, 2011).

Whilst most people self-medicate using over the counter (OTC) medicines, it is estimated that up to half of people do not take as directed their prescription-only medicines (POMs) for long-term illnesses. This results in a significant waste of medicines worth more than £100 million every year, not to mention the significant negative impact on service user health (McKee 2010). Clearly, therefore, it is evident that a person-centred approach to medicine management can benefit the individual, as well as organizations and society as a whole.

What are prescription-only medicines?

Prescription-only medicines require a prescription issued by a hospital doctor, GP or other suitably qualified healthcare professional, including nurses or midwives, in order for the service user to obtain the medicine legally. Currently, there are two types of nursing or midwifery prescriber – the community nurse prescriber and the independent and supplementary nurse and midwife prescriber. Information about nurses and midwives as prescribers can be obtained from the Nursing and Midwifery Council web pages on medicines management and nurse prescribing (NMC 2008).

Relevant legislation governing prescription-only medicines

It is important when supporting service users with their prescription medicines that healthcare professionals are aware that there are two main statutes regulating the availability of medicines in the UK: the Misuse of Drugs Act (1971), which regulates the three classes of controlled drugs, and the Medicines Act (1968). The Medicines Act (1968) governs the manufacture and supply of medicine and divides medical drugs into three categories –POMs, Pharmacy medicines, and the General Sales List medicines. POMs can only be sold or supplied by a pharmacist on the production of a valid prescription; Pharmacy medicines can be sold without a prescription but only by a pharmacist, whereas the General Sales List medicines (also referred to as OTC medicines) can be sold by any shop, not just a pharmacy, although advertising, labelling and production restrictions apply. For more information about the legislation governing medicines, the Medicines and Healthcare Regulatory Agency (MHRA) provides valuable information as does the British National Formulary (BNF).

What are the main reasons service users take prescription medicines?

Reader activity

Think about people that you know or service users that you have encountered and the reasons why they needed to take prescribed medicine.

Now 'put to one side' the specific clinical condition or health issue and try to identify common themes that underpin the reasons why service users need to take their prescribed medicines.

There are six main reasons why service users may need to take prescription medicines:

- To relieve symptoms – for example pain, breathlessness or low mood
- To treat overt disease – for example diabetes, psychosis or cancer
- To prevent disease – for example tuberculosis, measles or influenza vaccination
- To reduce risk factors or the process of an occult disease – for example cardiac, renal or respiratory disease
- To replace failed or failing body systems – for example the endocrine system (thyroid or adrenal glands)
- In anticipation of changing or deteriorating symptoms – for example terminal care at home, rescue courses of steroids for asthma, adrenaline for anaphylaxis

In many instances service users may be prescribed a combination of medicines that fulfil more than one of the reasons above, in addition to combating some of the unwanted side effects of the prescribed medicines. The excerpt below from Connor, a 21-year-old student who lives with Cystic Fibrosis, explains some of this:

A key factor in maintaining a healthy weight is my overnight feeds, delivered via a PEG tube (gastronomy) inserted when I was 9. This allows me to take in 2260 calories overnight. This often causes me to vomit in the mornings through coughing; I have now been prescribed anti-sickness medicine and acid reflux medicine to reduce or stop the vomiting. The mornings can often be painful and stressful, as I try to fight the urge to vomit. It has become standard routine in the mornings that I cough heavily and attempt to not vomit; this often goes on for two to fifteen minutes.

Service users and their prescription

It is important that service users understand the type of prescription that they have been given and what their responsibilities are in relation to completing the course of prescribed medication, or obtaining further medicine if a longer term or lifetime course is prescribed.

Prescriptions can be issued either electronically or by hand. It is possible with the advent of technology for prescriptions to be sent directly to a pharmacy of the service user's choice without them having to attend the GP or Nurse Practitioner (NP) surgery, depending on individual health circumstances. There are advanced plans to have electronic only systems in the community and do away with written prescription forms (EPS2) (see http://systems.hscic.gov.uk/eps). It is claimed this has advantages in terms of safer prescribing while maintaining service user choice of pharmacy, but may create problems for the 'information poor' carers and institutions who are used to the more traditional prescription.

Single prescription

This is generated either when there is a short course of medicine for an acute problem, for example antibiotics for acute infections, or for medicines requiring regular review in both type and dosage.

Repeat prescription

Repeat prescriptions are normally used for service users with a relatively stable long-term condition(s). The prescription can be supplied for a period of time on a regular basis without a review appointment being made with the health professional. Repeat prescriptions are normally authorized for a period of three to twelve months but this may vary with the type of medicine and at the prescriber's discretion. A clinical review is normally required every six to twelve months so that the medicine regime can be adjusted as required.

Repeat dispensing prescription

Repeat dispensing is a type of repeat prescribing which allows community pharmacists to dispense regular medicines to suitable service users without the direct involvement of the GP surgery on each occasion the prescription is needed. This is done according to an agreed protocol for service users with stable conditions for periods of time up to one year. The service user is given a batch of prescriptions to take to the pharmacy to be dispensed at regular intervals over the agreed period of time.

Common scenarios regarding the nurse and person-centred medicine management

Nurses will commonly encounter service users requiring prescription only medicine management in one of four care situations:

- a person who takes medicine episodically to treat a short-term illness, for example an infection, and usually consults with health professionals via walk in centres or their GP services:
  - a person living with a long-term condition who commonly takes one or more medicines for extended periods of time/their lifetime and is usually managed via their GP/nurse practitioner services;
  - a person accessing inpatient hospital services in response to an acute health issue (planned or emergency) who does not live with any pre-existing medical conditions;
  - a person accessing inpatient hospital services (planned or emergency) due to an exacerbation of a long-term health condition/with a superimposed acute condition, who will require medicines to manage their current illness in addition to ongoing therapy for their long-term health condition.

What is person-centred medicine management care?

Person-centred care means providing care that supports the service user to achieve the health outcomes that give them the best opportunity to lead the life that they want (The King's Fund 2014). Failure to treat service users as individuals results in them feeling disempowered and can lead to them feeling like spectators in their own care. Collins (2014) identifies four useful key elements for patient-centred (person-centred) care as shown in Figure 10.1.

A PCC approach to medicine management, whatever the underpinning reason that the service user requires the medicine, can incorporate the above elements through a range of care principles as outlined by Taylor (2014) – see Figure 10.2.

Whilst the above principles should be considered in relation to the role of the nurse and any situation where prescription medicines are required, the remainder of this chapter will focus on how the nurse can use Taylor's (2014) principles in two of the more complex areas of medicine management:

- a person living with a long-term condition who commonly takes one or more medicines for extended periods of time/their lifetime and is usually managed via their GP services;
- a person accessing inpatient hospital services due to an exacerbation of a long-term health condition/with a superimposed acute condition who will require medicines to manage their current illness in addition to ongoing therapy for their long-term health condition.

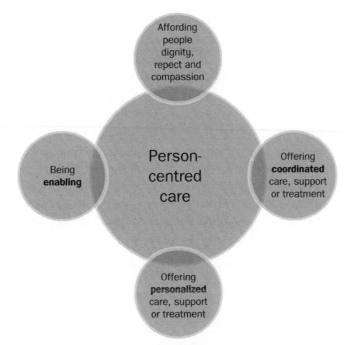

Figure 10.1 Principles of person-centred care
Adapted from Collins (2014).

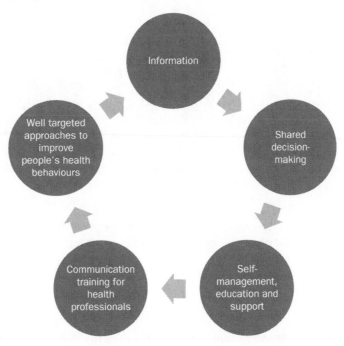

Figure 10.2 Principles of care
Adapted from Taylor (2014).

Medicine management and the service user living with a long-term condition

Reader activity

Think about people you know – family or friends who take long-term medicine(s)

> What activities do they need to consider every day to remember to take their medicines and to monitor the effects?

- How might this impact on their day-to-day life and plans for the future?
- How could you take this into consideration when caring for someone taking long-term medicine?

For many people, regular medicine is essential not solely to optimize their health but – as has been highlighted earlier – to keep them alive. This means they must remember to have sufficient medicine available, which in turn means ensuring they keep an eye on their prescriptions and that they keep the medicines safely stored and remember to take the medicine with them when at work, socializing, going on holiday or meeting new people. This is not always easy as the excerpt below from Catherine, a 62–year-old business woman, demonstrates:

> They say that this is a shared decision, how to manage my health. However, in reality I am prescribed the medicine that they (the health professional) recommends, and if I don't take it then my health will deteriorate – so in a way I don't really have any choice in this. Even the side effects – there's not really anything that can be done about that either. I know that I have to take the medicines, but it requires a lot of organization – remembering to put in the prescription, collect the medicines, take the medicines with me – holidays are particularly challenging as I am out of my usual routine, and I find that a routine helps me stay on top of remembering my medicine regime.

Using the principles of PCC, the nurse and other healthcare professionals can support service users in integrating safe and effective medicine management into their daily life as will now be discussed.

Information

'Information is effective therapy' (Coulter 2014). Access to good quality health information – written or electronic – can increase people's knowledge, understanding and ability to cope. The impact is greater when the written information is targeted, personalized and reinforced by verbal information from clinicians. There are a number of ways in which information can be provided, both face to face and remotely. The NHS has invested considerably in the development of electronic resource such as NHS Choices with the aim of helping people to take charge of their own healthcare (http://www.nhs.uk/aboutNHSChoices). Information is provided about a range of health conditions, treatments and therapies with details of effects, side effects and contra-indications of medicines. As Catherine reminds us, in taking medicines there is potentially a lot to consider:

> I do need to take medicines quite often now for my knee pain, painkillers that I was prescribed. I worry about becoming dependent on them so I only take them when necessary. No one seems really prepared to comment on that when I ask. Also they do have a number of adverse effects, they are quite strong so I need to think about driving and alcohol, and I also need to remember to eat before I take them. I am not sure where best to get the information and support . . .

The cost of prescription charges is often seen by service users as prohibitive. Service users need to be aware of prescription charges that currently operate in England. The current charge (as of 1 April 2015) is £8.20 per item. Prescription prepayment certificates (PPC) are also available. PPCs allow the service user to pay a fixed charge up front for either three or twelve months for all prescriptions. For example a three-month PPC saves the service user money if they need four or more prescription items in the three- month period.

Some service users are entitled to free prescriptions – this includes people who:

- are 60 or over , or under 16, or who are 16–18 and in full-time education;
- are pregnant or have had a baby in the previous 12 months and have a valid maternity exemption certificate (MatEx);
- have a specified medical condition and have a valid medical exemption certificate (MedEx) – this includes cancer, diabetes and thyroid disorders;
- have a continuing physical disability that prevents them from going out without help from another person, and have a valid medical exemption certificate;
- hold a valid war pension exemption certificate and the prescription is for their accepted disability;
- are an NHS inpatient;
- are entitled to (either self or partner) an NHS tax credit exemption certificate or a valid HC2 certificate (full help with health costs), or receive either:
  - Income Support
  - Income-based Jobseeker's Allowance
  - Income-related Employment and Support Allowance
  - Pension Credit Guarantee Credit
  - Universal Credit.

Decision-making

Service user involvement leads to better clinical decisions, especially when these are supported by evidence-based decision aids for service users, and effective decision support by specially trained staff. This leads to better communication, more accurate risk perceptions and therefore more appropriate medicine choices.

Ahmad *et al.* (2014) view shared decision-making as an important person-centred activity as it is enabling, allowing people to develop their own capabilities to manage their condition and therefore improve service user satisfaction with their care. Central to shared decision-making is the belief that both clinicians and service user have expertise; the knowledge and experience they bring to decisions are different but equally important (Coulter and Collins 2011). Shared decision-making in medicine management is clearly reflected in NICE guidelines (CG76) (2009) where it is noted that health professionals should: 'Offer all patients the opportunity to be involved in making decisions about prescribed medicines. Establish what level of involvement in decision-making the patient would like' (2009). Reasonably, this should include establishing what level of involvement in decision-making the service user would like to have, and that increased involvement may mean that the service user decides not to take, or to stop taking, the medicine (NICE 2009).

Coulter and Collins (2011) acknowledge that sharing decision-making with service users may be challenging. They propose that the health professional needs to be 'curious, supportive, and non-judgemental' and to present unbiased evidence about benefits and risks (p. 25). They suggest following the simple model of 'ask-tell-ask' when sharing complex information. This model is described more fully in Chapter 8.

Self-management education and support

Providing service users with the resource to manage their medicines is pivotal in enhancing adherence. Most service users are more confident when they have some control over the regime. Health professionals must start with ensuring that service users have simple to follow medicine regimes that are acceptable to them. This may include considering the drug form that is prescribed – for example oral, injectable or rectal; that they have the financial resources to purchase the medicine, including access to free prescriptions, if eligible; or that they have aide memoirs to ensure that they take their medicine as prescribed, for example the use of Dosset boxes or similar.

As Connor explains:

Up until very recently the IV medicine was very time consuming at home as I had to mix all the medicine and prepare everything, now, however, the home delivery service has taken over and I now receive the medicine in prefilled syringes that need to be kept in the fridge. This has eradicated mixing times but it is still time consuming to administer the drugs. IV medicine also means I must be in the house at certain times of the day for a fairly long period of time; this does impact on my social life as I may not be able to meet friends for very long or at all due to time constraints. Recently the portacath has stopped working and can no longer be used. This means when I am in need of IV antibiotics a line needs to be placed. This is very stressful and makes the prospect of having IVs again a daunting prospect, something I wish to avoid.

Engagement with and ability to self-manage care is often referred to as patient activation (Wallace *et al.*, 2012). Individualized care planning and shared decision-making are fundamental to the process of maximizing activation and are also central to a range of initiatives introduced to help people manage their medicines successfully.

One further factor to consider is the adaptation that service users may be required to make in order to continue with the regime. Many service users can find the reaction of members of the public challenging, for example if they need to take their inhalers when out and about or inject medicines. For some service users the constant reminder of their need to take medicines can lead to a change in behaviour, with potentially a sense of isolation or of being an outsider. Connor shares his feelings when describing the impact of his PEG on how he joins in with activities his friends and family pursue:

The PEG itself has caused me some issue over the years, namely at beaches or swimming pools or anywhere where its common practice to remove your shirt. The PEG attracts stares and comments from people. As a child I simply shrugged it off but as I have become older I have become more conscious of the looks I receive and often opt to leave my shirt on. To protect the PEG when swimming I have to cover it with a protective patch, this is often difficult to apply and does not last long in the water. It has become very rare that I enter the water now and often sit on the side and watch.

Communication training for professionals

In order to ensure involvement of the service user in their medicine management regime, it is essential that health professionals responsible for both prescribing and ongoing monitoring interact appropriately with each individual service user. The health professional needs to look at the situation from the perspective of the service user in terms of their ideas, concerns and expectations and match this with a coherent and practical medicine management strategy.

To do this, it is imperative that they listen to the service user and hear what they have to say about their medicine – how they are feeling, the effects (expected and unexpected) that the medicine is having, and the strategies that the service user uses to ensure they have taken the medicines as prescribed.

Medicine management is usually approached through a structured consultation which might occur in a hospital setting, the GP surgery or in the service user's own home. An effective consultation becomes a two-way interaction between the health professional and the service user that has as its goal an effective therapeutic relationship that will maximize the

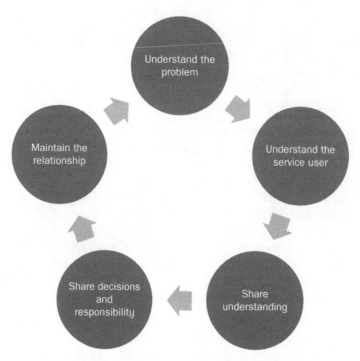

Figure 10.3 Components of Pendleton *et al.* (1984, 2003) consultation model

service user's health and wellbeing. Pendleton *et al.* (1984, 2003) popularized a five-stage partnership model derived from research into the work of GPs. The five stages are as shown in Figure 10.3:

Communication is clearly the key skill in any consultation. It is important to keep in mind the steps shown in Figure 10.4 to optimize the communication that takes place regarding medicine management. This will minimize the likelihood of misunderstanding and confusion and increase the possibility of full engagement of the service user in their medicine care.

Communication about medicine management may be provided verbally or in writing – the use of diagrams or pictures as well as words should be considered. The use of translators may be necessary, and/or the involvement of carers depending on the cognitive ability of the service user. It is best practice to follow up any verbal advice with written information. The service user may be anxious, which will reduce their ability to remember new or complex information.

Improving people's health behaviours

Service users' ability to adhere with their prescribed medicine regime may vary, often due to the reason that they are required to take the medicine. For example, if the medicine is required for a symptom that is impacting on daily living there is often greater adherence than for a medicine prescribed for an occult disease or a risk factor which, by its very nature, may not be overtly impacting on the service user's daily routine.

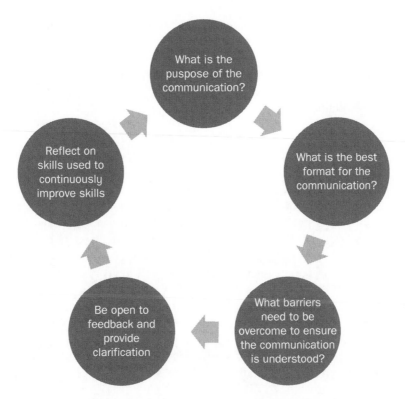

Figure 10.4 Components of effective communication in a consultation model

The term adherence has been recently introduced as a more person-centred term in place of compliance or concordance with medicine regimes. Compliance was felt to suggest a paternalistic approach, that service users were solely acting in accordance with advice (Aronson 2007), whereas concordance, whilst suggesting a more mutual agreement between patient and professional, was still seen as health professional led. Adherence in contrast is felt to be more realistic, to convey the idea of sticking with a medicine regime – acknowledging therefore that this may not always be straightforward.

There are a number of traditional barriers to any service user's adherence to a medicine management regime. These can be intentional and unintentional, perceptual or practical and include, but are not limited to, each service user's:

- Insight into their health issue
- Understanding or recall of what is required of them
- Personal motivation
- Cognitive ability
- Social situation
- Financial situation
- Regimen complexity (the number of medicines, the frequency of administration and length of time the medicine must be taken for)

- Ability to make lifestyle changes to accommodate a recommended regimen of treatment
- Beliefs or preferences
- Challenges in managing the medicine routine in public

Connor goes on to explain:

> I am now 21 and have suffered with Cystic Fibrosis since birth and have undoubtedly struggled with many aspects for it; this in turn means I have to take a multitude of long-term medicines. Most of my long-term medicine tackles theproblems I have with gaining and maintaining weight and how my body processes food. Due to pancreatic insufficiency and having half of my bowel removed at birth, I have to take a number of supplements to simply keep my weight up. Most of these, such as Creon (taken every time I eat) and vitamin supplements, I have taken all my life so I honestly know no different, and I know that whenever I eat I must take the Creon. This does mean that I must carry them wherever I go, which sometimes can be an issue, I may merely forget them or even when leaving the house decide I do not want to carry them with me and make the conscious choice not to eat till I get home. Due to the amount of medicine I am taking alcohol is avoided at all costs, something that can be difficult at university, prompting questions and strange looks when I tell someone that I do not drink, a prospect foreign to most students.

Adherence to medicine regimes can be improved if they are tailored to the individual's lifestyle, so this needs to be taken into account in developing interventions to improve adherence. Comprehensive interventions combining cognitive, behavioural and affective components are more effective than single-focus interventions (Roter *et al.*, 1998).

The simple guide in Figure 10.5, which can easily be used with a range of service users, has been developed by Bergman-Evans (2006) to support medicine adherence in older people:

A: Assessment – Assess all Medicines
I: Individualization – Individualize the regimen
D: Documentation – Provide written communication
E: Education – Provide accurate & continuing education tailored to the needs of the individual
S: Supervision – Provide continuing supervision of the regimen

Figure 10.5 AIDES Framework

Medicine management for people needing hospital admission when living with a long-term conditions

Many service users who take long-term medication may have to access hospital care either as an emergency or planned admission.

Information

An important area of attention when a service user is admitted to hospital is to ensure that the medicines prescribed on admission correspond to those that the service user was taking before admission, unless clinical diagnosis mitigates against this. It has been reported that a quarter of all hospital prescribing errors are the result of incomplete medication histories (Tam *et al.*, 2005). Medicine reconciliation has been defined as:

> the process of identifying the most accurate list of the service user's current medicines including the name, dosage, frequency and route and comparing them to the current list in use, recognising any discrepancies, and documenting any changes, thus resulting in a complete list of medicines accurately communicated.

> (IHI 2009)

NICE, together with the National Patient Safety Agency (NPSA), have worked to produce detailed guidance for both service users and health professionals on medicine reconciliation. Healthcare organizations are now obliged to have policies in place for medicine reconciliation on admission (NICE 2007).

On admission health professionals are required to record details of the name of the medicine(s), dosage, frequency and route of administration that the service user was taking prior to being admitted to hospital. Establishing these details involves discussion with the service user or carers, and the use of records from primary or community care. It is imperative that a thorough medicine history is obtained as part of the admission process. The nurse (or midwife) is strategically placed to be able to do this.

Reader activity

Reflect on interactions between people taking long-term medicine and health professionals that you have observed.

- Can you think of examples where there was shared decision-making?
- What were the characteristics of the interactions that facilitated shared decision-making?
- Where did these interactions take place?

Knowing what medicines a service user was taking prior to hospital admission (whether these are POMS, or other medicines and remedies), enables informed decisions to be made including whether the service user can carry on taking their medicines as usual, that they receive the correct medicines and that they can take any new medicine safely. Whilst it is reasonable to assume that when someone is admitted to hospital they may be in a position where it is difficult for them to make decisions, either due to acuity of their condition or anxiety about their condition, that does not mean that they should not be involved in decisions about their care. Participation in care has been varyingly defined but Brearley's (1990) early explanation that participation is about being involved, or being allowed to become involved in decision-making processes, is helpful. In relation to medicine management the service user must be afforded the opportunity to be included in the decisions made about their care, as they are likely to be experts on this subject matter. In addition they must be consulted on what is to happen to the medicines that they have brought into hospital with them, and whether changes are to be made to their medicine regime. Many service users are not eligible for prescription exemptions and therefore may be financially compromised if medicines are changed unnecessarily on discharge home.

Self-management education and support

Whilst most service users, or their carers, administer medications unsupervized at home, regulations governing the storage and administration of medicines are different in a hospital setting (RPS 2005).

This may lead to service users having their independence in medicine administration removed if admitted to hospital. Recommendations and guidance from the Audit Commission (2001) highlights that self-administration in hospital allows service users greater independence and enables them to participate in their own care, making decisions about their treatment in partnership with clinical staff.

Many hospitals now recognize that service users should be given the opportunity to administer their own medications in hospital provided this can be done safely, and have specific guidance available to support this taking place. Self-administration has many benefits as the Audit Commission (2001) noted including:

- enabling the medicine to do its job – service users can take analgesics when they are in pain, sedation when they want to sleep, and tablets that need to be taken before, with or after food, at the correct time;
- simplifying the medicines regime – self-administration leads to simpler and better medicine regimes because fuller assessment of all the service user's medication is required. In turn this improves compliance. Simplification improves compliance with the medication regimen;
- allowing service users to practise taking medicine under supervision;
- alerting healthcare staff to any problems the service user may experience with their medicines.

Increasingly service users therefore may retain or assume responsibility for some or all of their own medicines during their stay in a hospital. The context of care and service user individual health status are also important considerations. Any transfer of responsibility should occur on the basis of an assessment of their ability with their agreement and should be recorded with the date and time (RPS 2005). As Connor notes:

I also had a Portacath inserted at age 9 as my need for IV antibiotics increased and my veins became more difficult to place any form of line into. I self-administer the IV antibiotics both in and out of hospital, mainly due to the fact that many of the nurses I interact with are not trained on Portacaths or have very little knowledge on them. I find that I struggle to trust the nurses in these instances and feel it is simply easier and safer for me to do it myself.

Communication training for professionals

It is recognized that when service users move from one setting to another, there is considerable potential for things to go wrong in relation to their medicines (RPS 2006). Medicine management is a crucial element in the preparation of service users' transfer/discharge. In turn, this has an impact on the recovery and/or maintenance of their conditions following discharge. Therefore, discharge planning following admission to hospital for a service user on long-term medicine management, whose medicine regime may have changed, requires particular attention.

Whilst there are many important facts for service users to be aware of regarding their individual medicines, it is essential that they understand how to take their medicines, the drug type and mode of working, the effect, side effects and contra-indications as well as how to safely store and dispose of their medicines. The health professional has a key role in ensuring that service users have the required knowledge and skills to be able to take their medicines appropriately. It is essential that an inter-professional approach to discharge planning from the perspective of medicine management takes place, and that there is timely and effective communication across the traditional care boundaries of hospital and community, particularly if a medicine regime has changed. For effective teaching and assessment of the service user's comprehension and recall, a service user-centred communication approach employing the 'teach-back method' (Kripalani *et al.*, 2008) is particularly helpful. Teach-back confirms that the service user understands the information the health professional has given them, closing the communication gap between clinician and service user while enhancing the service user's knowledge. During a teach-back session, the service user's understanding is confirmed by them explaining the concept accurately back to the health professional.

One particular area of confusion for service users on discharge is commonly the name of their medicine. *The same medicine can sometimes be called different things.* Many medicines have two names:

- the brand name given to a medicine by the pharmaceutical company it is developed by (a medicine may have several brand names if manufactured by several companies);
- the scientific or generic name for the active ingredient of the medicine that is decided by an expert committee.

One of the commonest examples of a medicine that is known by both names is paracetamol (generic name) and Calpol® (brand name). Prescribers are encouraged to prescribe medicines by their generic name and should they change a service user's regular prescription from a branded medicine to a generic version, they should discuss this with the service user. This can be problematic, as the pharmacist can substitute, at their discretion, equivalent generic versions of the same drug. A few drugs are recommended to be prescribed only by specific formulation due to known bioavailability issues, for example, Priadel for generic lithium and several anticonvulsants. This is to ensure that they understand that although their medicine may have a different name, it will still contain the same active ingredient. It is important to note that the medicine may look different and there will be a different name on the label. However, it will contain the same active ingredient as the medicine they used before.

As Catherine notes:

> I was really worried when one of my medicines was changed. Well, it was only the name that changed apparently. It looked different, so my natural assumption was that it was different. I really didn't understand, despite many thoughtful explanations, why this was necessary. It really knocked my confidence initially because I had been reasonably stable for quite a long period of time and I was worried that might change.

Improving people's health behaviour

Reader activity

List factors that might make it difficult for a person on long-term medicine to manage their condition safely and effectively.

What are the challenges for health professionals in providing PCC to people who find their medicine management challenging?

The use of medicines to sustain health and relieve symptoms is increasing. Many service users will be taking a number of different medicines, quite appropriately, to manage their condition. This is particularly evident in the older age group who characteristically suffer from a number of chronic diseases. The risk of drug interactions increases with multiple medication, as does the risk of non-adherence. The evidence supporting polypharmacy and complex regimes is actively being challenged (Moynihan 2002), as is the applicability of the majority of NICE recommendations in the GP or out of hospital clinical setting (Steel *et al.*, 2014). A high proportion of hospital admissions and readmissions is due to adverse reactions to medicines or incorrect medicine taking, perhaps due to service users reverting to taking medicine previously taken but still stored in the home (MHRA/NHSE 2014).

Adverse drug reactions are frequently serious enough to result in admission to hospital and place a significant burden on the health service accounting for 1 in 16 hospital admissions, and for 4 per cent of hospital bed capacity (Pirmohamed *et al.*, 2004). Notably these figures are on the increase (Wu *et al.*, 2010). It is therefore essential that health professionals work with service users to ensure that they can safely store and retrieve their own medicines for their own use. Taking control of their medicine management is more likely to lead to a sustained change in health maintenance.

Polypharmacy is common as people live longer with multiple health conditions and it is not unusual for several members of one household to be taking medicines. Each service user should ensure that their medicines are stored separately from other members of the household and not shared. Medicines that are no longer being used should be safely disposed of via a local pharmacy. Health professionals have a pivotal role in ensuring service users are prompted to do this.

Summary

This chapter has discussed a number of issues that health professionals need to consider when working in partnership with service users to deliver person-centred medicine management. Medicines are the commonest intervention provided by the NHS, and nurses are the main body of workforce that the NHS employs. It stands to reason therefore that a considerable amount of nursing time is spent delivering medicine-related care. Through a person-centred approach, the nurse is in a pivotal position to coordinate the service users' medicine management care and to enable and support service users in working this into their life, thereby enabling them to maximize their health status.

References

Ahmad, N., Ellins, J., Krelle, H. and Lawrie, M. (2014) *Person-centred Care: From Ideas to Action*. London: The Health Foundation.

Aronson, K. (2007) Compliance, concordance, adherence, *British Journal of Clinical Pharmocology*, 63(4): 383–4.

Audit Commission (2001) *A Spoonful of Sugar*. London: The Audit Commission.

Bergman-Evans, B. (2006) AIDES to improving medicine adherence in older adults, *Geriatric Nursing*, 27: 174–82.

Brearley, S. (1990) *Patient Participation*. London: RCN.

Collins, A. (2014) *Measuring what Really Matters: Towards a Coherent Measurement System to Support Person-centred Care*. London: The Health Foundation. Available at: www.health.org.uk/sites/default/files/MeasuringWhatReallyMatters.pdf (accessed 6 November 2015).

Coulter, A. (2014) Person centered care – what works? *British Medical Journal*. Available at: http://blogs.bmj.com/bmj/2014/06/16/angela-coulter-person-centred-care-what-works/ (accessed on 26 October 2015).

Coulter, A. and Collins, A. (2011) *Making Shared Decision-making a Reality: No Decision About Me, Without Me*. London: The King's Fund.

DH (Department of Health) (2004) *Building a Safer NHS for Patients: Improving Medicine Safety.* London: Department of Health.

Duerden, M., Millson, D., Avery, A. and Smart, S. (2011) The quality of GP prescribing. London: The King's Fund.

IHI (Institute for Healthcare Improvement) (2009) www.ihi.org/ihi (accessed 5 November 2015).

Kripalani, S., Bengtzen, R., Henderson, L.E. and Jacobson, T.A. (2008) Clinical research in low-literacy populations: using teach-back to assess comprehension of informed consent and privacy information, *Journal of Empirical Research on Human Research Ethics,* 30: 13–19.

McKee, S. (2010) RPSGB urges greater focus on medicines adherence, *Pharma Times.* vailable at: www.pharmatimes.com/Article/10-01-21/RPSGB_urges_greater_focus_on_medicines_adherence.aspx?rl=1&rlurl=/10-09-09/NHS_money_wasted_on_unused_drugs_study.aspx (accessed 5 November 2015).

MHRA/NHSE(2014)*StageThree:DirectiveImprovingMedicationErrorIncidentReportingand Learning.* Availableat:www.england.nhs.uk/wp-content/uploads/2014/03/psa-sup-info-med-error.pdf (accessed 1 August 2014).

Moynihan, R. (2002) Too much medicine. Available at: www.bmj.com/too-much-medicine (accessed 5 November 2015).

NICE (National Institute of Clinical Excellence) (2007) Technical patient safety solutions for medicines reconciliation on admission of adults to hospital (PSG001). Available at: www.nice.org.uk/guidance/psg001 (accessed 5 November 2015).

NICE (2009) Medicines adherence: involving patients in decisions about prescribed medicines and supporting adherence. Available at: www.nice.org.uk/guidance/cg76/chapter/6-related-nice-guidance (accessed 5 November 2015).

NMC (Nursing and Midwifery Council) (2008). Standards for medicine management. Available at: www.nmc-uk.org/Nurses-and-midwives/Regulation-in-practice/Medicines-management-and-prescribing/ (accessed 5 November 2015).

Pendleton, D., Schofield, T., Tate, P. and Havelock, P. (1984) *The Consultation: An Approach to Learning and Teaching.* Oxford: Oxford University Press.

Pendleton, D., Schofield, T., Tate, P. and Havelock, P. (2003) *The New Consultation.* Oxford: Oxford University Press.

Pirmohamed, M., James, S., Meakin, S. *et al.* (2004) Adverse drug reactions as cause of admission to hospital: prospective analysis of 18 820 patients, *British Medical Journal,* 329: 15–19.

Prescribing Support Unit (2010) Available at: www.hscic.gov.uk (accessed 1 August 2014).

Roter, D.L., Hall, J.A., Merisca, R. *et al.* (1998) Effectiveness of interventions to improve patient compliance: a meta-analysis, *Medical Care,* 36: 1138–61.

RPS (Royal Pharmaceutical Society) (2005) *The Safe and Secure Handling of Medicines: A Team Approach. A revision of the Duthie Report (1988).* Available at: www.rpharms.com/support-pdfs/safsechandmeds.pdf (accessed 5 November 2015).

RPS (2006) *Moving Patients, Moving Medicines, Moving Safely: Guidance on Discharge and Transfer Planning.* London: RPS. Available at: www.wales.nhs.uk/sitesplus/documents/829/Medicines%20Management%20-%20Moving%20Patients%20Moving%20Medicines.PDF (accessed 5 November 2015).

Steel, N., Abdelhamid, A., Stokes, T. *et al.* (2014) A review of clinical practice guidelines found that they were often based on evidence of uncertain relevance to primary care patients, *Journal of Clinical Epidemiology*, 67(11): 1251–7.

Tam, V.C., Knowles, S.R. and Cornish, P.L. (2005) Frequency, type and clinical importance of medication history errors at admission to hospital: a systematic review. *Canadian Medical Association Journal*, 173: 510e15.

Taylor, J. (2014) Person-centred care. Available at: http://personcentredcare.health.org.uk/resources/five-top-tips-how-make-person-centred-care-really-work, (accessed 5 November 2015).

The Kings Fund (2014) Patient and Family centred toolkit. Available at: www.kingsfund.org.uk/projects/pfcc?gclid=CMyBseqR3MECFW3JtAodvmAAxg (accessed 5 November 2015).

Wallace, L.M., Turner, A., Kosmala-Anderson, J. *et al.* (2012) *Co-creating Health: Evaluation of First Phase*. London: Health Foundation. Available at: www.health.org.uk/publications/co-creating-health-evaluation-phase-1/ (accessed 5 November 2015).

Wu, T-Y., Jen, M-H., Bottle, A. *et al.* (2010) Ten-year trends in hospital admissions for adverse drug reactions in England 1999–2009. *Journal of the Royal Society of Medicine*, 103(6): 239–50.

Part

4

INTELLECTUAL DISABILITY, GENETIC DISORDER AND MENTAL HEALTH

Chapter

11

Person-centred care and people with intellectual disabilities

Issues and possibilities

Michael Brown and Zoë Chouliara

Introduction

In this chapter the focus is on PCC and people with intellectual disabilities, where we consider their health and care needs and what PCC means to and for them as high level and frequent consumers of health and social care services. Their health needs and the need to access care and support will be considered and related to the evidence regarding poor care and treatment, where PCC has been found to be lacking, further contributing to their disadvantage. The benefits and challenges to delivering PCC for people with intellectual disabilities will be explored and possible solution highlighted. The voice and experiences of people with intellectual disabilities and their carers will be included throughout the chapter, thereby setting out what does and does not work from their perspectives.

After reading this chapter the reader will be able to:

- understand PCC from the perspective of people with intellectual disabilities and their carers;
- have an appreciation of the scope of health needs and inequalities experienced by people with intellectual disabilities;
- have an understanding of the benefits and opportunities to delivering PCC for people with intellectual disabilities;
- have an understanding of the issues that need to be overcome to enable PCC for people with intellectual disabilities;

- consider a model of PCC relevant to people with intellectual disabilities and the implications for improving their care and support to ensure it is person centred.

I need to go to hospital sometimes because I have epilepsy and take fits. I don't like going but I need to. When I do go to hospital I want the nurses and doctors to ask me about my fits and what I want to happen and not talk over me as though I'm invisible and not there. I don't like it when they do that, it really annoys me. . .

(Service User 3)

People with intellectual disabilities

The term intellectual disability is used to refer to people who are cognitively impaired, with the level of impairment often being described as mild, moderate, severe and profound. For a diagnosis of intellectual disability to be made, three core components need to be present:

1   Onset during childhood and remaining lifelong
2   A significant global intellectual impairment, with a functional IQ of < 70
3   Impairment of adaptive behaviour and in independent living skills

People with intellectual disabilities comprise some 1-3 of the population with Maulik *et al.* (2011), suggesting a prevalence rate of 10.37 per 1000 population. There are therefore some 1.5 million people across the spectrum of intellectual disability in the United Kingdom, set within the context of a general population of 65 million, with more males with intellectual disabilities than females. The intellectually disabled population is changing as life expectancy is improving with a greater percentage living into older age; however life expectancy remains significantly shorter, by 20 years or more, when compared to the general population, and is shorter as the level of impairment and disability increases (Scottish Government 2013). As the intellectual disability population ages and increases, there will be a range of complex comorbidities, presenting new challenges for the future (McCarron *et al.*, 2013). The increase in the number of children, adults and older people with intellectual disabilities is a global phenomenon which means that all care providers such as education, social care, healthcare and non-government organizations (NGOs) will need to provide more care and support for this population in the future.

Health inequalities and health needs

The past three decades have seen the closure of long stay institutions for people with intellectual disabilities across the developed world (Scottish Executive 2000; Department of Health 2001). The closures have been accompanied by the development of community-based services where the majority now live in local communities and use universal services, accessing specialists when required. With the move to community-based care, there has been a focus on the health inequalities and health needs experienced by people with intellectual disabilities (Slevin *et al.*, 2007). There is a growing and developing evidence base that clearly highlights the significant health inequalities that exist and the unidentified and unmet health needs that exist that impact on life expectancy and quality of life (Krahn and Fox 2014).

Accompanying these inequalities is a range of complex and interrelated factors that contribute to the poor health of people with intellectual disabilities (Haveman *et al.*, 2010; Cooper *et al.*, 2011). Many experience health inequalities as a consequence of wider determinants of health, such as poor housing, unemployment, poverty, discrimination and social isolation (Emerson and Baines 2010; Cooper *et al.*, 2011). Those with specific syndromes such as Down's Syndrome have associated health conditions including heart disease, obesity, dementia, hypothyroidism and those with Fragile X-syndrome experience mental illness and behaviour challenges while those with Prader-Willi Syndrome experience obesity, mental illness and behaviour challenges (Emerson 2011). As a population many people with intellectual disabilities have a poor diet and experience obesity and sedentary lifestyles with limited physical activity, increasing the risk of cardiovascular disease, diabetes, hypertension, strokes and metabolic syndrome (De Winter *et al.*, 2011). Mental illness is common by way of depression, anxiety disorder, schizophrenia and bipolar disorder and many also present with comorbid physical health conditions (Whitaker and Read 2006; Kwok and Cheung 2007). As a result of their health needs, people with intellectual disabilities are high and frequent consumers of healthcare services, yet many experience barriers to access to care and treatment appropriate to their needs in line with the non-intellectually disabled, with their presentation being attributed to their disability rather than clinical need, resulting in diagnostic overshadowing (Mason and Scior 2004; Redley *et al.*, 2012; Heslop *et al.*, 2013).

Reader activity

Pause now and think about a person with intellectual disabilities that you know.

What are their physical and mental health needs and what are the challenges that they may face when accessing health services?
What are the implications of the barriers they experience when accessing health services?

People with intellectual disabilities and models of care

It is important to recognize that the majority of people with intellectual disabilities have always lived at home with their family in the community; for a minority their care was provided in institution settings. Across the developed world there have been significant changes and developments since the mid-1980s with a shift away from institutional congregated care settings that have resulted in people with intellectual disabilities moving back into their community. These changes have been informed by new government policies that have been heavily influenced by the principles of normalization, social inclusion and citizenship (O'Brien and Tyne 1981) and Social Role Valorisation (Wolfensberger 1983). Central to these developments has been the 'Social Model of Disability' that recognizes the needs of the individual and the negative impact of attitudes and behaviours within society that leads to marginalization and stigmatization of people with disabilities. As a result of these changes people with intellectual disabilities are increasingly supported in community settings, with access to additional support from specialists when required.

More recently there has been an interest and a focus on the 'Capabilities Framework' to address the health needs and inequalities experienced by some people with intellectual disabilities (Emerson and Hatton 2014). The central focus of the framework is on the individual and what they *can* do and what they *want to do and achieve,* as well as the identification of the opportunities needed to enable change and personal development (Nussbaum 2009). Emerson and Hatton (2014) go on to suggest that there are four main characteristics of the Capabilities Framework:

1   Social justice is central and applies to all people with intellectual disabilities by enabling individuals to exceed minimum levels of functioning as opposed to seeking to eliminate health inequalities.
2   All domains of capabilities and functioning are of equal importance in their own right and cannot be represented as a single concept.
3   People with intellectual disabilities must have the right to live in a just and equal society and can exercise freedoms and make autonomous decisions regarding their lives, such as health.
4   People with intellectual disabilities need to experience capability security whereby they feel secure that social supports and conditions necessary to sustain freedoms will not be withdrawn.

The framework is therefore concerned with ensuring that each individual with an intellectual disability has the opportunity and necessary supports to exercise self-determination through choice and freedom to make decisions about their care. Previous literature recognizes injustices experienced by some people with intellectual disabilities in relation to the legal system, rights, respect and care. The need to exercise responsibility and address these issues in practice is also recognized (Carlson and Kittay 2009).

Emerson and Hatton (2014) suggest that the Capability Framework is compatible with the Social Model of Disability and offer a way to address the complex inequalities experienced by many people with intellectual disabilities. Wolff (2009) suggests that ways forward such as providing state cash compensation, enabling personal enhancement, supporting status enhancement and targeted resources and the provision of self-directed payments will start to address the status of people with intellectual disabilities as equal citizens and ensure that their individual needs are met in a way that is person centred. It is possible therefore to see how the framework is closely related to the notion of person-centredness.

Person-centred care and people with intellectual disabilities

Person-centred care is generally defined as providing care and treatment that is responsive to and respective of individual personal preferences, needs and values and assuring that patient values guide all clinical decisions. This definition however overlooks the undeniable relational aspects of PCC. In England the White Paper, *Liberating the NHS: Equity and Excellence,* emphasizes the importance of giving people more autonomy and control over their healthcare. The principle of 'No decision about me without me' underpins the NHS reform plans. Person-centred care is one of the three core tenets of care in NHS Scotland focusing on delivering 'Person-centred, safe and effective care' to all. It is also an important part of the Government's agenda with the recent publication of the Patient Rights (Scotland) Act 2011. Person-centred care is also one of the key drivers for Scotland's healthcare quality strategy (NHS Education for Scotland 2012).

Previous evidence is largely supportive of the effectiveness of PCC especially for patients with chronic physical and mental health conditions, including those with intellectual disabilities. It appears that PCC is effective in improving both treatment and patient outcomes and therefore is cost effective (O'Donnell *et al.*, 1999; Ashby and Dowding 2001; Stewart 2001; Kwan and Sandercock 2002). Barriers, which are consistent across patient groups and conditions, include, time (Chan and Leung 2002), dissolution of professional power (Ashby and Dowding 2001), lack of autonomy to practise in this way (McCormack 2003), client communication difficulties (Sim 1998) and the constraining nature of institutions (McCormack 2001), including impoverished environments of care (Nolan *et al.*, 2004). Important gaps in the literature so far seem to include a lack of understanding of highly vulnerable groups' definitions of PCC, such as people with intellectual disabilities, and a lack of empirical evidence on the effectiveness and effective application and operationalization of the approach when meeting their needs.

There is growing research evidence of the benefits of health screening to identify unidentified and therefore unmet health needs within the intellectually disabled population, thereby offering inclusion in and access to public health programmes, health promotion, health education and preventative services that improve quality of life and reduce health burden (Mencap 2007; 2012; Robertson *et al.*, 2005). Despite the need to access universal health services, many people with intellectual disabilities continue to be disadvantaged notwithstanding the legal duty to make adjustments to care to enable assessment and treatments and for interventions to be provided (DH 2008; Turner and Robinson 2011). Despite the drive to promote PCC, there is evidence of poor care when people with intellectual disabilities attend for investigations and treatments in the acute care environment. Failure to meet the needs of people with intellectual disabilities has attracted significant attention due to issues related to poor care and access to healthcare that have contributed to avoidable premature deaths (Heslop *et al.*, 2014). The Mencap (2007; 2012) *Death by Indifference*, Sir Johnathan Michael's report *Healthcare for All* (DH 2008) and the Confidential Inquiry report by Heslop *et al.* (2014) are examples of this and they set out the legal duty in the UK to make reasonable adjustments and provide PCC. The key points arising from these reports include those listed in Box 11.1:

Box 11.1 Adjustments required to promote PCC in the acute care environment

Supporting families as partners in care of their family member with intellectual disabilities

- Including people with intellectual disabilities and their families in service planning and delivery

- The identification of needs through Strategic Joint Needs Assessments
- Compliance with disability legislation to ensure that reasonable adjustments are made to enable the provision of PCC
- Systems to collect data to identify people with intellectual disabilities within general health services
- Establishing Intellectual Disability Liaison Nursing services in all general hospitals to provide access to experts with knowledge and skills of the needs of people with intellectual disabilities
- Education at undergraduate level on the needs of people with intellectual disabilities and the reasonable adjustments required to enable access to healthcare
- Postgraduate education and CPD opportunities for health professionals about the needs of people with intellectual disabilities

The findings from these reports highlight that people with intellectual disabilities are one of the most vulnerable groups receiving care services. One of the mechanisms of operationalizing PCC for this group which has been recommended by the World Health Organization and in government reports is the role of intellectual disability acute hospital liaison nurses with specialist knowledge and skills about the care needs of people with intellectual disabilities (Brown *et al.*, 2006; DH 2008; Gibbs *et al.*, 2008; World Health Organization 2010; Mencap 2012; Brown *et al.*, 2012; Bradbury-Jones *et al.*, 2013; Heslop *et al.*, 2013). Due to the innovative nature of the role of liaison nurses, it presents an ideal window through which it is possible to gain valuable insight into the realities and challenges of PCC in action.

In a recent study the authors have analysed narratives of the main stakeholders – that is, service users with intellectual disabilities, their carers and professionals – on the role of liaison nurses by using the lens of PCC and the impact when it is both present and absent (Brown *et al.*, 2014). The study sought to understand the role as a mechanism of enabling and facilitating PCC and also considered definitions and experiences of PCC and the impact of the lack of it from a service user and carer perspective. The study provided 'an anatomy' of PCC for people with intellectual disabilities, which could be useful in a wider sense too for developing our understanding of PCC for many other vulnerable groups in health and social care. The findings from the study suggest vulnerable groups such as those with intellectual disabilities present with a number of challenges, including high comorbidity and complex needs, as well as individual and specific informational needs about care services and their condition and the treatment options and risks. Such challenges often lead to critical points in their care, when risks of morbidity, low satisfaction with services and mortality are high. Providing PCC can therefore potentially act as a buffer by preventing poor care for individuals with intellectual disabilities and by facilitating better resolution when these points do occur.

The Benefits of PCC

Evidence on definitions and effectiveness of PCC has been growing over the last 15 years, although it remains by comparison a new field of research. Based on our research and

PERSON-CENTRED CARE AND PEOPLE WITH INTELLECTUAL DISABILITIES

review of the wider evidence, we believe that PCC for people with intellectual disabilities *is the provision and maintenance of a consistent, trusting, safe, competent, and perceptive personal-professional relationship in times of heightened psychological and physical vulnerability for the service user and their carer(s).* Given the issues experienced by some people with intellectual disabilities when accessing and receiving healthcare, specific characteristics which form the essence of PCC come into play. In the following section we outline the benefits of PCC.

Reader activity

Pause now and think about a person with intellectual disabilities that you know or know of and what their individual care needs are when attending for acute hospital care.

How can person-centred approaches to care and support meet their needs?

Is personal

It is highly **relational**. It relies heavily on forging and maintaining a personal connection with the individual with intellectual disabilities and for some may involve drawing on the knowledge and expertise of their family and carers. It is based on knowing who the person is, their strengths and vulnerabilities, preferences and fears. It relies on using this connection and personal knowledge to protect their interests at all times and treat them in a respectful and considerate manner, in other words, as a unique individual. Without the personal connection, the professional's knowledge and practices alone will not achieve PCC. Person-centred care bridges the personal and professional aspects of care seamlessly to create the optimal psychological and physical environment for care and recovery. Such issues are central to providing PCC for people with intellectual disabilities in both universal and specialist health services, due to their high vulnerability, and comorbidity.

> She (the liaison nurse) told me she'd be coming to see me . . . yes, that was even more personal, coming to see me and she couldn't believe I was sitting up and it was like having a cup of tea, that's how quick it was
>
> (Service User with intellectual disabilities)

Person-centred care is consistent

It develops and depends upon consistent presence and reliable action. The individual with intellectual disabilities needs to feel that they have not been abandoned or failed at their most vulnerable time. Consistency relies on appropriate, timely and effective communication and information sharing between people with intellectual disabilities and their families and carers and between and amongst health professionals. Therefore effective PCC is based on the concept of care being consistent, which is central to the care of people with intellectual disabilities where issues such as communication and capacity to consent to care and treatment may be impaired and additional individualized approaches and adjustments may be required.

> He (the service user) was involved with (this hospital) since he was a tiny baby, so sort of twenty years. . . . I think it was quite difficult and daunting, and they had to get used to us, and we had to get used to them. But after twenty years so many staff knew him and his sort of little quirks. . . . I mean there were only seven wards, but we've visited them all and felt quite comfortable. And I knew it would be hard moving on, and I knew it had to happen.
>
> (Family Carer of individual with intellectual disabilities)

Person-centred care promotes safety

Safety in the acute care environment may be psychological, and can also be physical. Person-centred care reduces morbidity and mortality and manages risks, especially so in vulnerable groups, such as those with intellectual disabilities in healthcare. It promotes a psychological environment which is not threatening and therefore encourages the individual to function rather than 'dys-function'. A person-centred context allows the emotional and physical care needs of people with intellectual disabilities to be heard and met within a safe and accepting environment and therefore then allows recovery and growth. Given the evidence of preventable premature deaths of people with intellectual disabilities when accessing universal healthcare, promoting a safe care environment is central to PCC.

Person-centred care builds interpersonal trust and trusting relations

It relies on trust and promotes trust, thus preventing communication breakdown that leads to a poor patient experience and complaints. Trusting relations are a key component of PCC and are defined as:

> A state of positive expectations regarding both the competence and benevolence of intentions of the professional. During this state the service user holds the unwavering belief that the professional is both able and knowledgeable as well as willing to act to the service users benefit. (Calnan and Rowe 2004: 2–4). These expectations need to be developed, valued, and maintained and require consistency of care behaviours and personal resources on behalf of the professional. Due to the nature of an intellectual disability and the issues related to comprehension and processing information, such as during a hospital admission, trusting relationships with healthcare professionals providing care and treatment are essential to ensure person-centred outcomes that recognize and respond to the needs of the individual, their family and carer.

> There was an element of frustration from all of us (carers and liaison nurses). And we did pursue a formal complaint . . . and we got our complaints addressed, and great promises of how it will be different the next time, but I take it all with a pinch of salt.
>
> (Family Carer of service user with intellectual disabilities)

Person-centred care is competent and perceptive

It relies on good knowledge of the person and 'know-how' of how the system works. It is also sensitive to the needs of the individual with intellectual disabilities and how these change in different interactions and environments. It is in other words how 'in tune' professionals are with the person with intellectual disabilities and their family and carers. Therefore for PCC to be a reality for people with intellectual disabilities, engaging with families and carers throughout the care journey is important to support decision-making and communication, as taking into account their wealth of knowledge and expertise related to their family member can help prevent avoidable premature deaths.

> There have been confusions there (in communication). That does seem to be an area where things have often slipped. I can think of several instances with different service users at different times where that has slipped. One of my service users has epilepsy and his consultant . . . the information form had not been relayed to the GP, 'cause when he went back for his appointment, the consultant worked on the basis that his instruction had been passed to the GP and it hadn't. Oh, there does seem to be perhaps a grey area there, gaps that things can slip through.
>
> (Carer of service user with intellectual disabilities)

Challenges to PCC

There are various challenges in operationalizing PCC in day-to-day clinical practice to ensure that people with intellectual disabilities receive the care and support they require and that the knowledge and expertise of families and carers are recognized and exploited positively. If these challenges are managed efficiently and in a timely way they can become opportunities of facilitating and ensuring PCC. Service user-related challenges include their high level of vulnerability and therefore the risk and potential to reach critical points in care. If, however, they are not managed efficiently, they can undermine PCC and increase risks of distress, dissatisfaction and contribute to morbidity and mortality.

Reader activity

Pause now and think about a person with intellectual disabilities that you know or know of and identify the potential challenges to meeting their individual care needs are when attending for acute hospital care.

Set out the approaches necessary to provide PCC to ensure they get the right care and support throughout their care journey.

Vulnerability

PCC is not only important for people with intellectual disabilities, it is important across patient groups and care settings. However, it takes a paramount importance here as people with intellectual disabilities face additional challenges in terms of their impaired cognitive functioning, communication disorders, reduced capacity and increased risk of mortality. Their physical, psychological and cognitive vulnerability predisposes many to higher levels of distress and potential complications, which compromises their ability to voice their concerns, understand and retain information and for some to participate actively in care and treatment decisions.

Critical points

As part of the challenges faced by people with intellectual disabilities, care delivery can reach critical points. Such critical points consist of a health crisis, often a sudden and unforeseen acute illness, which escalates into the need to access primary and acute care services for assessment and diagnosis and with multiple or consecutive referrals across and between services. Some people with intellectual disability and their carer enter a state of high distress and confusion that if not recognized and responded to can lead to hopelessness, disappointment and mistrust of individual health professionals and the health system as a whole. Such distress may escalate to increased risks for the safety of service users, leading to medical complications and deterioration of already compromised physical state. Prevention, if possible, and timely, effective management of critical points is a crucial factor in operationalizing PCC for people with intellectual disabilities.

Transitions

Multiple transitions within and across healthcare services are one of the most common challenges faced by people with intellectual disabilities and present a major challenge in operationalizing PCC. Developmental transitions between children and adult health services lead to changes in professionals providing care and to new referrals, all part of the referral system and health protocols. The latter are unavoidably linked to government imposed standards of care and measurable outcomes and resource allocation. Transitions imply change and adjustment for the individual with intellectual disability and their family and carers and also for the healthcare system. They therefore bring high levels of uncertainty and potentially distress. They demand risk management and flexibility on behalf of the system and health professionals and if not managed appropriately can reveal the 'cracks' in the system, leading to confusion and additional distress for service users, their family and carers.

Choice and involvement in decision making

As a result of all the above challenges faced by people with intellectual disabilities, especially so their often compromised decision-making capacity, patients and their professional and non-professional carers often have to make various decisions about investigations, treatment and care. Such decisions are often critical and have to be made within a specific time frame and under high levels of stress and uncertainty. They can impact on the wellbeing, safety and even the life of the patient with intellectual disabilities. In a system that does not operate in ways that promote PCC, such decisions fall on the carers, who often feel unqualified to make

Table 11.1 Person Centred Care – What it is and what it is not

Person-centred care is	Person-centred care is not
• Relational to the needs of the individual • At the centre of the Human Interface - working on the edge of personal and professional practice • Consistent • Safe • Trustworthy • Competent, particularly at critical care points • Communicative and transparent	• A quick fix solution and set of new 'buzz words' for health services • Passive participation by the individual in decision-making about their care • Simply about offering choice • Simply about attempting to 'empower' individuals within healthcare settings • Simply outcome driven without considering the experience of care and organizational adjustments needed to meet individual needs

them with a detrimental effect on their emotional wellbeing and that of their family member with intellectual disabilities.

By consciously analysing and reflecting on individual practice and the healthcare systems in place and operationalized, it is possible to start to identify and consider what PCC is and what it is not from the perspective of people with intellectual disabilities. Table 11.1 sets out what PCC is and is not. Box 11.2 provides a case study that illustrates the challenges of providing PCC.

Box 11.2 A case study from practice

Paul is a 45 years old and lives at home with his elderly mother and their two dogs. Paul has a moderate earning disability, autism spectrum disorder and communication problems.

Over several days Paul complained to his mother of abdominal discomfort which his mother initially thought was due to constipation. When the abdominal discomfort did not settle, she took him to see a GP who following examination referred him to the accident and emergency department of the local general hospital. Following a wait of eight hours in A & E, Paul had become increasingly anxious and distressed and complained to his mother of increasing abdominal discomfort. He was eventually seen by a junior doctor in A & E and following examination he was diagnosed with suspected appendicitis. During the examination Paul became increasingly distressed and his mother attempted to advise doctors and nursing staff on how best to understand his non-verbal communication, his difficulties in 'being touched' due to his autism and how he found the busy A & E department noisy and frightening and that providing a quiet, more isolated environment was necessary. Paul's mother was told that this was not possible as the department was very busy and he would need to wait until a bed could be found for him. She felt she was not listened to as his legal welfare guardian and that no one valued her opinion or experience of Paul and how best to meet his needs.

Following a further wait in the busy A & E department, Paul was transferred to a dermatology ward as there were no beds available in the acute surgical receiving unit. Paul was admitted to the dermatology ward and his mother told that he would be kept under observation and transferred to a surgical bed at some point. She was advised to go home and that the ward would contact her if there were any change. Paul was later transferred to the surgical unit where his anxieties increased. Doctors attempted to canulize him and start antibiotics and provide fluids to prevent dehydration. Paul became distressed and staff in the ward decided that a sedative was required which he refused to take orally. The medication was administered by intramuscular injection administration and involved staff holding him down. His mother was shocked when she learned of this the next day and voiced her concerns that she had not been told of his transfer to the surgical ward or of the decision to administer medication by intramuscular injection. She made a request for Peter to be assessed by the Intellectual Disability Liaison Nurse, however the doctor made a referral to the Liaison Psychiatric Team who work with patients with mental health problems.

Paul's mother was annoyed and questions the confusion about the care of people with intellectual disability and autism spectrum disorder and tried to explain that she had worked with Paul's community intellectual disability nurse and speech and language therapist to develop a communication passport that explained how to understand his communication style and meet his care needs. Paul's mother was concerned that communication was poor and that as his legal welfare guardian she has not been involved in decisions about his care. She was also concerned that the attitudes and skills of staff were not what Paul required and about the lack of appropriate support and reasonable adjustments for him.

Reader activity

Reflecting on Paul's care, consider the following points and identify possible barriers and solutions to providing PCC:

What are the barriers that ought to have been addressed to ensure that Paul received appropriate PCC?

How should Paul's mother have been supported and her expertise utilized to contribute to Paul's care?

What are the organizational barriers and solutions that need to be addressed to ensure that the needs of people with intellectual disabilities are addressed in the future?

Making PCC for people with intellectual disabilities a reality

Person-centred care in policy reports and in research is often portrayed as a-theoretical, individualistic, or even as a new concept; however, it is neither. Person-centred care is well rooted in the humanistic and person-centred tradition and approach. It is much more than involvement, participation, empowerment and compassion. It is more relational and interpersonal and therefore more complex and the 'human interface' is the crux of PCC and lies at the heart of any attempt to define and apply it in practice.

The ability to connect with another human being in a vulnerable state within an environment of heightened uncertainty and anxiety by using both the human side as well as professional competence is the essence of PCC. It is at its heart and has to be embedded at all levels across the organization and in all types of professional practice. The application of PCC demands that professionals are able to work on the edge of the personal and professional realms within a system that acknowledges the human experience and the vulnerability that comes with it and are able to manage crisis and vulnerability in an efficient, respectful and transparent way. Working with people with intellectual disabilities at the human interface demands a high level of competency, personal development and authenticity, as well as a system that respects and facilitates the development and maintenance of a safe, flexible, consistent and trusting care environment. Therefore, PCC and meeting the needs of people with intellectual disabilities is not an easy, 'quick-fix' solution or buzz word; it must be viewed as a long-term investment, necessary to the distinct health needs with which many present and need to be met. The effectiveness of PCC and people with intellectual disabilities although taxing on resources in the short term, is cost effective in the long term. Person-centred care for people with intellectual disabilities can prevent revolving doors, promote patient safety, reduce likelihood of overload and burnout in professionals, and increase patient satisfaction and concordance with treatment. It is not realistic to claim that professional practice health systems are quite there yet in relation to providing PCC for people with intellectual disabilities, as evident in the accounts of the main service users with intellectual disabilities, their families and carers and the professionals involved in their care.

Over the years there have been significant paradigm shifts from the Biomedical Model to the Social Model of Disability and Biopsychosocial Model, to new ones such as the Capabilities Framework set out earlier in this chapter, through to those that emphasize patient empowerment and more recently to PCC and compassionate care. Culture changes take a long time and they require long-term investment as well as interim solutions, especially so within an already financially compromised healthcare system, growing demands for care and treatment, the burden of ageing populations, migration and what feels like constant change. With all these challenges it is vital that PCC becomes embedded within professional practice and organizational culture, thereby improving the care experiences of people with intellectual disabilities and other vulnerable groups.

To effect pragmatic and tangible change, the operationalization of PCC needs to include a strong focus within aspiring professionals' education and preparation as well as organizational adjustments and long-term developments. For the professionals delivering care, education, training, supervision and consultative support are all key factors that must be developed and integrated across the organization. This does not detract from the importance of the role of individual professional who has a responsibility to take charge of their own personal and professional development and take steps to operationalize PCC for people with intellectual disabilities in their day-to-day practice and find solutions to the challenges in their own practice, however small. In some areas and for some patient groups who are more vulnerable than others, such as people with intellectual disabilities, there are a number of strategies that can be adopted and developed to support and facilitate PCC, including:

- providing access to specialist Intellectual Disability Liaison Nursing to provide additional expert and skilled resource within the acute care environment, necessary to help minimize increased risk and uncertainty;
- making adjustments in communication channels and information sharing with the individual with intellectual disabilities;
- reviewing care pathways and having more comprehensive and efficient referral procedures to ensure PCC to facilitate smoother care journeys for people with intellectual disabilities;
- sharing 'red flag' information with other services about chronic health conditions, previous relapses and supports needs;
- developing and tailoring information to cognitive ability and emotional state;
- utilizing families' and carers' expertise about the needs of their family member with intellectual disabilities;
- developing accessible information about the organization and particular common health conditions associated with people with intellectual disabilities such as epilepsy;
- choosing appropriate times and place to provide information and facilitate informed decision making based on the needs of the individual.

Summary

There is currently a strong focus on quality control, expressed in measurable targets and outcomes within health services. Maintaining and evaluating quality of care is important for an effective healthcare system; however, is the obvious still being ignored? Person-centred care principles and the human interface in healthcare should not be assumed, and in reality, it is the most important factor from the perspective of the service user. By ignoring the human interface no system seeking to meet the needs of vulnerable individuals can work effectively; this is what PCC is fundamentally all about.

Vulnerable groups such as those with intellectual disabilities present with a number of challenges, including high comorbidity and complex needs, as well as individual and specific informational needs arising from their cognitive impairment. As a result, they require multi-professional involvement, due to the frequent number of transitions between and across health and social care services and the high risk associated with poor communication and information sharing which contribute to their premature and avoidable deaths. Providing PCC can potentially act as a buffer by preventing poor care for people with intellectual disabilities and by facilitating better resolution when these points occur. The absence of PCC through the complexities of healthcare pathways can lead to confusion, manifesting in patient and carer dissatisfaction, anxiety and broken trust, unclear roles and decision-making challenges, risk and muddled care pathways. Such confusion reinforces the vulnerability of people with intellectual disabilities within healthcare systems and care environments and their susceptibility to avoidable harm.

In this chapter, we have provided a practice-oriented definition of PCC, rooted in the experience of service users, their family and carers. We have identified and highlighted new challenges and barriers in the application of PCC in the care of people with intellectual disabilities and have set out meaningful strategies for its application when working with this and other vulnerable service users. This chapter has raised questions about the importance of adopting PCC across healthcare systems if we are to fulfil policy directives, improve the patient experience and achieve quality, efficiency and safety of care. It also raises questions about the training and consultative support of professionals, necessary to facilitate changes in care culture and shifts in care models towards PCC. Despite the challenges and barriers, PCC is the way forward for long-term change and positive, safe and effective care experiences, particularly for people with intellectual disabilities.

References

Ashby, M.E. and Dowding, C. (2001) Hospice care and patient's pain: communication between patients, relatives, nurses and doctors. *International Journal of Palliative Nursing*, 7(2): 58–97.

Bradbury-Jones, C., Rattray, J., MacGillivray, S. and Jones, M. (2013) Promoting the health, safety and welfare of adults with learning disabilities in acute care settings: a structured literature review, *Journal of Clinical Nursing*, 22(11–12): 1497–509.

Brown, M. and MacArthur, J. (2006) A new research agenda: improving health care in general hospitals, *Journal of Clinical Nursing*, 15(11): 1361–9.

Brown, M., Chouliara, Z. and MacArthur, J. (2014) A Model of Compassionate, Person-Centred Care: The perspectives of stakeholders of intellectual disability liaison nurses, *Journal of Clinical Nursing* (under review).

Brown, M., MacArthur, J., McKechanie, A. *et al.* (2012) Learning Disability Liaison Nursing Services in south-east Scotland: a mixed-methods impact and outcome study, *Journal of Intellectual Disability Research*, 56(12): 1161–74.

Calnan, M. and Rowe, R. (2004) *Trust in Health Care: An Agenda for Future Research*. London: The Nuffield Trust.

Carlson, L. and Kittay, E.F. (2009) Introduction: rethinking philosophical presumptions in light of cognitive disability, *Metaphilosophy*, 40(3–4): 307–30.

Chan, S.W. and Leung, J.K. (2002) Cognitive behavioural therapy for clients with schizophrenia: implications for mental health nursing practice, *Journal of Clinical Nursing*, 11(2): 214–24.

Cooper, S-A., McConnachie, A., Allan, L. *et al.* (2011) Neighbourhood deprivation, health inequalities and service access by adults with intellectual disabilities: a cross-sectional study, *Journal of Intellectual Disability Research*, 55(3): 313–23.

De Winter, C., Magilsen, K., van Alfen, J. *et al.* (2011) Metabolic syndrome in 25% of older people with intellectual disability, *Family Practice*, 28(2): 141–4.

DH (Department of Health) (2001) *Valuing People: A New Strategy for Learning Disability for the 21ˢᵗ Century.* London: HMSO.

DH (2008) *Healthcare for All: The Independent Inquiry into Access to Healthcare for People with Learning Disabilities.* London: HMSO.

Emerson, E. (2011) Health inequalities and people with learning disabilities in the UK, *Learning Disability Review*, 16(1): 42–8.

Emerson, E. and Baines, S. (2010) *Health Inequalities and People with Learning Disabilities in the UK: 2010.* Lancaster: Learning Disabilities Observatory.

Emerson, E. and Hatton, C. (2014) *Health Inequalities and People with Intellectual Disabilities.* New York: Cambridge University Press.

Gibbs, S., Brown, M. and Muir, W. (2008) The experiences of adults with intellectual disabilities in general hospitals: a focus group study, *Journal of Intellectual Disability Research*, 50(12): 1061–77.

Haveman, M., Heller, T., Lee, L. *et al.* (2010) Major health risks in aging persons with intellectual disabilities: an overview of recent studies, *Journal of Policy* and *Practice in Intellectual Disabilities*, 7(1): 59–69.

Heslop, P., Blair, P., Fleming, P. *et al.* (2013) *Confidential Inquiry into the Premature Deaths of People with Learning Disabilities.* Bristol: Norah Fry Research Centre.

Heslop, P., Blair, P., Fleming, P. *et al.* (2014) The Confidential Inquiry into premature deaths of people with intellectual disabilities in the UK: a population-based study, *The Lancet*, 383(9920): 889–95.

Krahn, G. and Fox, M. (2014) Health disparities of adults with intellectual disabilities: what do we know? What do we do? *Journal of Applied Research in Intellectual Disabilities*, 27(5): 431–46.

Kwan, J. and Sandercock, P. (2002) *In-hospital Care Pathways for Stroke.* Cochrane Database Systematic Reviews CD00292.

Kwok, H. and Cheung, P. (2007) Co-morbidity of psychiatric disorder and medical illness in people with intellectual disabilities, *Current Opinion in Psychiatry*, 20: 443–9.

Mason, J. and Scior, K. (2004) 'Diagnostic Overshadowing' amongst clinicians working with people with intellectual disabilities in the UK, *Journal of Applied Research in Intellectual Disabilities*, 17(2): 85–90.

Maulik, P., Mascarenhas, M., Mathers, C. *et al.* (2011) Prevalence of intellectual disability: a meta-analysis of population-based studies, *Research in Developmental Disabilities*, 32: 419–36.

McCarron, M., Swinbourne, J., Burke, E. (2013) Patterns of multimorbidity in an older population of persons with an intellectual disability: results from the intellectual disability supplement to the Irish longitudinal study on aging (IDS-TILDA), *Research in Developmental Disabilities*, 34: 521–7.

McCormack, B. (2001) Autonomy and the relationship between nurses and older people, *Ageing and Society*, 21 (4): 417–46.

McCormack, B. (2003) A conceptual framework for person-centred practice with older people, *International Journal of Nursing Practice*, 9(3): 202–9.

Mencap (2007) *Death by Indifference: Following up the Treat me right! Report.* London: Mencap.

Mencap (2012) *Death by Indifference: 74 Deaths and Counting.* London: Mencap.

NHS Education for Scotland (2012) *People at the Centre of Health and Care.* Edinburgh: NHS Education for Scotland.

Nolan, M.R., Davies, S., Brown, J. *et al.* (2004) Beyond person-centred care: a new vision for gerontological nursing, *Journal of Clinical Nursing,* 13(3a): 45–53.

Nussbaum, M. (2009) The capabilities of people with cognitive disabilities, *Metaphilosophy,* 40(3–4): 331–51.

O'Brien, J. and Tyne, A. (1981) *The Principle of Normalization: A Foundation for Effective Services.* London: Campaign for the Mentally Handicapped.

O'Donnell, M., Parker, G. and Proberts, M. (1999) A study of client-focused case management and consumer advocacy: the Community and Consumer Service Project, *Australian and New Zealand Journal of Psychiatry,* 33(5): 684–93.

Redley, M., Banks, C., Foody, K. and Holland, A. (2012) Healthcare for men and women with learning disabilities: understanding inequalities in access, *Disability & Society,* 27(6): 747–59.

Robertson, J., Roberts, H. and Emerson, E. (2010) *Health Checks for People with Learning Disabilities: A Systematic Review of Evidence.* Lancaster: Improving Health and Lives.

Robertson, J., Emerson, E., Hatton, C. *et al.* (2005) *The Impact of Person Centred Planning for People with Intellectual Disabilities in England: A Summary of Findings.* Lancaster: Lancaster University, Institute for Health Research.

Scottish Executive (2000) *The Same as You? A Review of Services for People with Learning Disabilities.* Edinburgh: The Stationery Office.

Scottish Government (2013) *The Keys to Life: Improving the Quality of Life for People with Learning Disabilities.* Edinburgh: The Stationery Office.

Sim, J. (1998) Collecting and analysing qualitative data: issues raised by the focus group, *Journal of Advanced Nursing,* 28: 345–52.

Slevin, E., McConkey, R., Truesdale-Kennedy, M. *et al.* (2007) Community Learning Disability Teams: perceived effectiveness, multidisciplinary working and service user satisfaction, *Journal of Intellectual Disability Research,* 11 (4): 329–42.

Stewart, M. (2001) Towards a global definition of patient centred care, *British Medical Journal,* 322 (7284): 444–5.

Turner, S. and Robinson, C. (2011) *Reasonable Adjustments for People with Learning Disabilities: Implications and Actions for Commissioners and Providers of Healthcare.* Lancaster: Learning Disability Health Observatory.

Whitaker, S. and Read, S. (2006) The prevalence of psychiatric disorders among people with intellectual disabilities: an analysis of the literature, *Journal of Applied Research in Intellectual Disabilities,* 1(9): 4330–45.

Wolfensberger, W. (1983) Social role valorization: a proposed new term for the principle of normalization, *Mental Retardation,* 21(6): 234–9.

Wolff, J. (2009) Cognitive disability in a society of equals, *Metaphilosophy,* 40(3–4): 402–15.

World Health Organization (2010) *Better Health, Better Lives: Children and Young People with Intellectual Disabilities and their Families* EUR/51298/17/PP/7. Geneva: WHO Regional Office for Europe.

Families affected by an inherited genetic condition

The need for family-centred care

Alison Metcalfe and 'Anne'

Individuals do not exist

(Minuchin 1974)

Introduction

Between two and three million people in the UK are affected by an inherited genetic condition that is caused by a single gene mutation. The gene mutation can occur spontaneously in rare cases but more often is inherited from one or both of the parents, depending on whether the gene is autosomal dominant, autosomal recessive or is sex linked (Skirton and Patch 2009). For every person affected by an inherited genetic condition around four family members will be at risk (Genetic Alliance UK 2015). This is risk of being affected by the genetic condition now, or in the future if not already affected, or at risk of carrying the gene mutation that they will pass to their children. Therefore all inherited genetic conditions have implications for the individual and their family – not only because they are long-term conditions but also because of the heritability and risk for other family members, and these factors present some unique challenges for good healthcare.

Most of the chapters in this book focus on the 'person' or 'person-centred care'. However, as Chapter 4 has also pointed out, a person does not exist in isolation, and most are members of a biological and social structure called 'a family'. Throughout our lives, we are influenced by our family in how we cope and adapt to health and illness, the way in which we talk about it and the decisions we make to receive or reject health screening or treatment of diseases.

The family is often described as a system, and the relationships between the individual members are fundamental to ensuring how well the system functions. If one part of the system changes the way it functions, it has repercussions throughout the system. Similarly if an individual within the family experiences problems, family systems theory (Bateson and Ruesch 1951) shows that there are impacts on all other family members, changing the rules and expectations by which the family members live and relate to each other. As the family responds to change this is called adaptation and coping, and good communication between family members plays a fundamental role (Rolland 2006). All healthy-functioning families experience change and learn to adapt to changing circumstances, and the emphasis in family systems theory is on the relationships between individuals, rather than the individuals themselves.

A family affected by an inherited genetic condition face all the same expectations and challenges that most other families face however they have to cope with the long-term health problems caused. When a family member becomes ill, much of the attention is focused on that person, finding ways to make them well or help them live with their disease or disability and still achieve their fullest potential. Serious or long-term illness for one person places significant demands on their family; there are repercussions for all other family members, in taking decisions to assist the person affected, the need for extra resources, the financial implications and the socio-psychological consequences. In inherited genetic conditions, there is also the additional dimension that other family members might be affected or at risk from developing the same disease, including any future children of those family members that carry the genes that cause that genetic condition. Therefore as a family, being affected by an inherited genetic condition has more and different types of challenges than long-term conditions more generally.

What is a family?

Despite appearing simple this question is complicated by emotional and politically-charged rhetoric. The term 'family' can reflect a different discourse depending on the context in which it is used. Until relatively recent times, the Western idea of a 'normal family' was a man, a woman and their joint child or children. This is a highly mono-cultural and heterosexist view, which allows for little variation despite the many variations in family formations and constituencies we now observe in a multi-cultural society. Therefore to intentionally move away from any predefined or prescriptive definition of family, we developed our own psychosocial definition of 'family'; building on suggested definitions of Degenova and Rice (2002: 2) and Koerner and Fitzpatrick (2002), we define family as:

> any group of individuals united by the legal ties of marriage or partnership, blood or adoption in which the people are committed to one another in an intimate interpersonal relationship where the members see their individual identities as importantly attached to the group they call 'family' which has an identity in its own right through a shared history and shared future, and the adult(s) cooperate emotionally and financially to support dependent individuals (and each other).

(Metcalfe *et al.*, 2008)

This definition underpins all our research, as we make no assumptions about 'who' is or is not a family member; that is defined by family members themselves.

To illustrate some of the issues that families face, we are going to provide you with Anne's own story as a case study. You can also read further about the issues families face in our other studies (Metcalfe *et al.*, 2008, 2011; Plumridge *et al.*, 2010, 2011; Rowland and Metcalfe 2013, 2014). We have observed throughout our research that many of the socio-psychological effects are likely to be similar across any family affected by an inherited genetic condition, with some slight variations in relation to the symptoms the disease causes. It is therefore important for nurses and midwives to make assessments and observations based on the whole family perspective, taking into account other extraneous factors that may also be affecting or impinging on a family's coping with, and adapting to, living with the genetic condition.

Anne's story

The narrative Anne provides is not unusual; it is one heard many times during the course of our research with families affected by genetic conditions. Therefore we have not named the genetic condition, which also protects Anne's anonymity. We provide only a brief overview about Anne's experience and the effect she observed on her family members and the family's functioning but it will provide a good background for the discussion in the main text.

Anne and her husband David were married in their early 20s and decided they wanted to have a child. Despite a difficult pregnancy initially Caroline was eventually born at full term and via normal delivery, and had a normal development until aged 4 years old. Caroline was taken ill just before her fourth birthday and went on to have episodes of acute symptoms with increasing frequency. The symptoms affected Caroline's intellectual development and by her seventh birthday Caroline's intellectual abilities were still that of a 4-year-old. However Caroline was cheerful and enjoyed the company of others – she enjoyed being with friends, although did not have many because she had difficulty understanding their games and play. Jane was Caroline's younger sister by three years and once Jane had reached 3–4 years of age, Caroline's difficulties were very apparent when the two sisters were compared side by side. Physically Caroline was developing but not intellectually, and it took several years to diagnose the genetic condition affecting her.

Anne explained that she and her partner David noticed that their daughter Caroline was experiencing problems with development. Teachers however, described Caroline as simply naughty or as 'manipulative'. On meeting clinicians when seeking help or reassurance, Anne was told quite literally that she was a 'paranoid mother', and many did not even try to engage with Caroline to ascertain the level of her difficulties. Caroline was admitted to hospital a number of times due to acute exacerbations of her rare symptoms, but even when Anne tried to explain what was wrong with her daughter and what treatment she required, nurses and doctors did not listen and wasted significant time testing Caroline for other illness, rather than hearing Mum's explanations or phoning the paediatrician responsible for treating Caroline.

The genetic condition had significant repercussions for Caroline's physical and mental health and also all her family.

Mum and Dad felt and still feel a huge sense of guilt and responsibility. Anne said 'I could write a whole chapter on blame and guilt . . . it must have been our fault'. Caring for a child who is so dependent and who was frequently hospitalized affected both parents and their relationship. Time needed to care for Caroline meant limited time to spend together as a couple, and the pressures of caring for an ill child where no one knew what was happening and there had been no diagnosis had psychological effects, particularly for Anne, where she experienced anxiety and depression because of the pressures and developed agoraphobia. Anne and David had to cope with caring for Caroline, not knowing exactly what was wrong and what they should be doing, and at the same time receiving little or even unhelpful assistance from health professionals.

Mum and Dad's relationship with Caroline was also tested because they felt their parenting skills were being questioned and they were expected to do more to push their daughter's development, which it subsequently became clear was inappropriate. Anne describes how she felt she made life miserable for Caroline as a child because she tried to force her to do things that she was simply unable to do because of her condition. Whilst their relationship with their younger daughter Jane was close, Anne feels that Jane had to learn to be independent much sooner than other children of her age and help out around the house to support the care of her older sibling. Caroline often wanted to join in games with Jane and her childhood friends but she did not always have the intellectual capacity to do so, and Jane would get upset with her sister for spoiling her game. In younger adolescence Jane often felt uncomfortable about bringing her friends home because of her sister's problems. However as an older teenager Jane became very protective of Caroline and they have grown closer as they have got older.

Eventually getting a diagnosis was a large step forward in assisting the family in coping.

Grandparents were heavily involved, caring for Jane whilst Caroline was in hospital, and they provided significant support to Anne and David. However the grandparents too experienced feelings of guilt and self-blame that they might have passed on the gene that caused Caroline's genetic condition. When the condition was diagnosed as genetic there was variation in grandparents' responsiveness to providing information about other family members, with some able to provide comprehensive information but for others it was too difficult to talk because of family bereavements. Grief often affects when and how family members discuss those deceased, and sometimes the deceased person is the main person who 'held' the family history of illness and disease.

Anne felt unsupported by her own and David's siblings through the early years of Caroline's illness. Anne felt her siblings only became interested once they learnt it was a genetic condition and then they became concerned and were worried for their own children. Also Jane recognized that she too might be at risk from carrying the gene mutation that caused her sister's condition, and after some time decided she wished to undergo genetic testing to find out because of the potential consequences for her own children. Therefore there were anxieties about decisions for family members to undergo genetic testing to see if they carried the gene that caused the genetic condition.

Whilst the genetic condition has caused its issues and challenges for the family, Anne also emphasizes there are positive aspects. Anne explained that the family has been strongly supported by close friends. The friends' children have grown up to care for Caroline, and recognize her strengths; Caroline has been a uniting force in all their lives and her peers focus on the positive aspects of their own lives and their relationships. Jane has chosen a career which involves caring for others with learning difficulties and her experiences in her own family have made her very good at acknowledging others' need for care and support.

When asked what helped Anne in healthcare settings and caring for her daughter and her family, several things emerge as being essential for nurses providing care to note to help them improve family and patient experiences:

- **The effects of the illness impact not just on the person with the illness but there is a ripple effect outward to the whole family and all their relationships.** In nursing, the rhetoric of 'family-centred care' is often used when the reality shows a different story. In families affected by genetic conditions there is often little assistance from health professionals in assisting all family members' coping with and adapting to living with the genetic condition (Metcalfe *et al.*, 2011; SPRinG collaborative 2015)
- **Better support for families is essential.** Anne described how the family muddled through with little assistance or advice about how to cope with Caroline's condition or the repercussions it had for their family relationships. Even without knowing what the condition is, it is important that the effect of trying to cope with a child who is experiencing any kind of difficulty will affect the parents' relationships with their child, with each other, their other children and their wider friends and family.
- **Listening to the parents and the children is vital.** Too often Anne feels dismissed or judged, and often her daughter Caroline was barely acknowledged or spoken to.
- **Clear explanations are required.** Health professionals often speak in jargon, and both Anne and Caroline had difficulty understanding what was happening. On occasions if Caroline was spoken to, she was patronized. Having written explanations is very helpful for Anne and for her to share with Caroline and the wider family, as well as assisting her own understanding.
- **The power of language should always be considered**. Anne still recalls with heartfelt emotion the words used to describe her as a 'paranoid mother' or labeling her daughter Caroline as 'manipulative'; those words still hurt 20 years later.
- **Health professionals' should recognize their power where families are facing emotional situations; empathy and compassion is required.** Anne often felt judged by health professionals and they did not take time to establish relationships with Anne or Caroline nor the wider family. There was often a lack of continuity in care provision. Nurses should focus on building a relationship with all family members through valuing and understanding their relationships and the contribution they all make to family life, and assisting the family's coping and resilience.
- **Being prepared is important when meeting families for the first time: health professionals should have read the family history.** Anne described the frustration and anger she felt at having to repeat Caroline's story several times over, (sometimes in the same day). It meant continually reliving painful memories, which were compounded by the stress and worry that the current consultation was adding, particularly when Caroline was acutely unwell.

How can nurses and midwives work with families?

An important aspect of nursing is to recognize the effect of the genetic condition on the family and their relationships. This is regarded as family systemic practice and generally is not part of care. However, it is essential that nurses increasingly take a systemic approach to care because it is only by assisting the family in coping and adapting to the genetic condition that they will stand their best chance of succeeding as a family unit with least impact on their individual mental health. In the longer term a well-functioning family reduces the use of health resources including GPs, emergency admissions, hospitalization and mental health services.

By assessing the impact of the genetic condition on the family you can begin to understand what socio-psychological resources family members can draw up to support each other and assist their coping. Families often learn to manage the genetic condition and to become resilient over time but health professionals can assist their coping and adaptation more quickly by assisting them in identifying their family's strengths. In doing so, this has enormous benefits for the individuals involved, assisting them in maintaining their mental health, through increased resilience to the effect of the genetic condition.

One of the ways to assess the family's resource is to prepare a genogram. Genograms are used in family therapy but in genetics, a similar device is called a family pedigree or family history chart. The genogram provides information of the family's socio-psychological relationships whilst the family pedigree focuses on the biological relationships. In this situation the family genogram/pedigree has a double function. First, used as a pedigree it quickly identifies individuals who are affected by or at risk from the genetic condition, which genetic counsellors and nurses need to know and communicate to the family. Secondly, used as a genogram it can be used to map family relationships, who is close to whom, on who do family members rely and how well do the family communicate? Using the genogram you can also map in important friendships or equally less productive relationships that might impact on the family. The genogram allows you opportunities to explore the family's belief and understanding about illness and disease, and will provide important insight into what can increase the family's resilience and adaptability to living with the genetic condition.

Figures 12.1 and 12.2 show Anne's family pedigree and her genogram. Family pedigrees are used in genetics to assess the risk of an inherited genetic condition (see Figure 12.1). Usually pedigrees include three to four generations indicated by the roman numerals on the left side of the figure, with lines indicating relationships to partners and children. Where a genetic condition is present the disease will often be present in more than one generation. Caroline's condition however is caused by a 'spontaneous' gene mutation. Mainly biological relationships are included.

Family genograms are used to review and understand family relationships but are very similar to the pedigrees used in genetics, as you can see in Figure 12.2. The main difference is that non-generational lines are used to denote the psycho-social relationships between the family members. Close friendships are also acknowledged and any other important individuals or groups who are working with the family such as health and social care workers will also be included; for example we could include Caroline's care workers. It gives you a 'picture' of the family and their relationships at a single time point.

There is no reason why both the genogram and family pedigree should not include lots of information, as a diagrammatic representation can provide so much information on a single page. They can provide a good and quick assessment about who is at risk from the genetic condition and quickly provide clues about the family's functioning, rather than having to read many pages of notes.

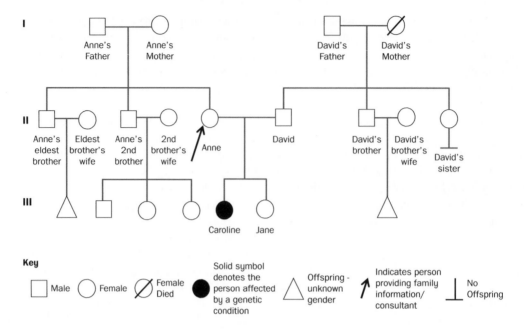

Figure 12.1 Anne's Family Pedigree: 3 August 2015 (always include date and time taken)

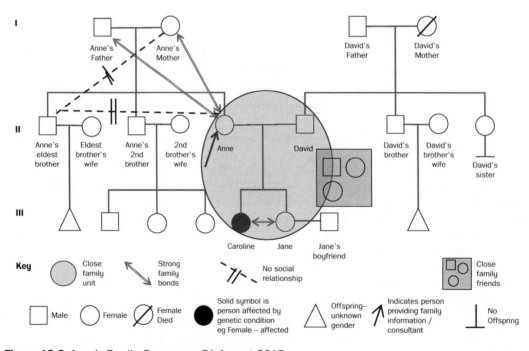

Figure 12.2 Anne's Family Genogram: 31 August 2015

Family members' perspectives on genetic conditions affecting their family

Ourselves and others (see reference list) have carried out research that has explored families' experiences of living with and coping with a genetic condition. Using Family Systems Theory to guide our work we have now interviewed more than one hundred families as a whole, and many hundreds of parents, children and young people separately. Here we provide a summary of our research findings but please revisit our original work too, provided in the references (Metcalfe *et al.*, 2011).

Parents

Many parents experience feelings of shock, anger, disbelief and guilt when they first learn that their child is affected by a disease or long-term condition, and these emotions are often intensified if there is an inherited genetic condition. Parents feel responsible, despite having no control about why or how a disease develops. In some of the life-threatening and life-limiting illnesses, it can be up to two years before parents can even begin to discuss the diagnosis with each other let alone talk openly with other family members. The reasons for this response are highly complex and multi-factorial and often men and women respond differently (Metcalfe *et al.*, 2011).

Many mothers report wanting to talk about the information, to try to make sense of it with their family and friends. By contrast fathers describe wanting to suppress and prevent any discussion. Trying to assist the couple in finding the right balance can be difficult at such an emotional time for the family, and nurses caring for the family play an important role in supporting both parents and ensuring their relationship remains intact. Many couples do divorce. The pressure of caring for a sick child and the worry experienced can leave little time for partners to spend together for emotional and sexual intimacy. As a result their relationship suffers and the partners can drift apart.

By recognizing the effects of caring for a child affected by a serious illness, nurses working with the family can support the partners and their relationship by asking couples how they are coping, making them aware that there is a risk to their relationship and encourage them to find ways of managing their relationship within their family life. A strong parental relationship will provide a good basis for the family to cope with the pressures they face and the unpredictability and uncertainty of the illness (Rolland and Williams 2005; Rolland 2006).

At different stages of their life cycle, parents face a number of important decisions. Whilst still at a reproductive age, there is a risk that parents will have another child affected by or at risk from the same genetic condition. Therefore parents will need genetic counselling and possibly genetic testing. Future pregnancies will require testing, and parents describe the joy of the pregnancy being removed; instead many feel it is a 'rollercoaster of emotion', waiting to find out whether the foetus is affected, which affects their bonding with their unborn child (Downe *et al.*, 2009; Dheensa *et al.*, 2012, 2013). Midwives therefore have an especially important role at this time, caring for the woman and baby, whilst also recognizing the needs of fathers, which can be overlooked (Williams *et al.*, 2011).

As children grow, parents are excited as they watch them go through the various developmental milestones, eagerly anticipating their child's achievements. When a child is affected by a genetic condition, development might be slower either as a direct result of the disease, for example cognitive impairment as part of the genetic condition, or because of the consequences of the disease. Frequent hospitalization and complex treatment regimes can sometimes affect a child's learning educationally and socially compared with their peers.

If the genetic condition has serious consequences for a child's development or the disease is degenerative, there is a decline in the individual's capacity to live independently. Many parents report a sense of anticipatory grief that their child will not grow up to be independent and may not have families of their own. Parents also express fears about who will care for the child once they are no longer able to (Rolland 2006).

Mothers are often the main carers, providing the physical care for their child and the emotional care for the family unless they are also affected by the genetic condition. Fathers tend to have more difficulty with providing the same level of emotional input and often focus on the practical tasks. Whilst this divides the labour between the parents both have different emotional support needs and Mums can complain of emotional fatigue and fathers can feel too distant and removed from the family (Metcalfe *et al.*, 2008; 2011).

Siblings

Siblings of an ill child are often overlooked, or one parent tends to take more responsibility in caring for the ill child and the other parent looks after the siblings. This can cause a schism within the family and is often observed by children and young people but can go unexpressed unless they have the opportunity to do so. As a result many children and young people can become overly protective of their ill sibling or if they do not understand what is happening, they can become jealous and eventually get very angry. The jealousy and anger leads to resentment, which results in poor behaviour, and on occasions this is directed towards the affected child (Plumridge *et al.*, 2010).

Children and young people who are the siblings of a child affected by a genetic condition, or indeed have a parent affected, can often feel confused about what is happening in their family until someone explains it to them. Between 50 and 60 per cent of families affected by an inherited genetic condition do not talk about it, even when the symptoms are very apparent in the family affected (Biesecker and Erby 2008). However children learn from an early age, approximately 7 to 8 years, not to ask questions that they fear might upset their parents. Parents decide against discussing the genetic condition with their children because they have not asked any questions, and a vicious cycle of non-communication is reinforced between parents and child (Metcalfe *et al.*, 2008).

Depending on the birth order of the children, there might also be differences in the amount of information shared with siblings. Older siblings tend to be given more information about what is happening, whereas parents can overlook discussing the genetic condition with siblings younger than the affected child. Several parents have observed that younger children are more jealous and behave more naughtily towards their affected sibling but when asked how they had explained the genetic condition to the child and the need for treatment, parents suddenly realize they have told them very little. There is an assumption that because the younger child has grown up always witnessing their older sibling's treatments, they will know about the disease and the reason why more attention is focused on them. Parents often report that after realizing and correcting their omission their younger child's behaviour towards their ill sibling changed overnight (Metcalfe, personal communication).

Facilitating parents in age- and developmentally appropriate conversations with their children about what is happening in their family, and trying to answer their children's questions honestly once they fully understand what the child is asking, are so important for a more harmonious and cohesive family. Young people who do not understand what is happening in their family and who are unable to discuss it with their parents or other close family members can sometimes find it useful to talk to a member of the extended family such as grandparents, aunts or uncles.

Children affected by the genetic condition

Children we have spoken to describe a wide range of experiences. Many children resent being affected by the genetic condition but even from a relatively young age they explained that they tried to make sure their illness was not the focus of their lives, only a part of it. The child or young person wanted to be included in family discussions about their illness and many wanted to make their own decisions about treatment and care from a relatively young age, usually from about 9 to 10 years depending on their developmental stage: occasionally it might be slightly older (Metcalfe *et al.*, 2011). The young people said their decision was usually guided by their parents' advice but having the choice made them more likely to comply with the treatments and recommendations of their parents and health professionals. Therefore there was an expectation that parents and health professionals will talk to children and young people in an age- and developmentally appropriate manner to explain the genetic condition and treatments (Metcalfe *et al.*, 2011).

Grandparents

Little work has taken place with grandparents' experiences generally. Grandparents can find understanding the genetic condition quite difficult and can want to challenge the diagnosis, and may want to try many alternative treatments. Grandparents will vary widely in the level of physical and psychological support they are able to offer parents and grandchildren but will also experience feelings of guilt and blame. If appropriate and parents agree, it can be very beneficial to work with grandparents as part of reviewing the family's ability to cope and adapt to living with the genetic condition as they can play a significant role in helping the family (or on occasion hindering it).

Trans-generational effects

Beliefs about family, health and disease will have been handed down across the generations, so even family members that have died may provide useful insights into how a family copes. For example, in clinics talking to families affected by a genetic condition a widely held belief is that a disease can 'skip' a generation and the family can wrongly believe that if a parent has the genetic condition, then their children will be free from it. This is of course untrue and there are likely to be several similar family 'myths' that whilst being very real to that family are actually falsehoods that have developed and handed down the generations. At other times family members assume that if you share the same physical characteristics as another family member, for example tall stature, then you will share the same hereditary disease, which of course is untrue unless the characteristic is actually part of the genetic condition. As a nurse you can work with the family to review these beliefs, and assist them in developing a better understanding or reframing the less useful notions.

Lifecycle model

From the cradle to the grave, families face many stressors related to the inherited genetic condition that affect how they experience their relationships and life transitions. Whilst it is not possible to go through all life transitions in detail here, by being open to discussion, and assessing the family before them, nurses and midwives can recognize which parts of the life-cycle are particularly pivotal for family relationships based on the history family members provide. (Rolland and Williams 2005 and Rolland 2006 provide detailed overviews).

Conception and birth

Prior to conception of a child, a person in a family affected by a genetic condition might consider attending genetic counselling to ascertain their risk of carrying the gene mutation. This may have consequences for the prospective parents' relationship. Undergoing genetic testing during pregnancy can affect the parents' relationship with their unborn child, which can result in them not bonding so closely initially (Downe *et al.*, 2009; Dheensa *et al.*, 2013) and potentially has repercussions once the child is born.

Irrespective of whether parents have a child who is affected or unaffected by the genetic condition, the parents often report feelings of guilt and stigma. Parents' blame themselves if their child is affected but equally parents whose child is unaffected may feel guilty because their child is well but their sibling's child is not.

Childhood and adolescence

Many children and young people describe experiencing difficulties talking to their parents and asking them questions, so that from the age of eight years they learn to stay silent about the genetic condition (Metcalfe *et al.*, 2008). Therefore, nurses working with families may need to assist and support parents in talking to their children and explainingthe genetic condition in developmentally appropriate terms. Giving parents the reassurance and confidence to talk to their children can significantly enhance family relationships because parents will often have experienced secrecy surrounding the condition during their own childhood. Parents who discuss the genetic condition usually have stronger relationships with their children, and this makes the family more resilient (SPRinG Collaborative 2015).

Adulthood

In adulthood parents are caring for each other if one of them is affected by the genetic condition, and they may also be caring for grandparents and children affected by the condition. Therefore parents may experience significant pressures from three generations requiring care. Nurses and midwives will need to observe the many ethical dilemmas an adult might be facing, including reproductive choices, care decisions and their own health screening when faced with the genetic condition. There are also many ethical dilemmas faced by health professionals in caring for families affected, not least not divulging information from one family member to another by assuming a shared history may represent a shared view.

End of Life

Grief and bereavement significantly affecting families is one the biggest problems we observed for those affected by life-limiting and life-threatening genetic conditions. There has been little research into the area but we do know that if people die at what is perceived as a relatively young age or if there are multiple deaths within a short space of time in one family, this can cause complicated grief reactions. With many genetic conditions there are often multiple deaths in one generation *and* the people dying are considered relatively young for death to occur. It is not unusual to observe some very complex grief reactions within the family (Sobel and Cowan 2003; Lillie *et al.*, 2011; Metcalfe *et al.*, 2010; 2011).

As you can observe, each family member will be at a different life stages. Therefore assisting families in recognizing different members' needs when they are under pressure requires skilled health professionals who can make the difference between assisting a family to adapt and cope, or to break apart. Often it is nurses and midwives who will come into closest contact with the family, which means they need the skills to facilitate the communication required to ensure the family adapts and copes.

Summary

Nurses and midwives have a pivotal role to play in providing family-centred care. Even if not all the family members are physically present, the effects of family relationships will be present in every single patient that you meet. As such it is important to always bear in mind how the family members at different life stages might be coping with and adapting to the situation. Anne's story provided some insights into the struggles faced by many families affected by inherited genetic conditions but further reading as recommended below can assist in developing these perspectives and insights further.

Increasing use of genetic risk information following the sequencing of the human genome will necessitate better consideration and care of the wider family. More family-focused healthcare will also lead to better health and social outcomes for a wide range of health problems. Families that have healthy and well-functioning relationships are more likely to have a better quality of life, and fewer mental or physical health problems. People in strong caring relationships are also more likely to care for each other when they become ill or infirm due to the genetic condition, or age and frailty. Families, in whatever form or shape they take, are therefore worthy of care and assistance, and as nurses and midwives we have a duty to provide this if we wish to contribute to a flourishing society that values all its members.

Acknowledgements

A special thank you to Anne for sharing her story. Obviously all names are pseudonyms and her genome/family history has been disguised too.

Useful resources

Telling stories – National NHS Genetics Education Centre www.tellingstories.nhs.uk/
100,000 Genomes Online Education Resource https://www.genomicseducation.hee.nhs.uk/

References

Bateson, G. and Ruesch, J. (1951) *Communication: The Social Matrix of Psychiatry.* New York: Norton.

Biesecker, B. and Erby, L. (2008) Adaptation to living with a genetic condition or risk: a mini-review, *Clinical Genetics*, 74: 401–7.

DeGenova, M.K. and Rice, F.P. (2002) *Intimate Relationships, Marriages and Families*, 5th edn. Boston, MA: McGraw Hill.

Dheensa, S., Metcalfe, A. and Williams, R. (2012) Men's experiences of antenatal screening: a meta-synthesis of the qualitative research, *International Journal of Nursing Studies*, 06/2012. DOI:10.1016/j.ijnurstu.2012.05.004

Dheensa, S., Williams, R. and Metcalfe, A. (2013) Shattered schemata and fragmented identities: men's experiences of antenatal genetic screening in Great Britain, *Journal of Family Issues*, 34(8) 1081–103. DOI 10.1177/0192513X13484274

Downe, S., Finlayson, K., Walsh, D. and Lavender, T. (2009) Weighing up and balancing out': a meta-synthesis of barriers to antenatal care for marginalised women in high-income countries, *British Journal of Obstetrics and Gynaecology*, 116(4): 518–29.

Genetic Alliance UK (2015) Available at: www.geneticalliance.org.uk/education3.htm Accessed 25 September 2015.

Koerner, A.F. and Fitzpatrick, M.A. (2002) Towards a theory of family communication, *Communication Theory*, 12: 70–91.

Lillie, A.K., Metcalfe, A. and Clifford, C. (2011) The missing agenda: caring for patients with a family history of cancer, *Palliative Medicine*, 25(2): 117–24. DOI: 0269216310383738.

Metcalfe, A., Pumphrey, R. and Clifford, C. (2010) Hospice nurses and genetics: implications for end of life care, *Journal of Clinical Nursing*, 19: 192–207.

Metcalfe, A., Coad, J., Plumridge, G. *et al.* (2008) Family communication between children and their parents about inherited genetic conditions: a meta-synthesis of the research, *European Journal Human Genetics*, 16: 1193–1200.

Metcalfe, A., Plumridge, G., Coad, J.*et al.* (2011) Parents' and children's communication about genetic risk: qualitative study learning from families' experiences, *European Journal Human Genetics*, 19(6): 640–6. DOI:10.1038/ejhg.2010.258.

Minuchin, S. (1974) *Families and Family Therapy.* Harvard, MA: University Press.

Plumridge, G., Metcalfe, A., Coad, J. and Gill, P. (2010) Family communication about genetic risk information: particular issues for Duchenne muscular dystrophy, *American Journal of Medical Genetics Part A*, 152A(5): 1225–32.

Plumridge, G., Metcalfe, A., Coad, J. and Gill, P. (2011) Parents' communication with siblings of children affected by an inherited genetic condition, *Journal of Genetic Counselling*, 20(4): 374–83.

Rolland, J.S. (2006) Genetics, family systems, and multicultural influences, *Family Systems Health*, 24: 425.

Rolland, J.S. and Williams, J.K. (2005) Toward a biopsychosocial model for 21st-century genetics, *Family Process*, 44: 3–24.

Rowland, E. and Metcalfe, A. (2013) Communicating inherited genetic risk between parent and child: a meta-thematic synthesis, *International Journal of Nursing Studies*, 50: 870–80. DOI.org/10.1016/j.ijnurstu.2012.09.002

Rowland, E. and Metcalfe, A. (2014) A systematic review of men's experiences of their partner's mastectomy: coping with altered bodies, *Psycho-oncology*. DOI: 10.1002/pon.3556

Skirton, H. and Patch, C. (2009) *Genetics for Health Sciences*. Oxford: Scion Publishing.

Sobel, S. and Cowan, C.B. (2003) Ambiguous loss and disenfranchised grief: the impact of DNA predictive testing on the family as a system, *Family Process*, 42: 47–57.

SPRinG (Socio-psychological Research in Genetics) Collaborative (2015) Developing an intervention to facilitate family communication about inherited genetic conditions, and training genetic counselors in its delivery, *European Journal of Human Genetics*.

Williams, R.A., Dheensa, S. and Metcalfe, A. (2011) Men's involvement in antenatal screening: a qualitative pilot study using e-mail, *Midwifery*, 27: 861–6.

Person-centred approaches for people with long-term mental health problems

Ian P.S. Noonan

Introduction

This chapter will explore the core values that underpin a person-centred approach to working with people who have long-term mental health problems. The emphasis will be on adapting models of and approaches to person-centred mental health care to different stages in a person's recovery from, or life with, a long-term mental illness. In order to adapt how we work with people during transition from an acute phase of illness in to recovery, during recovery, whilst maintaining wellness and during relapse it will be proposed that it is our responsibility as practitioners to be flexible, to fulfil different roles in the relationship and to respond to the person's needs rather than expect the person with mental illness to fit in with prescribed professional roles and teams. This will require the reader to accept two things: first, that healthcare services exist within complex systems and that it may be a challenge to adapt some of these principles to the context in which they work; and second, that the therapeutic relationship is fundamental to all of our work with people with long-term mental health problems. We must first invest in the relationship with our clients so that any of the models or organizational frameworks might be employed effectively.

In order to have the chapter centred on the experience of people with long-term mental health problems, it is illustrated by a letter from Jonathan, a service user with schizoaffective disorder. It is a reasonable critique of service user involvement that one or two voices do not represent the experience of all and that it is not possible to generalize from the narratives of, in this case, Jonathan, and to translate his experience to others. However, there is power in his narrative and as you will see below, Jonathan acknowledges "'I can only tell you what

I need and this may be different from the next person, but at least it is a start.' His narrative will be used to link theory to practice and to explore different approaches to PCC.

Hitchen *et al.* (2009) identify the strong emotional content of service user experiences, power imbalances and both the difference and distance created by professional language barriers. Furthermore the principles identified in other studies exploring service user and carer needs in long-term mental health care, such as developing therapeutic relationships that share universal goals, respecting diverse needs, and encouraging recovery (Lloyd and Carson 2012), have a universality that is congruent with person-centred models such as Peplau's Interpersonal Model of Nursing (Peplau 1952), The Recovery Approach (Repper and Perkins 2003) and the Tidal Model (Barker and Buchanan-Barker 2005). Therefore Jonathan's contributions will be used both to capture something of his voice and narrative and to illustrate core principles within these person-centred approaches.

The learning aims of the chapter are in line with a relationship-based approach to mental health care. These are most clearly reflected in and have been modelled on the values of the Tidal Model applied to the principles of recovery (Barker and Buchanan-Barker 2005):

- to value the person's voice and make it central to the foundation of our therapeutic relationships with people with long-term mental health problems;
- to be able to adapt flexibly through transitions, in different stages of relationship, with people with long-term mental health problems by fulfilling different roles in the therapeutic relationship;
- to be able to structure creative and supportive work with people with long-term mental health problems and consider how this might be evaluated;
- to maintain therapeutic optimism in our work with people with long-term mental health problems and work hopefully, with a future focus 'crafting the step beyond';
- to support people and their carers if relapse occurs and reflect on how to maintain the therapeutic relationship in a return to an acute phase of illness.

Developing PCC in practice

Person- or client-centred approaches are core to most mental health nursing models. In an increasingly consumerist healthcare system, this term has come to mean more than the value that underpins our work, or the assumption that people have the resources within them to recover, and includes the organization and political context of care delivery. De Silva (2014: 2) defines it as follows:

A person-centred health system is one that supports people to make informed decisions about, and to successfully manage, their own health and care, able to make informed decisions and choose when to invite others to act on their behalf. This requires healthcare services to work in partnership to deliver care responsive to people's individual abilities, preferences, lifestyles and goals.

However, we need to focus on the therapeutic relationship in practice in order to avoid PCC being merely rhetoric to describe our intent in service organization. This chapter will therefore, focus on the interpersonal skills, values and theories that support working in partnership, responding to clients' transitions and helping to shape their goals.

Jonathan

Jonathan is a former teacher who now works as an administrative assistant in a bank in London. Soon after he started a new teaching job in his early 20s, he became mentally unwell and was diagnosed with a condition called schizoaffective disorder. He was experiencing very unusual thoughts, heard voices that no one else could hear and also felt more excited and high in mood. He heard what his students were thinking about him and the bad things that they thought about him. He has been admitted to hospital on four occasions to a specialist unit for early onset psychosis. Now in his late 30s, he is well and continuing to receive treatment and support from a community mental health team.

Jonathan has used both his teaching experience and first-hand knowledge of mental illness to help with some ideas for our curriculum review and development, and is keen that future nurses have a good understanding of how he perceives his needs. In order to do this, he has written a letter addressed to you as a potential future carer for him.

Jonathan has given his permission for his letter to be used in this book, but has chosen not to use his full name. When asked how he would like to be acknowledged in the chapter, he chose 'Jonathan: banker, lover, artist, living with schizoaffective disorder'.

Jonathan's letter

Dear Future Nurse

It feels odd to be writing a letter to a stranger, or even lots of strangers, but that is where we all start off in mental health. When you meet your first patient, you are strangers to each other and it is really important that you don't assume to know this person and that you don't assume that they will trust you. This all takes time, but if we don't get to know each other, if we don't want to know each other, then nothing else – the drugs; the therapy; the social stuff, just won't work.

So, hello – I'm Jonathan and you are someone who might be my future mental health nurse; nice to meet you! There, we've started the ball rolling. Thank you for wanting to be my nurse – we do need you. I need you. Even though I may not always express it that clearly. You have chosen something that I imagine is hard work but I doubt is ever as hard as being ill. . .

I have been asked to write to you to explain what it is I need from a mental health nurse and it is really hard to answer. Sometimes I need to be left alone and at others, listened to. Sometimes I need to just be believed and at others, challenged. Sometimes I need someone to make decisions for me (like to come in to hospital before it's too late), and at other times to respect the decisions I make for and about myself. So, ultimately – I need a nurse who can tell the difference between each of these times and who is flexible enough to adapt and to keep on trying.

I need a nurse who is open to me. Someone who accepts me as I am, where I am and is willing to work on what I want to work on. I don't need someone to tell me what I'm doing wrong – I do that enough to myself. I need a nurse with imagination:

Imagination to think, consider, try to feel what it is like to be woken up at night by a voice warning me that one of my neighbours has broken in and wants to kill me.

Imagination to wonder – how I cope, how I survive, to be interested in my story, not interested in what has gone wrong, but how I exist in amongst all of that chaos.

Imagination to see possibilities – what I can achieve, how I can achieve it, to be hopeful, to have fun working with me and to enjoy moving each step forward.

There are of course, some things I don't want you to imagine.

You need to know the law so you can protect my rights; know about the side effects of medication so you can help me choose what is right for me; know how to work with someone who is distressed and not give up on them and know how to manage yourself – it's not my fault if you've had a bad day or don't want to be at work – you are paid to be here and get to go home at the end of the day.

I hope this works out well for you and thank you for reading my letter. I can only tell you what I need and this may be different from the next person, but at least it is a start. If you have got to the end of this and still think it is for you – then best of luck!
Jonathan.

Reader activity

Having read Jonathan's letter, take some time to notice your response to what he asks for. Start by just noticing what you think and feel about what he has said. Then try to answer the following questions:

What does Jonathan suggest is needed before any treatment can work?

What different things does Jonathan want you to be able to a) imagine? b) know?

Jonathan describes some things he wants from a nurse that conflict with each other. Does this mean he is changing his mind or is unclear about what he wants?

What can you identify in Jonathan's letter that suggests he may have had difficult relationships with, or felt criticized by carers in the past?

How would you summarize Jonathan's overall message? You could acknowledge this by writing a reply to him, imagining you are being asked to care for him, to show that you have understood his letter to you.

Getting to know you – engagement is the key

In his letter, Jonathan challenges us not to assume that we either know the person we are working with or that they will automatically trust us. This echoes the principles of engagement outlined by Ryan and Morgan (2004) who propose that engagement underpins everything that we do. They suggest that 'without meaningful engagement we have nothing' (p.139). In order to get to know each other and to build the trust which Jonathan suggests is required we need to apply some key theoretical principles that explain the concept of therapeutic relationships. Horvath (2001) explains that the therapeutic relationship in counselling or helping relationships is founded in the psychodynamic phenomena outlined by Freud and others. Interpersonal dynamics fuel the processes of transference and countertransference, create resistance in relationships and can lead to the development of an alliance between the client and therapist or patient and nurse. However, it is not our role or intention in nursing to analyse the patient, but rather to be aware of the impact of these processes on the formulation of our relationship with them. Horvath (2001) suggests that the development of the concept of therapeutic relationship can be traced through the work of Carl Rogers in a humanistic approach to person-centred counselling. The qualities of a therapeutic relationship in this approach are as follows:

- Special, accepting, empathic and genuine relationship at the core of the healing process.
- All other aspects required (to heal or recover) are found within the client.
- People are unique, creative, responsible and need to make choices with a tendency to self-actualize.

These tenets seem particularly closely aligned to what Jonathan is asking for. In addition to not assuming that you know him or that he trusts you, he also states, 'I need a nurse who is open to me. Someone who accepts me as I am, where I am and is willing to work on what I want to work on. I don't need someone to tell me what I'm doing wrong – I do that enough to myself.' It seems clear that Jonathan is asking for us to take a humanistic approach to our relationship with him: to accept him unconditionally.

What are transference and countertransference and why are they relevant to nursing?

The terms transference and countertransference come from a psychodynamic or psychoanalytic approach to therapy and they explain unconscious processes that impact on the formulation, quality and maintenance of relationships between a client and their therapist. Transference means that the client responds to the therapist in a way that communicates something of how they feel and think about someone else in their lives, of whom the therapist reminds them. The client may not be aware of this connection and it may not be anything as obvious as a physical resemblance, but rather they are reminded of a core feeling or belief about the role the therapist may represent, in that moment in time, in their therapy. In psychotherapy, the therapist may also experience an unconscious response to the client feeling anxiety, hope, frustration or even desire for the client. This unconscious process from the therapist to the client is countertransference. In some types of therapy a distinction is made between the unconscious, *personal* countertransference (which the therapist addresses in their own therapy and supervision) and *diagnostic* transference of which the therapist is aware and may explore or even respond in the role in which the client sees them so that the client can address unresolved issues that relate to the person or role of whom they are reminded.

So, why is this relevant to nursing? When we first meet someone, there can either be a seemingly instant connection or distance between us. The people we work with may well have had invalidating experiences in their past from their families, in other relationships, and from other mental health professionals. This can obviously impact on the formation of the trust between us, that Jonathan acknowledges is required but should not be assumed. It is not our role to exploit personal or diagnostic countertransference, but these concepts may help us to understand that we need to adapt, be flexible and work through any initial hostility or disinterest someone may have about working with us. Equally, we need to ensure that when there seems some sort of instant alliance or attraction we remain aware of the purpose and intent of our therapeutic relationship so that we are able to recognize our similarities and differences; accept the person's response to us; and build a working relationship so that we are in a position to help the client. This may involve us noticing our own irritation or pleasure in being disliked or liked by someone so that we can manage *ourselves*, our own personal countertransference (rather than exploit or use diagnostic countertransference) to help us continue being with the client and open to them. We need to understand the concept of countertransference in order to manage ourselves and our own reactions to the client within a person-centred therapeutic relationship. These concepts underpin Peplau's Interpersonal Relations Theory model of nursing.

Peplau: Interpersonal Relations Theory

Peplau (1952) viewed the process of nursing in different stages or phases of relationship: orientation, identification, exploitation and resolution. These stages are usually presented as linear: we move from orientation to identification and so on. It may be more helpful to think of them as inter-related and progressive. If, for example the exploitation stage is not working well, it may be that we neither have identified a truly shared goal nor genuinely engaged the client in their care. Whilst working forward through the stages of her model, we may have to be mindful of needing to step back.

Orientation is when we engage the client in a therapeutic relationship with us. We need to make efforts to get to know them, acknowledge that we are strangers, facilitate building trust by acting as a resource, answering questions, being available. Once we have come to know and trust each other, specific things that client may want to work on can be identified.

Identification starts to occur when the client is able to express how they feel and what they want. They may demonstrate more independence in the relationship alongside a willingness to work with you. If you have established a trusting working relationship they will be able to identify what is important to them. The reason someone needs to trust you to do this is that by identifying something they want to work on, they are also revealing something in their life that is currently a problem or that they are unhappy with. Clients need to trust us to be able to take this risk.

Exploitation is neither about us nor the client exploiting each other, but about being able to exploit or use the relationship and resources available to achieve what they want: To use the trust they have established, and the security of a therapeutic relationship, to risk trying something new and to try out whatever interventions you may have agreed upon. It is a phase where the client is working, with our support.

Resolution marks the end of the therapeutic relationship. If the client is able to work independently and use their own resources to address future stresses and strains, our relationship with them is no longer needed.

Getting to know you – *again*: transitions in long-term mental healthcare

In long-term PCC we may need to think about these phases as both a model for working on specific problems or goals identified by the client and as a longer arc spanning our therapeutic relationship and including relapse prevention work to shore up someone's coping strategies before the resolution phase. Different transitions in someone's recovery journey may require us to restart or refresh these processes as our clients get used to us in the context of different relationships.

When Jonathan was in hospital, his care plans often focused on getting 'well enough' to go home and he recalls feeling confused as to why that was a goal and what he would do when he got home. It may be more helpful to think of PCC as dynamic and fluid in response to the transitions experienced by the client rather than as progressive through any particular model. Schumacher and Meleis (1994) describe four types of transition: developmental; situational; health-illness and organizational. Each of these can be seen in the recovery journey of people with long-term mental health needs. Table 13.1 defines the different types of transition people may experience and gives an example of possible transitions in Jonathan's care.

These transitions require the individual to be able to make meaning of the anticipated transition, to be clear about their expectations and have the knowledge, skills and resources to be able to maintain emotional and physical wellbeing. Schumacher and Meleis (1994) go on to suggest that wellbeing of relationships is a key indicator of a healthy transition. It is therefore up to us to develop the skills required to adapt and 'get to know again' the person in our care even if that means rebuilding the relationship or renegotiating the focus of our goals in the identification stage.

Peplau suggested that we all have psycho-biological experiences which can lead to either constructive or destructive responses to each other (both the nurse and the client) or to situations in life. These psycho-biological experiences include: needs, frustration, conflict and anxiety. One way to think of these experiences is as the fuel that drives tension and change within the nursing relationship – a relationship in which Peplau views the nurse and client as partners, rather than the active nurse delivering care to the passive patient.

This tension can be seen in Jonathan's letter where he describes several continua of what he needs from a nurse (see Figure 13.1).

Jonathan challenges us to know the difference between these times and to be flexible enough to adapt. He is asking us to fulfil a number of different roles at different times rather than to adopt one fixed nursing role. This view illustrates Peplau's approach well. In 1952, Peplau wrote,

> the nursing process is educative and therapeutic when nurse and patient can come to know and to respect each other, as persons who are alike, and yet, different, as persons who share in the solution of problem . . . [and] the kind of person each nurse becomes makes a substantial difference to what each patient will learn as s/he is nursed throughout his/her experience with illness.

Table 13.1 Definitions and examples of transitions

Transition	Definition	Example
Developmental	Developmental transitions are typically described in terms of biological changes, like adolescence and becoming a parent, where there are both developmental and sociological changes in role	Jonathan's transition from adolescence to adulthood saw his first experience of mental illness. His transition from student to teacher felt overwhelming. This may leave him with anxiety about other transitions and guilt or regret that he was not able to stay in that role. We might assume that Jonathan would feel excited about developmental transitions which in fact leave him feeling frustrated or fearful
Situational	Situational transitions often involve changes in employment; in family relationships; or location	Jonathan has had several admissions to hospital and the way in which services are organized with separate community and inpatient teams means he is often experiencing situational transitions where he has to restart the process of engaging with different people and different teams
Health-Illness	Includes transitions from states of health to illness, and from illness to recovery as well as transitions between acute, primary and community care	This type of transition can be seen in Jonathan's various contacts with inpatient, home treatment and community mental health services as well as with his lifelong management of his illness. Within recovery, relapse may be anticipated and Jonathan may experience health to illness to health transitions in quick succession and within a longer recovery journey
Organizational	Transitions in the environment (rather than the intra-personal) and in the socio-political organization of care	Jonathan has seen firsthand the impact of financial cuts and reduced in-patient beds. He describes an anxiety that part of his relapse drill is to be able to identify when he might need to come in to hospital, but that if that happens, beds may not be available and he may be managed by the home treatment team instead

After Schumacher and Meleis (1994).

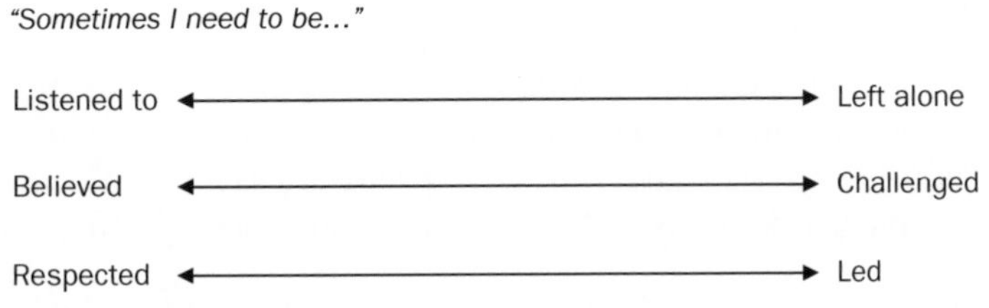

"Sometimes I need to be..."

Listened to ←———————————→ Left alone

Believed ←———————————→ Challenged

Respected ←———————————→ Led

Figure 13.1 Continuum of needs

This coming together in partnership, to know and respect each other, meets the 'orientation' stage of Peplau's model. As Jonathan observed, we are strangers and in order to fulfil the other roles suggested by Peplau (1952), we need to learn, through our clients and through our experience of nursing, how to switch between the different roles of:

- Stranger
- Resource person
- Teacher
- Leader
- Surrogate
- Counsellor

Although Peplau's theory was first published in the 1950s it still underpins person-centred practice today. Stockmann undertook an extended literature review to explore how interpersonal relations theory was being used in nursing practice in an attempt to answer whether Peplau was still relevant to mental health nursing practice. Largely based in Forchuk's work, Stockmann (2005) found the following:

- Clients perceived nurse attitude and the nature of nurse-client interactions as being the most influential on relationship progress.
- Clients described nurses as facilitating the movement of the relationship through their availability, consistency and trustworthy actions.
- Clients described closeness, genuine liking and trust, with the focus remaining on client needs as typical of the working phase.

Furthermore, the different roles are reflected in the Nurses in Society report (Maben and Griffiths 2008) which identified the role of nurses as practitioner, partner and leader.

Different types of relationship

It is clear that Jonathan is asking for us to be flexible and to recognize the times when we need to adopt different roles in order to establish and maintain different types of therapeutic relationship. Ellis and Day (2013) identify five characteristics of effective therapeutic relationships:

- Supportive
- Connected
- Facilitative
- Influential
- Purposeful

They go on to define engagement as 'the active and emotional involvement of a client in their care' and distinguish it from other forms of participation such as acceptance of or rejection or refusal of treatment (Ellis and Day 2013). These characteristics can variously be seen in the different types of relationships experienced by clients that fall short of a partnership relationship:

- The expert relationship – where the nurse is perceived by him/herself and/or the client as having some professional knowledge and insight;

- The friendship – often occurs in inpatient units where formal and informal time together blurs boundaries;
- The dependent relationship – nurse takes on excessive responsibility; acts on behalf of the client;
- The adversarial relationship – characterized by antagonism and hostility; overt or covert disagreement; inability to reconcile differences;
- The avoidant relationship – emotional and intellectual detachment; distant and uninvolved (Ellis and Day 2013).

A partnership relationship is characterized by:

- the nurse and client having opportunity to discuss openly and mutually agree aims and purpose;
- the opportunity to identify, negotiate and explicitly resolve difficulties and conflicts;
- shared processes respect complementary roles, expertise and knowledge;
- mutual trust and respect;
- active and ongoing commitment.

It is possible to cross reference the different types of relationship and the characteristics of effective therapeutic relationships proposed by Ellis and Day (2013) to identify which types support which therapeutic aims (see Table 13.2).

In Jonathan's letter, he explains that he needs a nurse who can tell the difference between his different needs and role in the relationship, and who can adapt to these needs. One way to think about adaptation is to consider where you and the client are on a helping continuum in order to know whether you should take a leading 'expert' type role or work with the client as expert in their care (see Fig. 13.2).

Table 13.2 Characteristics and types of therapeutic relationship

	Supportive	Connected	Facilitative	Influential	Purposeful
Expert	X	X	X	✓	✓
Friendship	✓	✓	X	X	X
Dependent	X	X	X	✓	✓
Adversarial	X	X	X	X	✓
Avoidant	X	X	X	X	X
Partnership	✓	✓	✓	✓	✓

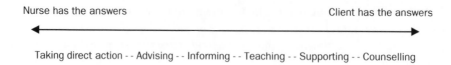

Figure 13.2 Continuum of helping relationships

The issue of choice

Weinstein (2009) provides a thoughtful summary of the debates about choice in mental health-care. On the one hand individual service users and service user groups have made consistent requests for choice in terms of 24-hour crisis services, greater access to talking therapies, advance care directives and increased help with things that risk or contribute to social exclusion; and on the other, there are moral and philosophical questions about an individual's autonomy, or ability to action their choices; when they may be detained or treated against their will; questions over funding of services which vary across the country; and even questions about how individual practitioners promote one intervention over another for reasons of available expertise, experience or convenience (Weinstein 2009). Whilst there is a clear policy agenda to promote choice (DH 2000; Care Services Improvement Partnership 2006), there is a risk that a misinterpretation of the principles of choice enshrined in the Recovery approach (Repper and Perkins 2003) and Tidal model (Barker and Buchanan-Barker 2005), may lead to a tokenistic view or application of patient choice – we record choices that are made by default and only allow choice over issues that are less significant. However, if we accept Jonathan's challenges, shown below in Table 13.3 mapped against the core principles of recovery and the Tidal model, there is a way in which we can deliver PCC that shifts between being directive and facilitative.

So Jonathan's choice is to have his opinion and experience recognized and accepted; to have someone work with him with hope and imagination; to be included, empowered, recognized as an individual and given time and possibility within a secure relationship. This doesn't mean however that he always wants to lead his care. Part of his expertise is his recognition that 'Sometimes I need someone to make decisions for me (like to come in to hospital before it's too late), and at other times to respect the decisions I make for and about myself'. He asks us, at times, to be directive. This need not mean he has no choice and his care can still be carried out in a person-centred way. John Heron's (2009) work *Helping the Client* explains the different types of facilitative and directive interventions we might try in order to adapt to: the direction the client wants and the place on the helping continuum that the client finds themselves with their current problem or goal.

Heron's six-category intervention analysis

In order to be able to understand whether or not we are getting this right, we need to examine both the intent and outcome of our therapeutic interactions. Heron (2001) devised a conceptual framework to help us analyse our intent in any verbal and/or non-verbal communication that is part of our work with and for our clients. The forms of intervention can be therapeutic (or valid), degenerate or perverted. Degenerate interventions are ones which are misguided

Table 13.3 Jonathan's narrative and the Recovery and Tidal Models

Jonathan's narrative	Recovery model principles	Tidal model commitments
This all takes time, but if we don't get to know each other, if we don't want to know each other, then nothing else – the drugs; the therapy; the social stuff, just won't work.	Secure base	Give the gift of time
Imagination to see possibilities – what I can achieve, how I can achieve it, to be hopeful, to have fun working with me and to enjoy moving each step forward.	Hope	Craft "the step beyond", Know that change is constant
I need a nurse who is open to me. Someone who accepts me as I am, where I am and is willing to work on what I want to work on. I don't need someone to tell me what I'm doing wrong – I do that enough to myself.	Self	Value the voice, Respect the language
You need to know the law so you can protect my rights; know about the side effects of medication so you can help me choose what is right for me; know how to work with someone who is distressed and not give up on them and know how to manage yourself – it's not my fault if you've had a bad day or don't want to be at work – you are paid to be here and get to go home at the end of the day.	Supportive relationships	Develop genuine curiosity, Be transparent
Thank you for wanting to be my nurse – we do need you. I need you. Even though I may not always express it that clearly. You have chosen something that I imagine is hard work but I doubt is ever as hard as being ill. . .	Empowerment and inclusion	Become the apprentice
I need a nurse with imagination. Imagination to wonder – how I cope, how I survive, to be interested in my story, not interested in what has gone wrong, but how I exist in amongst all of that chaos.	Coping strategies	Use the available toolkit
Sometimes I need to be left alone and at others, listened too. Sometimes I need to just be believed and at others, challenged. Sometimes I need someone to make decisions for me (like to come in to hospital before it's too late), and at other times to respect the decisions I make for and about myself. So, ultimately – I need a nurse who can tell the difference between each of these times and who is flexible enough to adapt and to keep on trying.	Meaning	Reveal personal wisdom

and lack both awareness and experience. Perverted interventions are inappropriate, deliberate and malicious attempts to harm someone, leaving them distressed (Heron 2009). In order to fulfil the different roles identified by Peplau, and shift between different parts of the helping continuum, above, we need to develop an awareness of, and ability to shift between, the following valid classes of therapeutic intervention.

Authoritative Interventions

These are:

- **Prescriptive.** You explicitly direct the person you are helping by giving advice and direction.
- **Informative.** You provide information to instruct and guide the other person.
- **Confronting.** You challenge the other person's behaviour or attitude. Not to be confused with aggressive confrontation, "confronting" is positive and constructive. It helps the other person consider behaviour and attitudes of which they might otherwise be unaware.

Facilitative Interventions

These are:

- **Cathartic.** You help the other person to express and overcome thoughts or emotions that they have not previously confronted.
- **Catalytic.** You help the other person reflect, discover and learn for themselves. This helps them become more self-directed in making decisions, solving problems and so on.
- **Supportive.** You build up the confidence of the other person by focusing on their competences, qualities and achievements.

Reader activity

The aim of this exercise is to broaden your range of approaches, responses and interventions so that you have a wider choice of ways of working within a person-centred approach.

Using Jonathan's narrative and the helping continuum, identify different times when he is looking for the nurse to take responsibility and when he wants to take the lead.

Choose an example of each and explore how you might respond in a prescriptive; informative; confronting; cathartic; catalytic and supportive way.

Then try to think how you might fulfil each of Peplau's roles in your work with Jonathan: stranger; resource person; teacher; leader; surrogate and counsellor.

Once you have identified an example of each type of intervention and each type of role, think why each one might be more or less acceptable and helpful for Jonathan.

How do we know if we are getting it right?

So far this chapter has explored ways in which we can engage with people who need long-term mental healthcare. It has been suggested that we need to adapt to different roles and different phases in the relationship in order to help support people through transitions from acute to community care and with their recovery journey. Furthermore, different forms and categories of intervention have been suggested so that we can responsively shift along the helping continuum in order to keep the client at the centre of what we do. Jonathan states that he needs a nurse who is able to tell the difference between the times when he wants a support-ive and directive approach to his care. So, now that we have a broad range of possibilities, how do we know if we are getting it right? In short, we can ask our clients, but there are also structured models that may help measure whether our care is person centred.

The Mental Health Foundation (2012) has devised a checklist of good practice devised in collaboration with service users. Eighty-one service users who had direct experience of the Care Programme Approach, contributed to the study and suggested a number of ways in which they would know that care is client centred and promotes recovery. In order to assess whether you are working in a person-centred way, ask yourself if you are doing the following:

1   Drawing on service users' personal descriptions of recovery?
2   Taking special account, too, of recovery concepts that service users from particu-larly disadvantaged groups and communities find meaningful and valid?
3   Helping service users to find the ways of understanding mental distress that make most sense to them, rather than offering medical explanations alone?
4   Putting as much emphasis on the warm, human qualities that service users want from professionals as on skills and knowledge that service users find support their recovery?
5   Recognizing in practice that medical treatment is useful only insofar as it assists service users with leading lives that they find meaningful and offering treatment accordingly?
6   Employing the full range of holistic approaches that are important to a particular service user?
7   Allowing for drawbacks that set recovery tools can have and varying tools to meet differing service user wishes?
8   Having adequate discussion with service users when medication is prescribed, acknowledging service users' concerns about distressing side effects and working actively with service users to keep these to a level that service users find acceptable?
9   Tackling any staff discrimination towards people with mental health problems, including the additional discrimination which may be experienced by service users from marginalized groups and communities?
10 Helping service users to feel safe, whilst avoiding a focus on risk that service users say is counterproductive to recovery?
11 Making active use of positive risk-taking?
12 Addressing the tension highlighted by a number of service users: between the use of compulsion under the Mental Health Act 2007 and the exercise of choice, control and citizen rights that is fundamental to most service users' concepts of recovery?

Table 13.4 Types of measurement of person-centred care

Type of measurement	Quality assessed
Examining how patients or professionals define the components of person-centred care	Definitions of person-centred care
Examining the type of care that patients want or professionals' attitudes and values	Preferences
Examining the extent to which care feels person centred	Experiences of person-centred care
Examining what happens as a result of person-centred care	Outcomes

Source: De Silva (2014).

13 Making sure that service users have involvement, influence and control in relation to their individual care plans?

14 Acknowledging peer support in practice when service users find that this helps to promote their recovery?

15 Providing opportunities for service users to influence the Care Programme Approach at a strategic level?

16 Employing resources as effectively as possible by listening to service users' expertise about useful recovery services, not to professionals alone, and by providing consistent and reliable support? (Mental Health Foundation 2012: 2)

There are a large number of tools available to measure whether care is person-centred at a personal, interpersonal and organizational level. De Silva (2014) has concluded that these fall broadly into three categories: surveys and interviews with people using health services; surveys of clinicians and observation of clinical encounters. Table 13.4 shows the different types of measurement and the aspect of PCC on which they focus.

Reader activity

Read De Silva's report *Helping Measure Person-centred Care* (De Silva 2014) available on the Health Foundation website http://www.health.org.uk/

Consider which tool assessing PCC might best fit your practice area. Think how you might introduce measurement of PCC preferences, experiences and outcomes in your field of practice.

Summary

This chapter has explored the interpersonal skills required to maintain flexible, person-centred engagement with people with long-term mental illnesses. We are required to adapt our practice in order to support people through the transitions from acute to community care, community to recovery, through relapse and onward with their recovery journey. To do this we need to be able to recognize what type of relationship and help the client wants and to be able to shift between facilitative and authoritative interventions. We also need to be mindful of how we know whether we are getting this right, and this can be achieved by reflecting on checklists or more formally measuring the experience, preferences and outcomes for people in our care.

References

Barker, P. and Buchanan-Barker, P. (2005) *The Tidal Model: A Guide for Mental Health Professionals*. London and New York: Brunner-Routledge.

Care Services Improvement Partnership (2006) *10 High Impact Changes for Mental Health Services*. London: CSIP. www.comfirst.org.uk/files/nimhe_10_high_impact_changes_.pdf (accessed 2 November 2015).

De Silva, D. (2014) *Helping Measure Person-centred Care: A Review of Evidence about Commonly Used Approaches and Tools Used to Help Measure Person-centred Care*. London: The Health Foundation.

DH (Department of Health) (2000) *Working in Partnership: Consumers in Research – Third Annual Report*. London: DH.

Ellis, M. and Day, C. (2013) Engaging clients in their care and treatment, in I. Norman and I. Ryrie (eds) *The Art and Science of Mental Health Nursing: A Textbook of Principles and Practice*, 3rd edn. Maidenhead: Open University Press.

Heron, J. (2009) *Helping the Client: A Creative Practical Guide*, 5th edn. London: Sage.

Hitchen, S., Watkins, M., Williamson, G. R., Ambury, S., Bemrose, G., Cook, D. and Taylor, M. (2009) Lone voices have an emotional content: focussing on mental health service user and carer involvement, *International Journal of Health Care Quality Assurance* 24, 164-177.

Horvath, A. O. (2001) The alliance, *Psychotherapy: Theory, Research, Practice*, Training, 38(4): 365–72.

Lloyd, M. and Carson, A. M. (2012) Critical conversations: developing a methodology for service user involvement in mental health nursing, *Nurse Education Today*, 32: 151–5.

Maben, J. and Griffiths, P. (2008) *Nurses in Society: Starting the Debate*. London: National Nursing Research Unit, King's College London.

Mental Health Foundation (2012) A Checklist of Good Practice from Service Users: The Care Programme Approach and Recovery. London: Mental Health Foundation. www.mental-health.org.uk/content/assets/PDF/publications/checklist-good-practice-approaches-recovery.pdf (accessed 6 November 2015).

Peplau, H. E. (1952) *Interpersonal Relations in Nursing*. New York: G. P. Putnam and Sons.

Repper, J. and Perkins, R. (2003) *Social Inclusion and Recovery*. London: Balliere Tindall.

Ryan, P. and Morgan, S. (2004) *Assertive Outreach: Strengths Approach to Policy and Practice.* London: Churchill Livingstone.

Schumacher, K. L. and Meleis, A. I. (1994) Transitions: a central concept in nursing, *IMAGE: Journal of Nursing Scholarship*, 26(2): 119–27.

Stockmann, C. (2005) A literature review of the progress of the psychiatric nurse-patient relationship as described by Peplau, *Issues in Mental Health Nursing*, 26(9): 111–19.

Weinstein, J. (2009) *Mental Health, Service User Involvement and Recovery.* London: Jessica Kingsley Publishers.

Chapter

14

Person-centred approaches in inpatient acute, emergency and intensive psychiatric care

Louise L. Clark and Jimmy Cangy

Introduction

This chapter will explore views of care and treatment from a person-centred patient perspective on acute psychiatric wards and psychiatric intensive care units (PICUs). These specialist services are where emergency, acute and intensive care is given to some of the most mentally unwell patients in an acute phase of illness. In both acute psychiatric wards and PICUs the common factor is that people are often detained against their will (under the Mental Health Act 2007), therefore providing the potential for problematic relationships between patient and nurse. This has an impact on care as the thoughts and feelings of the patient are not always considered especially regarding restrictive practices. This chapter will open with learning outcomes, a brief history and description of current service provision and then explore patient views and experiences of acute psychiatric wards and PICUs utilizing relevant literature and individual patients' comments. The chapter will conclude with recommendations to support the needs of patients and their families receiving care in these services.

LEARNING OUTCOMES

- To develop an understanding of the lived experience of being a patient on an acute mental health ward or PICU

> • To appreciate the need to reduce restrictive practices in order to improve patient care in these environments
> • To understand from patients' own accounts some of the long-term effects that may result from practices such as restraint, rapid tranquillization and seclusion
> • To appreciate the importance of individualized PCC in these clinical environments

A brief history

The traditional psychiatric system of asylums and certification of patients began a steady transformation in the 1960s. Often people diagnosed with a psychotic illness were said to have 'problems in living', being incarcerated for social rather than medical reasons.

The 'mental hospital' was an institution in which nurses attempted to defend themselves from stigma by social distancing from patients. Russell Barton (1976) formulated complex diagnostic criteria of physical and mental features displayed by long-term mental hospital residents which he termed 'institutional neurosis'; he attributed this to a depersonalizing regime and use of tranquillizing medication.

Mental health services have altered radically since the 1960s becoming more 'normalized' in the community with a less 'power-based' ethos. However, the ascendancy of the biomedical model of psychiatry has been reinforced by biological theories of mental disorder and the growing importance of modern medication. People who have mental health problems may lack an understanding of neurotransmitters, pharmacology and scientific methodology which can lead to feelings of exclusion, as their own wealth of experience and insights are not always considered as comprehensively as they could be by clinicians. Patient perceptions and understanding must therefore be at the forefront of therapeutic interventions and clinical practice.

The recovery approach and social inclusion

'Mind' is a charitable organization which gives support and advice to people experiencing mental health problems. It aims to improve mental health services, raise awareness and promote understanding. It has a long history in campaigning for the rights of the mentally ill; in 1986 an offshoot group known as 'Survivors Speak Out' was formed as advocates for the personal and collective rights of people with mental illness. The group's founding member Peter Campbell (in Repper and Perkins 2003) asserted that people with a diagnosis of mental illness have a contribution to make because of, and not in spite of, their life experiences. Campaigners have made major contributions towards a more positive attitude to mental illness and the service user perspective is now central to policy, research and clinical practice in the United Kingdom.

The recovery approach aims to empower people who have mental illness to develop a sense of identity, and to take responsibility for their lives rather than be mere recipients of services. The Sainsbury Centre's paper *Making Recovery a Reality* (Shepherd *et al.*, 2008) defined the meaning of recovery:

- Recovery is to engage in a meaningful and satisfying life, from the person's perspective, irrespective of mental health problems.
- It shifts the focus from pathology, illness and symptoms to the person and his/her strengths, goals and well-being.
- It emphasizes personal agency and self-management.
- Hope is the essence of recovery.
- Rather than assuming expertise and control, clinicians work with the person on a partnership basis.
- Recovery does not occur in isolation but relies on social inclusion.
- It promotes rediscovery of the self, separate from illness or disability.

Therefore, recovery recognizes the person as an individual expert travelling on their own unique journey. Promotion of social inclusion is at the core of this approach and the resourcefulness and views of the individual should be central to assessment, care planning, treatment and management processes, including risk assessment and its management.

The importance of families and social networks cannot be underestimated and a culturally sensitive approach is essential including sensitivity towards a diversity of views regarding mental illness.

Reader activity

With regard to a recovery approach consider some of the following situations that acutely ill patients may face:

Imagine what it would be like to be locked in a secure mental health unit against your will when you are at your most distressed and frightened.

How do you think it would feel to be physically held in a prone position on the floor by five nurses at the same time or secluded in a barely furnished locked room on your own? Would this add to your distress?

How would you react if you were forced to take medication against your will when you didn't know what it was for or what affect it would have on you?

The Mental Health and Social Exclusion Unit Report (2004) highlighted the fact that people with mental health problems are one of the most excluded groups in society. Exclusion has been attributed in some instances to stigma and subsequent discrimination towards people with mental health problems. The *National Service Framework for Mental Health* (DH 1999) called for Health and Social Services to tackle the stigma and discrimination experienced by

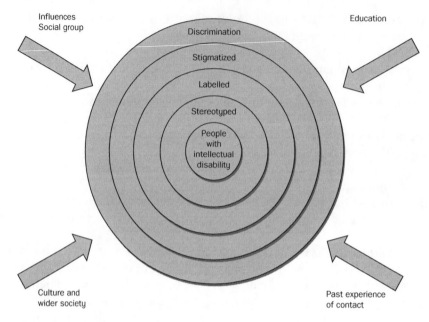

Figure 14.1 The origins of stigma and discrimination

people with mental health problems as this was seen as a barrier to positive mental health promotion and social inclusion.

Discrimination against people with mental health problems follows a pathway often underpinned by assumptions and fear of the unknown in addition to intolerance and exclusion of those who do not comply with social cohesion (Goffman 1963). The terminology and labelling (including diagnostic labelling) associated with the wide spectrum of conditions covered by the terms 'mental health' are often unhelpful and in turn lead to stereotyping whereby the individual is categorized and subsequently subject to the other person's knowledge base in this area, which may be positive or negative and is often dependent on previous exposure. Stigma and prejudice often occur when previous exposure to people with intellectual disabilities and/or mental health problems has been negative or absent (While and Clark 2009) (see Fig. 14.1).

Effective communication regarding mental illness is therefore essential if stigma and subsequent discrimination are to be prevented and social inclusion facilitated. Certain mental health conditions can be associated with stereotypes and prejudice; however, fear, aggression and dangerousness often dominate perceptions. Communication with people who have mental illness requires a person-centred approach in order to achieve optimum outcomes and should be aimed towards recovery and social inclusion from the outset. If there are shortfalls or omissions in communication between professionals this could result in substandard care for patients which ultimately may affect both short- and long-term goals in the recovery process.

What is acute, emergency and intensive psychiatric intensive care?

In the UK, the agenda for reduction of inpatient services was set out in the *National Service Framework for Mental Health* (DH 1999) and consequently Home Treatment teams (HTTs) were formed preventing many admissions to acute psychiatric services. Admission to hospital is determined by the HTTs who 'gatekeep' inpatient services and are influenced by risk and safety considerations, bed availability and what support the person has in the community.

A person may be admitted to hospital for assessment and/or treatment of a mental illness under the Mental Health Act (2007). The police can use section 136 of the Mental Health Act (2007) to take someone who appears to be suffering from a mental disorder from a public place to a 'place of safety'. The place of safety may be a special 136 suite within a psychiatric hospital, an accident and emergency department of a general hospital, or at a police station, a person may be conveyed from one place of safety to another under the Act. Detention under section 136 is for up to 72 hours and during this time mental health professionals will assess the person. Following assessment the person may be either free to go, sometimes with the support of HTTs or community mental health teams (CMHTs), or they may need to be admitted to hospital. This can be as an informal patient, or they may be detained under another section of the Mental Health Act (2007).

The majority of mental health care is now provided in the community and the number of inpatient beds continues to decrease. Acute psychiatric wards are reserved for the most vulnerable and seriously unwell (Health and Social Care Information Centre 2011) many of whom are detained under the Mental Health Act (2007). Acute psychiatric wards may be locked; even though not all patients are detained under the Mental Health Act (2007), inpatient services are still considered to be 'custodial' by many. People who are deemed to need closer supervision and more intensive care may need to be admitted to a PICU, however, this is generally only under extreme circumstances. Patients now admitted to inpatient services are therefore more acutely ill than ever before and some would argue that a large number of acute psychiatric wards resemble PICUs in many areas.

Psychiatric Intensive Units (PICUs)

The move away from closed to open wards in the 1970s benefitted the majority of patients (Crowhurst and Bowers 2002), however, concerns were raised about the minority of people whose acute mental health needs were not met on an open ward (Basson and Woodside 1981). The PICU was thought to be the solution to these issues, as the most severely unwell people could be nursed in a secure environment (Crowhurst and Bowers 2002).

Rachlin (1973) described the first locked psychiatric unit for patients in New York as a way of treating patients who did not respond to treatment or were more likely to abscond. Other authors reported the development of PICUs to treat people who were violent (Crain and Jordan, 1979), acutely severely mentally ill (Goldney et al., 1985) or suicidal (Warneke 1986). In the UK the first PICU was developed in Portsmouth in 1972 (Mounsey 1979) and treated patients referred from the rest of the hospital.

As PICUs have developed to match local needs there have been no objective criteria to describe the role of the PICU (Beer et al., 2008). However, certain characteristics of PICUs tend to be similar, and three core characteristics of a PICU have been identified:

- Patients are acutely disturbed with a loss of self-control, and subsequent increased risk that means they cannot be treated on an open ward. Additionally, more resources are required in order for a PICU to function effectively, these resources being both environmental and human (Beer *et al.*, 2008).

- PICU treatment needs to be patient centred, intensive, multi-disciplinary and to be able to respond swiftly (Pereira and Clinton 2002); the swift response to treatment is a key element of the PICU.
- The final characteristic concerns the need for staff to deliver care based on an agreed philosophy and one that is underpinned by risk assessment and management (Pereira and Clinton 2002).

Patients admitted to a PICU are most likely to have major psychosis, complex needs and to use illicit substances. PICU patients may range in age from 18 to quite elderly, however, a survey of patients in the 17 PICUs in London ($n = 172$) showed that 80 per cent were male with a mean age of 33, 50 per cent were black, 66 per cent had a diagnosis of schizophrenia and 55 per cent of admissions were due to physical aggression (Pereira *et al.*, 2005). Furthermore, patients are admitted to a PICU due to (1) risk to others; (2) risk of intentional harm to self; (3) risk of unintentional harm to self; (4) therapeutic benefit from the PICU environment; and (5) other problems in patient management in the acute care setting (Bowers *et al.*, 2003).

PICUs have an increasingly important role in the provision of care for people with acute mental health problems and often complex physical health issues which may complicate management of care. High quality assessment, treatment and proactive care of patients depend on a competent workforce that engages in continuous personal and professional development. In addition a person-centred bio-psycho-pharmaco-social approach to care (Clark and Clarke 2014) must be adopted throughout assessment and treatment which includes listening to the expert voice of the patient and involving them actively in all aspects of their care and treatment, especially care planning.

The management of acutely disturbed behaviour is a feature of PICUs and a wide variety of behaviours may present in a number of ways including threats or acts of violence, destruction of property, psychological distress, self-harm, verbal abuse, disorientation, confusion or extreme over-activity. Often disturbed behaviour is associated with the psychiatric problem; sometimes it may be the result of frustration through diminished communication or diagnostic over-shadowing, whereby signs and symptoms of a secondary condition are attributed to the primary condition and are not explored further.

High levels of nursing observations are performed on a PICU at varying degrees of intensity on each patient dependant on individualized risk assessment. Such supervision can cause distress and exacerbate behaviour if not carried out with skill and expertise by nurses; whilst engagement with the patient is essential this needs to happen without unnecessary intrusion. An advanced level of skill, knowledge and emotional intelligence is required by nurses in order to successfully maintain the therapeutic relationship without appearing 'custodial' to the patient.

De-escalation is a key factor in the prevention of serious incidents which could result in physical and emotional damage to either patients or staff if not handled with expertise. Advanced communication skills are essential in such situations and achieving the right balance of 'structure verses control' on a PICU is crucial; overly aggressive or power-based attitudes by staff will only result in confrontation, rapid tranquillization, restraint and/or seclusion, which should be avoided at all costs. Physical restraint and the use of seclusion can be distressing for all concerned and an extremely frightening, disempowering and humiliating experience for patients as described later in this chapter.

Restraint and seclusion in the management of psychiatric disorder can be traced back through the centuries. Seclusion, as defined by Needham and Sands (2010) involves the isolation of a patient in a room that they cannot freely exit. In recent decades the use of seclusion has fortunately been dramatically reduced: Beer *et al.* (1997) reported in a survey of PICUs ($n = 110$) that 40 per cent had no seclusion rooms.

A number of recent issues have been highlighted in the media regarding the use of physical restraint in healthcare settings including the *Mid Staffordshire NHS Public Inquiry* (2013) and the Winterbourne View scandal (DH 2012). Physical restraint is not defined in the Mental Health Act (2007) but guidance is given in the Code of Practice of the Act (DH 2008) explaining that it is a 'last resort' requiring adherence to hospital policy which must be in place regarding prevention, de-escalation, risk assessment/management, enhanced observation, physical intervention, rapid tranquillization and seclusion (DH 2008).

An insider view of inpatient care: admission and detention

Patients describe hospital as a place of safety (Gilburt *et al.*, 2008) and relief was expressed at having been admitted. Some patients especially articulated the relief of refuge from their own self-destruction (Thomas *et al.*, 2002). Patients see safety as a positive aspect of care although in some cases patients describe not feeling safe from other patients (Gilburt *et al.*, 2008).

Katsakou *et al.* (2012) explored involuntary patients' views retrospectively regarding their hospitalization, concluding that some patients view this positively saying that when acutely unwell they do not always recognize that they need help. In-depth, semi-structured interviews were conducted with 59 involuntary patients detained under the Mental Health Act (2007) in acute wards across 22 hospitals in England. Out of the total number of participants the majority expressed overall positive views of their detention and hospitalization ($n = 28$). However, most of this group ($n = 24$) initially considered their admission wrong but later changed their minds. Another group of participants ($n = 19$) continued to consider their admission 'wrong', whilst the third group always held negative views towards hospitalization ($n = 12$). One participant stated,' I was glad I was in hospital . . . I couldn't have been anywhere else at that time. . . I didn't think I was well enough to come out . . . I was scared of going out, frightened' (participant 27, p. 1177). Another said that, 'It went on for about a month, and then I said to God I'm going to kill someone soon . . . I'm glad I was (sectioned) in a way, 'cos I was, like collapsing down the street so I was glad I was picked up in a way' (participant 41, p. 1177).

Common themes emerged from the study (Katsakou *et al.*, 2012) which seemed to underpin participants' views of their detention including the knowledge that they were unwell or at risk before admission, feeling out of control during hospitalization, averting risk by being hospitalized and an unjust infringement of autonomy. One patient said, 'I needed to be sectioned because when I become high and elated it's very hard for me to recognize it myself. Probably at these times if I'd been able to take myself voluntarily then that would have been a better choice. But the problem is I'm not very good at going voluntarily . . . people talk about trigger factors, but I can only say I've never been really able to recognize that happening' (participant 13, p. 1177).

All participants with positive views (*n* = 28) believed that they needed to be admitted involuntarily as they were acutely unwell, most believing that medication was necessary. Of this group of participants 89 per cent retrospectively thought they had been a risk to themselves or others before being admitted. However, the same percentage (89 per cent) of the group with negative views (*n* = 19) stated that their involuntary hospitalization had a negative effect on their mental health. From this negative group 74 per cent considered their hospitalization an unnecessary disruption: 'I certainly didn't need to be sectioned. I was very anxious to get home, to find out where my dog was and get my business running. . .' (participant 40, p. 1174).

The most common themes regarding dissatisfaction by inpatients is detailed by Nolan *et al.* (2011) in their study of people who had previously been admitted (*n* = 44). Most dissatisfaction related to a lack of clarity regarding the aims of their admission (*n* = 16) and lack of involvement in the care planning process (*n* = 14). Tyson's study (2013) of mental health staff attitudes found that 100 per cent of participants thought that the admission process should involve giving the patient information as to why they had been brought to hospital and 48 per cent of them agreed that care plans were difficult to negotiate with patients in acute environments.

An insider view of inpatient care: environment and therapeutic perspectives

With regard to the physical environment some patients cited a lack of basic hygiene, old buildings and a lack of home comforts (Gilburt *et al.*, 2008). Patients' attitudes towards smoking and smoking areas were positive (Thomas *et al.*, 2002) and outside space was also prized (Gilburt *et al.*, 2008). One study investigated how mental health nurses could improve the inpatient experience. Patients said that they wanted meaningful activities whilst in hospital and would have preferred it if nurses spent more time with them and less time in the office (Brimblecombe *et al.*, 2007). Findings also showed that patients wanted to influence services and make decisions about their own care.

Structure and activities on acute inpatient wards are not highly rated by patients in the main with comments such as 'access to different therapies was non-existent' (Mind 2011: 22) and:

> on my ward care was a knock on the door at 10 am to go and get my meds, and a knock every few days to see a psychiatrist. I had no one-to-one conversations with any nurses or support workers except one when I spent a day on eyesight obs. I felt extremely safe on the ward, and benefited from speaking to others with mental health problems. I got more therapy from them than I did from the staff.
>
> (Mind 2011: 22)

Relationships with staff are not always considered perfect; one ex-patient reported: 'the quality of life on the ward was terrible, it was a violent place to be. I was repeatedly hit and had things stolen but most nurses did not care. The hospital was filthy and the staff stressed and overworked' (Mind, 2011: 22). Another Mind report quoted a patient as saying 'What's the point of complaining? They don't believe you and you know you'll see them (staff) again the next day. It's not worth it' (Mind 2013: 19).

Patients wanted to be shown respect by nurses and be known beyond the symptoms of their diagnosis (Raydon 2005). Nurses were also expected to be therapeutic and have good communication and listening skills (Raydon 2005; Gilburt *et al.*, 2008); links were made by patients between being listened to and being respected (Gilburt *et al.*, 2008).

The opportunity and ability to form relationships with other patients and staff were found to be one of the most significant factors in determining the success or otherwise of the inpatient experience (Nolan *et al.*, 2011). Such relationships were highly valued and many patients reported a void being created in their absence on discharge home (Nolan *et al.*, 2011).

For patients, issues such as finances and benefits and seeking employment dominated concerns prior to discharge ($n = 21$); obtaining permanent housing ($n = 9$) and improving relationships ($n = 9$) also featured. Recommendations from this study included that greater effort should be made to listen to patients' views and experiences and include them when planning services (Nolan *et al.*, 2011).

An insider view of inpatient care: physical interventions

Members of the CAPITAL project, a user-led research and training group, describe their experiences of restraint and seclusion (Ockwell and Capital Members 2007: 50) and how the trauma of it leaves lasting psychological scars. One member recalls an incident of trying to leave his room, when bleepers went off and 'six nurses jumped on me'. He said that if someone had explained what was happening it would probably have resulted in a different scenario. Another member describes seclusion, saying that people think it's about being alone, 'but it isn't, it's about power. . .what if someone did something frightening to me in this room? I had a mattress and nothing else and the power they had was that they could do this to me' (Ockwell and Capital Members, 2007: 50). Others describe wanting to be shown compassion and share beliefs that nobody should be restrained as staff don't take in to account people's experiences of being held down.

The Maat Probe Group, a Sheffield-based African Caribbean service user organization, conducted a monitoring exercise exploring the experiences of black people in mental health services (Mind 2011). Of those interviewed 46 per cent had been restrained by mental health staff. Of these people 79 per cent said it was aggressive with 34 per cent having been physically injured. One lady described having been restrained by male staff which resulted in further distress whilst others reported being pinned to the floor and feeling violated (Mind 2011).

Recommendations by the Matt Probe Group (Mind 2011) included the importance of effective communication between staff and patients in the prevention of difficult situations. If some form of physical intervention (restraint) was unavoidable, it would be preferable to be held facing upwards and not in a prone position. Safety for all was paramount and 'respect' was considered to be 'the best tool they've got' (Mind 2011: 25).

One mental health service user group in Gloucestershire administered questionnaires to a range of mental health staff regarding attitudes. From two hundred questionnaires, fifty-four were returned (Tyson 2013). Opinions were divided regarding physical interventions (restraint), with some staff (37.7 per cent) feeling that if this should occur in situations of non-compliance with medication or rapid tranquilization it should be as a last resort. Restraint was considered to be acceptable by 20.8 per cent of staff if patients were not compliant with leave status, however, 67.9 per cent disagreed and 11.3 per cent were undecided.

Prone restraint (face-down) has recently received renewed media coverage. It was identified as a contributing factor in the death of Ricky Bennett in 1998 and since then it has been claimed that there have been at least another thirteen restraint related deaths, with eight occurring in 2011 (Mind 2013: 3). In their report Mind (2013) claimed that there were inconsistencies across England in reported restraints by mental health trusts; one trust reported 38 incidents in 2012, whilst another reported 3000 for the same year (Mind 2013).

Key recommendations in the Mind report (2013) include an end to prone restraint, dictated by Government and for national standards for the use of physical restraint, and accredited training for staff. Currently there are a variety of different training packages available and utilized across trusts. Patient quotes from the report include 'It was like a rugby scrum. . . They got on top of me and held my face to the floor . . . with my arms behind my back. There was someone on every limb . . . it stayed with me' (Mind 2013: 15). Another stated: 'Four of them held me down on to a bed and gave me an injection. I kept saying that I didn't want it and I wanted a female nurse. No one listened to me. The younger staff members are the worst. They're new and excited by their training and get carried away with it' (Mind 2013: 15).

Findings from a qualitative study by Ezeobele *et al.* (2014) demonstrated that patients perceived seclusion as a punitive intervention and a means whereby staff could exert their control. Patients also reported that they believed that they had been secluded due to a lack of de-escalation skills in staff. One patient whose name had been changed to Latasha to protect anonymity, had a diagnosis of bipolar disorder and said:

> the nurse told me to take my medicines . . . the nurse did not explain the situation to e. . .rather. . .uh. . .the nurse called four big guys and they held me. . .the nurse refused to listen. . .uh. . .I was. . .um. . .I was afraid and powerless. . .I did not know what they were going to do to me. . .I did not have any family at this hospital and uh. . .you know. . .they outnumbered me . . . and I was not able to concentrate. . .I felt I was going to die. . .
>
> (Ezeobele *et al.*, 2014: 307)

Mary (pseudonym), a woman diagnosed with bipolar disorder stated: 'I felt violated. . .I felt everything had been stripped from me. . .I felt ashamed because I wanted to cooperate with staff' (Ezeobele *et al.*, 2014: 307*)*. However, due to the nature of their illness some patients failed to remember incidents of seclusion. Justin (pseudonym), who had a diagnosis of paranoid schizophrenia said: 'I don't remember. . .I must have been out of it and. . .um. . .well I may be um. . .really bad. . .what happened on the day I was secluded. . .I do not even remember what you are asking me. . .the seclusion. . .are you kidding me. . .' (Ezeobele *et al.*, 2014: 308).

Of a total sample (*n* = 20) in the study (Ezeobele *et al.*, 2014) 20 per cent (*n* = 4) viewed seclusion as a positive experience saying that it was a time to meditate or pray because they were alone. The fact that there were staff members outside the room and nearby monitoring them made them feel safe and secure. Mike (pseudonym) recalled that 'seclusion calmed me down. . .I guess it's a "cool down" room. . .um. . .hm. . .I felt good. . .and. . .I was praying to God to forgive my actions' (Ezeobele *et al.*, 2014: 309). However many patients interviewed in this study (60 per cent) perceived their time in seclusion as penalizing and a negative experience with some identifying a lack of communication skills in addition to provocation by staff as having led to their seclusion (Ezeobele *et al.*, 2014). Patients commonly reported negative feelings of seclusion due to poor interaction from staff before, during and post the event (Kontio *et al.*, 2012).

No recent media reports or person-centred research place physical interventions in an entirely positive light; however sometimes there is no option for nurses working in acute, emergency and intensive psychiatric services. An experienced PICU charge nurse tells his story:

> If someone were to ask me what part of my role as a nurse I find the most controversial it has to be that of physical intervention. The first training course I attended on 'control and restraint' was soon after I qualified as a mental health nurse 10 years ago, it was (and still is) a mandatory requirement for nurses working in a PICU. At that time it was hard to see it as being therapeutic, I was taught how to hold somebody. The emphasis of the training was on safe restraint and avoidance of harm or pain, however, after 10 years of working on PICU, I cannot guarantee that all physical restraints were perfect and pain-less. Nothing prepares you for the various scenarios you will experience and nobody can predict outcomes, errors, or the injuries to patients and staff. I have been to my GP and A&E often enough to know the damage it may have on someone's physical condition, let alone the long term psychological impact to both patients and staff.
>
> I have reflected that some incidents could have been dealt with differently, particularly those that could be prevented or predicted. Restraint is a last resort intervention, when everything else has been attempted and failed, but imminent risk of danger to the patient or others remains. Undertaking physical restraint is not always as simple and straight forward as the text book and training suggests. I have seen patients sustain injuries due to the fact that they were struggling (understandably) against restraint. Even though I know I handle these situations to the best of my ability with the patients' best interests at the fore, it does affect me, moreover, you cannot guarantee that the damage caused to the staff–patient relationship can always be repaired.
>
> I believe that physical restraint is sometimes necessary, but must always be performed with care, compassion and dignity. There are occasions where it can be the result of nurses' anxiety and uncertainty of what may happen, or because they lack good com-munication or de-escalation skills. I am always shocked when I see restraint written as part of a 'Care Plan'. If I were unwell it's the last thing I'd want to see on my care plan and I wonder to what extent patients have been included in writing it. I have seen patients' expressions during restraint: fear, anxiety, submission and sometimes utter terror. One patient said to me 'five men walked into the room, I did not know what was going on, of course I had to fight for my life'. No matter how much explanation I offered to the patient I still felt that he did not see us as nurses. Another patient said 'You guys are security officers, you ensure everybody's on their best behaviour'.
>
> I see the benefit of restraint in managing dangerous situations and know the damag-ing impact it can have on the relationship between patients and nurses, sometimes con-tributed to by nurses themselves. There is a world of difference between control and structure; however the wrong attitude can easily make nurses believe that that control is structure. Physical restraint is required in some instances and I have seen excellent

examples where its use has avoided incidents of serious and even fatal violence or self-harm. Patients have thanked me when they were better and despite some views, physical restraint is not a failed intervention. It is the intervention required when all other interventions have completely failed, or perhaps when we have failed the patient. For physical restraint to be less controversial there is a need to explore the understanding and attitudes of nurses more fully. If the real concept of physical restraint is grasped by all nurses working in acute, emergency and intensive psychiatric services, other health professionals, patient groups and the public will quite possibly have a better understanding of the reasons behind this intervention, patient safety must always be paramount'.

Reader activity

Consider how you may avoid restraint and what other possible interventions could be used.

> Reflect on what the difference is between 'control' and 'structure' and how you can ensure that the latter is evident in your own practice.
> If a restraint is unavoidable consider how you may preserve the patient's dignity during the process.

An insider view of inpatient care: discharge

Regarding discharge from an acute ward one female patient, aged 45 with four previous hospital admissions, said: 'I dread my discharge probably more this time than I have done on previous occasions. In the past, I had high expectations of what could be achieved but I know now that admission itself causes many problems. . .I feel on a merry-go-round and very negative about the future' (Nolan *et al.*, 2011: 363). Another female patient aged 38 who had been admitted twice before stated that 'they have no idea what my situation is like at home, the endless boredom, lack of social contact, it's intolerable' (Nolan *et al.*, 2011: 363).

One 54-year-old male who had three previous admissions described not realizing 'how much the ward routine had taken me over. It seems the needier I became the more eagerly I embraced the ward routine. Going home to my empty flat, I immediately missed a sense of belonging and having my needs met and feeling wanted. It did feel as if I was back to where I was prior to admission' (Nolan *et al.*, 2011: 363). A second male aged 38 with four previous admissions said that on admission he was told he was a risk to himself and others, however, 'on leaving nobody thought about how much risk I was at from others, especially my landlord and the neighbours, and the police' (Nolan *et al.*, 2011: 364).

Recommendations for good practice

Throughout this chapter it is evident that good **communication** is a key element of what patients want from staff. They want to be treated with respect and dignity and be listened to.

Power- based relationships should be avoided and units need to adopt a structured approach to care, not one of control. Nurses need to have high levels of emotional intelligence in order to pre-empt the needs of the patient to avoid difficult or even dangerous situations. Good body language and an understanding of 'trigger' factors by staff ensure that timely de-escalation can prevent serious untoward instances. Cultural sensitivity and non-judgemental attitudes are essential qualities for nurses working in these environments. Feedback from patients, families and carers needs to be encouraged, listened to and acted upon, including complaints, and staff also need to be able to give and receive constructive feedback.

The **environment** should be conducive to recovery with patients treated as guests enjoying high standards of hospitality regarding cleanliness, food and environment (Mind 2011). These essentials are sometimes overlooked and nurses need to ensure that the basics such as clothing, soap and towels are readily available as patients often come in via accident and emergency departments or Section 136 suites. The impact that the environment and staff may have on patient behaviour cannot be underestimated.

Outdoor space and activities are also important, and it would seem the latter are sometimes lacking from what patients report. Smoking is noted as being important to many patients; although this a contentious issue, patient choice cannot be ignored. Smoking bans have the potential for placing staff in potentially dangerous situations unnecessarily.

Teamwork and evidence-based practice rely on good clinical leadership from senior nurses who practise alongside more junior staff. Ongoing personal and professional development and good clinical supervision are also key to this. Clinical leaders are crucial in the development of positive staff attitudes, particularly around prevention of power-based relationships between staff and patients. Establishing an environment of structure as opposed to control needs to be encouraged, and continuity of staff including named nurses and support staff is important in the delivery of patient care.

Patients should be made to feel welcome on **admission**, information packs should be supplied and explained and the 'reading of rights' under Mental Health Act (2007) should be delivered with sensitivity along with the 'rules' and boundaries of the ward or PICU. A cup of tea and a chat go a long way, as do introductions to staff and other patients; not all interactions with patients need to be on a formal basis. Encouragement with hygiene, feeding and physical health care are paramount and need to be addressed in a timely fashion and nurses should be aware of issues around diagnostic overshadowing which could result in challenging behaviour.

Patients need to be partners in the **assessment, formulation and care planning** and not in a tokenistic way. Care plans need to be flexible, person centred and creative. They must also be constantly updated (sometimes several times through a shift if the patient is on PICU) and should always follow a bio-psych-pharmaco-social approach (Clark and Clarke 2014). Safety, security and **risk management** are crucial in acute wards and PICUs and all nurses need expertise in this area.

Trust and national policy should be adhered to in the **management of acutely disturbed/ challenging behaviour including rapid tranquillization, restraint and seclusion.** Team commitment to advancement of skills in de-escalation without the use of restraint/seclusion is essential as is the recognition of trigger factors in individual patients. Debrief following restraint or seclusion should take place with patients, not just staff, reassuring the patient all the time. Mentor support for newly qualified staff regarding restraint should be readily available and senior nurses should lead de-escalation situations and unavoidable restraint. Up-to-date training in de-escalation, restraint and the use of seclusion needs to include agency staff and there are calls to standardize physical intervention and bring an end to the use of prone restraint (Mind 2013).

Patients should have choice and the opportunity to access independent advocacy services; where possible advanced directives can be recorded and followed in the crisis situation. **Consent and capacity** are big issues in psychiatric services and nurses should have an in-depth understanding of relevant legislation.

Discharge planning should consider the views of the patient, family and particular home circumstances, the fear expressed by patients regarding discharge cannot be underestimated. **Recovery and social inclusion** need to be at the heart of every inpatient experience.

Reader activity

What knowledge, skills, attitudes and competencies do nurses need when working on acute psychiatric wards or PICUs in order to promote patient recovery and support the patient's family?

References

Barton, R. (1976) *Institutional Neurosis*, 3rd edn. Bristol: John Wright & Sons.

Basson, J.V. and Woodside, M. (1981) Assessment of a secure/intensive/forensic ward, *Acta Psychiatrica Scandinavica* 64(2): 132–41.

Beer, D., Paton, P., and Pereira, S. (1997) Hot beds of general psychiatry: a national survey of psychiatric intensive care units, *Psychiatric Bulletin*, 21: 142–4.

Beer, M.D., Pereira, S.M. and Paton, C. (2008) Psychiatric Intensive Care – development and definitions, in M.D. Beer, S.M. Pereira and C. Paton(2008) *Psychiatric Intensive Care*. Cambridge: Cambridge University Press.

Bowers, L. (2014) Safewards: a new model of conflict and containment on psychiatric wards, *Journal of Psychiatric and Mental Health Nursing*, 21: 499–508.

Bowers, L., Crowhurst, N., Alexander, J. *et al.* (2003) Psychiatric nurses' views on criteria for psychiatric intensive care: acute and intensive care staff compared, *International Journal of Nursing Studies*, 40:145–52.

Brimblecombe, N., Tingle, A., and Murrells, T. (2007) How mental health nursing can best improve service users' experiences and outcomes in inpatient settings: responses to a national consultation, *Journal of Psychiatric and Mental Health Nursing*, 14(5): 503–9.

Campbell, P. cited in Repper, J. and Perkins, R. (2003*) Social Inclusion and Recovery: A Model for Mental health.* Balliere Tindall.

Clark, L.L. and Clarke, T. (2014) Realising nursing: a multimodal approach to psychiatric nursing, *Journal of Psychiatric and Mental Health Nursing*, 21(6): 564–71.

Crain, P.M. and Jordan, E.G. (1979) The psychiatric intensive care unit – an in-hospital treatment of violent adult patients, *Bulletin of the American Academy of Psychatry and Law*, VII(2): 190–8.

Crowhurst, N. and Bowers, L. (2002) Philosophy, care and treatment on the psychiatric intensive care unit: themes, trends and future practice, *Journal of Psychiatric and Mental Health Nursing*, 9(6): 689–95.

DH (Department of Health) (1999) *National Service Framework for Mental Health: Modern Standards and Service Models*. London: Department of Health.

DH (2008) *Code of Practice; Mental Health Act 1983*: Safe and Therapeutic responses to disturbed behaviour, Chapter 15. London. DoH.

DH (Department of Health) (2012) *Transforming Care: A National Response to the Winterbourne View Hospital. Final Report*. London: DoH.

Ezeobele, I.E., Malecha, A.T., Mock, A. *et al.* (2014) Patients' lived experience in acute psychiatric hospital in the United States: a qualitative study. *Journal of Psychiatric and Mental Health Nursing*, 21(4): 303–12.

Gilburt, H., Rose, D., and Slade, M. (2008) The importance of relationships in mental health care: a qualitative study of service users' experiences of psychiatric hospital admission in the UK. Available at: www.biomedcentral.com/1472-6963/8/92 (accessed 6 November 2015).

Goffman, E. (1963) *Stigma: Notes on the Management of Spoiled Identity*. Englewood Cliffs, NJ: Prentice Hall.

Goldney, R. *et al.* (1985) The psychiatric intensive care unit, *British Journal of Psychiatry*, 146(1): 50–4.

Health and Social Care Information Centre (2011) *Mental Health Bulletin: Fourth Report from Mental Health Minimum Dataset (MHMDS) Annual Returns, 2010*.

Katsakou, C., Rose, D., Amos, T. *et al.* (2012) Psychiatric patients' views on why their involuntary hospitalizationwas right or wrong: a qualitative study, *Social Psychiatry & Psychiatric Epidemiology*, 47: 1169–79.

Kontio, R., Joffe, G., Putkonen, H. *et al.* (2012) Seclusion and restraint in psychiatry: patients' experiences on how to improve practices and use alternatives, *Perspectives in Psychiatric Care*, 48(1): 16–24.

Mental Health Act (2007) Available at: www.legislation.gov.uk/ukpga/2007/12/contents

Mind (2011) *Listening to Experience: An Independent Inquiry into Acute and Crisis Mental Healthcare*. London: Mind.

Mind (2013) *Mental Health Crisis Care: Physical Restraint in Crisis: A Report on Physical Restraint in Hospital Settings in England*. London: Mind.

Mounsey, N. (1979) Psychiatric intensive care, *Nursing Times*, 75: 1811–13.

Needham, H. and Sands, N. (2010) Post seclusion debriefing: a core nursing intervention, *Perspectives in Psychiatric care*, 46(3): 221–33.

Nolan, P., Bradley, E. and Brimblecombe, N. (2011) Disengaging from acute inpatient psychiatric care: a description of service users' experiences and views, *Journal of Psychiatric and Mental Health Nursing*, 18(4): 359–67.

Ockwell, C. and Capital Members (2007) Restraint: a necessary evil? in M. Hardcastle, D Kennard, S. Grandison and L. Fagin (eds) *Experiences of Mental Health In-patient Care*. Hove: Routledge.

Pereira, S. and Clinton, B. (2002) *Mental Health Policy Implementation Guide: National Minimum Standards for General Adult Services in Psychiatric Intensive Care Units (PICU) and Low Secure Environments*. London: Department of Health.

Pereira, S.M., Sarsam, M., Bhui, K. and Paton, C. (2005) The London survey of Psychiatric Intensive Care Units: psychiatric intensive care; patient characteristics and pathways for admission and discharge, *Journal of Psychiatric Intensive Care*, 1(1):17–24.

Rachlin, S. (1973) On the need for a closed ward in an open hospital: the psychiatric intensive care unit, *Hospital and Community Psychiatry*, 24(12): 829–33.

Raydon, S.E. (2005) The attitudes, knowledge and skills needed in mental health services, *International Journal of Mental Health Nursing*, 14:78–87.

Shepherd, G., Boardman, J. and Slade, M. (2008) *Making Recovery a Reality*. London: Sainsbury Centre for Mental Health.

The Mid Staffordshire NHS Foundation Trust Public Inquiry (2013) *Report of the Mid Staffordshire NHS Foundation Trust Public Inquiry, Chaired by Robert Francis QC*.

Thomas, S.P., Shattel, M. and Martin, T. (2002) What's therapeutic about the therapeutic milieu? *Archives of Psychiatric Nursing*, 7(3): 259–68.

Tyson, P.J. (2013) A service user initiated project investigating the attitudes of mental health staff towards clients and services in an acute mental health unit, *Journal of Psychiatric and Mental Health Nursing*, 20(5): 379–86.

Warnecke, L. (1986) A psychiatric intensive care unit in a general hospital setting, *Canadian Journal of Psychiatry*, 31(9): 834–7.

While, A. and Clark, L.L. (2009) Overcoming ignorance and stigma relating to intellectual disability in health care, *Journal of Nursing Management*, 18: 166–72.

OLDER PEOPLE AND CARERS' ISSUES

Chapter

15

Older people and person-centred care

The opportunities and challenges in everyday encounters

Corina Naughton, Nicky Hayes, Bridgit Sam-Bailey and Fiona Clark

This chapter provides an overview of PCC within the context of an older population. It combines academic literature with the real world experiences of older people.

At the end of this chapter the reader will be able to:

- Describe the key components of PCC within academic literature concerning an older population
- Examine the association between the construct of PCC within academic literature and narratives from older people who have experienced care environments
- Discuss the role of individual practitioners in creating and sustaining PCC planning and interactions with older people, families and carers

Introduction

Person-centred care has a particular meaning and significance in caring for older people. A person-centred philosophy of care partly provides a defence against stereotypical constructs of ageing such as old age as 'hardship', burden and dependency. In the acute care setting these stereotypical constructs can be manifest when older people are portrayed as 'bed blockers', 'delayed discharges', 'being in the wrong place' or a 'drain on scarce resources'. Such a discourse is a manifestation of societal, institutional and professional ageism where the inherent value of older people is diminished in what Phillips (2010) describes as an 'othering effect' whereby older people are categorized as different and inferior.

Focuses on preserving and promoting an individual's unique identity, dignity, self-respect and supportive independence (Nolan 2001; Calnan *et al.*, 2013). Thus PCC acts as a defence against disparaging external discourses as well as the physical and cognitive decline of the ageing process. However, PCC is a vulnerable construct and is pivotally dependent on the values, beliefs, skills and above all courage and compassion of the individual practitioner as well as an organizational culture that supports these attributes. In this chapter readers are asked to examine their beliefs and values around caring for older people and to promote a shared conceptual framework of PCC through engaging with the personal narratives of two of the co-authors. The overall aim is to encourage the reader to develop personal strategies to implement and sustain a person-centred approach to caring as well as the confidence to influence others.

Background

Successful old age is constructed as:

> a feeling of being embedded in social relationships, usually but not exclusively, within the family; being able to pursue personally meaningful activity and feeling needed; having a positive view of the past, the present and the future, and having a philosophy of life based on religious or other personal beliefs.

> (Nilsson *et al.*, 1998: 94)

Declining physical health, increased frailty and diminishing cognitive capacity threaten the essence of individuality, dignity and autonomy that underpin a conventional concept of successful ageing (Nolan 2001). It is not surprising then that the core concept of person-centredness emerged in the context of people with dementia. Kitwood (1997: 20) defined 'person-centredness as a standing or status that is bestowed upon one human being by another, in the context of relationships and social beings'. As dementia progresses an individual's personhood (that which defines the unique status and value as a person) is partly preserved by the family, informal and formal carers who support the person living with dementia. The concept of PCC was further operationalized by Brooker (2003) through the VIPS framework. VIPS emphasizes a person's inherent value, individuality, perspective and the creation of a social environment (see Table 15.1). Although this framework has a focus on dementia it reflects the parallel concepts on delivering dignified care (Commission on Dignity in Care for Older People 2012). A central pillar of dignified and PCC is the quality of the communication and interaction between the older person, the family or carer and the multi-disciplinary health and social care team. The quality of this communication is predicated on recognizing not just the health condition but also the unique life experience of the individual and his/her preferences in planning and receiving care.

Reader activity

Reflect on a recent occasion you had contact with an older person in a healthcare setting. Using the VIPS framework critique one of the interactions or conversations you had or observed with an older person.

Were there positive or negative examples of valuing, treating as an individual, understanding perspective or creating a social environment?
Did you notice the impact and reaction of the older person during the encounter?
Was the event typical or atypical of the culture of the care environment?

In the face of ongoing physical and or cognitive decline the role of external actors (such as nurses, doctors, physiotherapists, healthcare assistants etc.) and the organizational culture become central to the preservation of personhood, dignity and the continuance of 'living well'. Yet, there is a tension with health and social care environments that are dominated by a target-driven efficiency agenda coupled with insensitive implementation of quality and safety initiatives (Calnan *et al.*, 2013). This is compounded by inadequate staffing levels (Ball *et al.*, 2014) as well as under-skilled or inflexible healthcare staff, which combine to dehumanize vulnerable groups (Brown 2008; Francis Report 2013; CQC 2013).

Table 15.1 Domains of Person-Centred Care

	Positive examples	Negative examples
• **V: Valuing** a person with dementia or older person and family/carers	The person and carers are actively involved in decision-making and care planning	Frequently moving older people in acute or social care because they are perceived 'not to be in the right place'
• **I:** Treating people as **individuals (I)**	Using the person's preferred name, having insight into a person's social history and life experience as well as medical history	A person who only drinks coffee, being constantly offered tea. Using a person's first name without asking permission
• **P:** Looking at the world from the **perspective** of the older person or the person with dementia	Proactive plan to maintain a person's continence and mobility during hospitalization	Confining patients to chair or bed to reduce risk of falls, forcing an individual to use continence pads rather than providing assistance to use the toilet
• **S:** A **positive social environment** in which the person living with dementia or frailty can experience relative wellbeing (see Table 15.2)	Nurses showing flexibility in work practice, initiating conversations and interactions for emotional support, providing meaningful activity even during acute hospital admissions	Task focused, exchanges are functional and reactionary in response to physical care needs. Environment devoid of personal effects (e.g. photos, cards) due to infection control risks. People left for long periods of time without any interaction

Brooker (2003).

Complexity, diversity and frailty

The older adult population is among the most diverse and complex of any patient or client group (Meiner 2015). The ageing process, with or without specific pathologies, combined with life experience, social networks and economic circumstances creates a highly heterogeneous population. However, current health and social care systems were designed to manage single health conditions that relied on the majority of people being anchored in large family networks to provide care and support. Ironically these systems, although currently struggling to manage the complexity of the older population, have significantly contributed to the unprecedented levels of successful ageing seen in the latter half of the twentieth century.

This increased longevity has contributed to the emergence of frailty as a clinical and social phenomenon. Frailty is described as a 'non-specific state of vulnerability that reflects multisystem physiological change as well as psychological and social factors' (BGS 2014). It has been defined both in terms of phenotype (Fried *et al.*, 2001) and accumulated deficits (Rockwood and Mitnitski 2011). Frailty phenotypes describes functional changes such as slow gait speed, weight loss, impaired strength, exhaustion and low physical activity/energy expenditure (Fried *et al.*, 2001). In contrast the Frailty Index, based on an accumulate deficits model, suggests a minimum of 30 deficits should be used to assess the presence of frailty. A higher number of deficits correlates with a greater degree of frailty and associated adverse health outcomes (Rockwood and Mitnitski 2011). In addition to this medical construct of frailty, Nicholson *et al.* (2013) describes the older person's experience of living with frailty. This personal perspective is markedly different and focuses on the person's 'potential capacity' to maintain normality and make connections with those around them including formal carers and health and social care professionals. This striving for connection with healthcare staff is a particular feature and challenge for an older person during an acute hospital admission or Emergency Department attendance (Bridges and Nugus 2010; Bridges *et al.*, 2010). The response of staff at this highly stressful and disorientating period can have a profound impact on an older person's sense of worth and 'individual significance' (Bridges and Nugus 2010).

An understanding of frailty, with or without cognitive impairment, is essential to establishing communication and overcoming the barriers to PCC planning. A key aspect of this is the impact of frailty and/or dementia on the person's ability to communicate and to participate in decision-making. There is therefore a very practical dimension to delivering PCC for older people, which centres on the skill of nurses and other members of the MDT in assessing for physical, cognitive, sensory and social factors that impact on quality of life. One model of assessment and intervention recommended for older adults living with frailty and/or dementia is Comprehensive Geriatric Assessment (see Figure 15.1). CGA fundamentally recognizes the complexity of older age and the need to integrate information from all elements of a person's life in order to provide PCC (BGS 2014).

While undertaking a full CGA requires training and time, and is not always necessary, the underlying philosophy highlights the inadequacy of task focused, technical nursing and medical care to meet the needs of older people and their families. A crucial conceptual difference in a comprehensive assessment approach for an older adult is to acknowledge the deficit(s) but to focus on the individual's priorities and capability. The emphasis is on moderating the effect of the deficit(s) while maximizing the individual's capability across physical, cognitive,

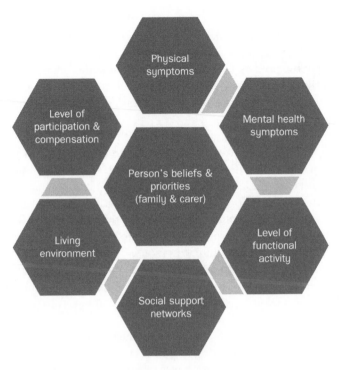

Figure 15.1 Domains of the Comprehensive Geriatric Assessment

psychological and social domains. A person-centred approach is fundamental to successfully integrating technical care with dignified and compassionate care.

Impact of care experiences

The experiences of older people and their families who come into contact with health and social care services are often ones of 'struggle' to maintain dignity and control. The preservation of identity, independence and autonomy are undermined by procedural bureaucracy to complete tasks (Taylor and Kelly 2006), fragmentation of services, specialization within nursing and medicine and crucially, inconsistency in the attitudes, practices and communication with nurses, doctors and others working in health and social care services (Calnan, Badcott and Woolhead 2006; Tadd and Calnan 2009, Bridges *et al.*, 2013; Prorok *et al.*, 2013).

As stated earlier the emotional impact of this experience on an older person can be profound. The Care Quality Commission (CQC) annually reports deficits in dignity of care in acute and long-term care settings (CQC 2013). Bridges and Nugus (2010) described how older people in urgent care environments were left questioning their legitimacy to be there and feeling they mattered little compared to other patients or medical tasks. These feelings occurred because of the unfamiliarity of the environment, lack of information, subordination of non-medical needs and above all the inability of some staff to engage with the person as an individual (Bridges and Nugus 2010). The generalizibility of these findings was reinforced in a meta-synthesis of qualitative studies of older people's experiences of acute care (Bridges *et al.*, 2010). The review identified a prominence of feelings of worthlessness, fear and lack of control especially in the presence of cognitive or communication impairment, Wwile Tadd *et al.* (2011: 10) described 'undignified care as that which renders individuals invisible, depersonalises and objectifies people, is abusive or humiliating, narrowly focused and disempowers the individual'.

Such reports dishearten the vast majority of health and social care staff who work with older people. There is ample literature testifying to the emotional and moral distress staff experience when they deliver unsatisfactory care or have become disengaged from the therapeutic relationship with their patients or clients (Maben *et al.*, 2012; Bridges *et al.*, 2013). This chapter focuses on the contribution that individual practitioners can make to promoting a person-centred and dignified care culture within their own practice and work environment through recognizing the everyday threats older people face to preserving their personhood. Central to a PCC philosophy is valuing a person's dignity which can be operationalized through constructing social environments that promote positive communication and interaction between healthcare staff and the individual and family. Table 15.2 outlines Kitwood's (1997) characteristics of a positive social environment compared to a malignant (negative) environment.

Creating a positive social environment is at the heart of Guidance on Best Practice for Older People in Acute Care Settings (Bridges 2009). This work is a blueprint for engaging and communicating with older people and emphasizes three core principles:

- Maintaining identity: 'see who I am' (what is important to the person and acknowledge the expertise of family and informal carers)
- Creating community: 'connect with me' (develop therapeutic not just functional relationships between healthcare staff and the older person and the family)
- Sharing decision-making: 'involve me' (understand what is happening, provide opportunities for meaningful involvement in decisions)

Recent publications echo and build on the three principles outlined above. Edvardsson *et al.* (2010) used qualitative studies to define the characteristics of PCC from the perspective of families. Promoting a continuation of self and normality was the overarching theme and involved knowing the person, welcoming families, providing meaningful activities, being in a personalized environment and experiencing flexibility and continuity, while Clissett *et al.* (2013) described opportunities and missed opportunities to construct a PCC in acute care settings. The observational study described staff and patient interactions in terms of attachment (relationships of trust and security), inclusion (feeling part of the group) identity (life story maintained by self or others), occupation (personally meaningful activity) and comfort (tenderness, soothing verbal and therapeutic touch). The authors noted that while healthcare staff promoted feelings of attachment and inclusion there was little evidence of preserving a sense of identity, occupation and comfort (Clissett *et al.*, 2013).

As a novice practitioner it can be difficult to visualize what the distinguishing characteristics are between functional care (doing the dressing, taking the vital signs, giving information) and person-centred interactions where the practitioner gives the person time, listens,

Table 15.2 Kitwood's (1997) characteristics of a positive and negative social care environments

Positive social environment	Negative (malignant) social environment
Celebration	Accusation
Collaboration	Banishment
Creation	Disempowerment
Facilitation	Disruption
Giving	Ignoring
Holding	Imposition
Negotiation	Infantilization
Play	Intimidation
Recognition	Invalidation
Relaxation	Labelling
Timalation	Mockery
Validation	Objectification
	Outpacing
	Stigmatization
	Withholding

recognizes and addresses communication barriers and views the situation from the individual's emotional perspective. The narratives from two of the co-authors, Mrs F.C. and Ms S-B, help to illustrate how the quality of the presence of the healthcare practitioner determines a person's experience of care. In the remainder of this chapter, the two co-authors share their experiences and wisdom with novice healthcare practitioners to enable them to communicate and behave in a way that brings PCC into each action and interaction especially with older people. It focuses on what you as an individual can control and on how you can choose to behave.

See my wisdom and life experience

Ms S-B was born in Guyana (formerly British Guyana) and taught commercial subjects before coming to London in 1960 where she initially worked as a Secretary and Personal Assistant in the Home Office. Whilst there senior staff were often surprised by her knowledge of British history and geography. She would laugh and say, 'of course I know about this. I studied the same curriculum as you.'

Asked about her experience of emigrating, Ms S-B felt 'coming to Britain was not as different as some people may think. There was already a shared language, education, legal and policing system.' Ms S-B later trained as a teacher and had a successful teaching career in the UK and Bermuda. Since retiring she has become an active older person's advocate and campaigner. Her Lewisham Pensioner's Forum was proactive in organizing the campaign to save Lewisham Hospital and has been an advocate for ethnic minority elders across a range of older people's issues in the UK and Europe. Ms S-B has personal experience of receiving healthcare following hip surgeries and through her advocacy role.

Mrs FC was born and has lived in London all her life. Although interested in medicine and her father being a surgeon, it was not viewed as a suitable profession for a woman at that time. Mrs FC studied law at university and worked for a legal publishing company where she met her husband. For four years Mrs FC ran the medical book shops in both St Thomas Hospital and Charing Cross Hospital. During this time Mrs FC was a sympathetic listener to many young students who shared their stories, trials and tribulations with her. Mrs FC became her husband's main carer as his health deteriorated due to diabetes, heart disease and cancer. As a carer Mrs FC acted as an advocate and mediator for her husband with healthcare staff. After his death she continued to work as an advocate for the elderly and today through her role as a Governor on the Board of a large teaching Trust she represents the views of all patients, especially older people.

What PCC means to me

Though the ladies come from different backgrounds and have different life experiences they share a similar understanding of PCC.

> Ms S-B: For me PCC is when they are going to treat me as a person, not a number; as an individual because my needs would not be the same as the other person's needs, and I always say the one size fits all analogy does not work with me. We are all different and we have to be seen as such.

> Mrs FC: I think I would call it integrated care . . . it is about putting the person themselves at the centre of what the medical treatment is, as opposed to the medical treatment being imposed on the person. When you go for medical care, particularly if you go from a GP to a hospital, my experience is of just being told what is going to happen to you and you don't get the chance, very often, to say what you feel and perhaps [what] is the best way for you to be dealt with. . . . The person receiving the care has not been in the picture very much.

Mrs FC reflects that the experience and insight of the older person or the family can be disregarded by professionals who focus on the illness. There can be a failure to recognize that PCC is a unique partnership based on trust, recognizing the individual, his/her life experience, and listening and responding to the person's perspective. The challenge is: how do you build individual partnerships when you are responsible for many patients at the same time with competing priorities? The experiences of the co-authors in this chapter suggest it is attention to the smaller details of everyday interactions that is the basis for creating a positive person-centred environment. Both authors experienced many of the same behaviours that can enhance or diminish a person's sense of self and dignity. The experiences recounted by the co-authors are often not deliberate or intended acts but omissions that stem from a lack of understanding and awareness of the unique impact you as a healthcare professional have on an older person's sense of worth and significance (Bridges and Nugus 2010).

Mrs FC describes it as:

> Not taking the time to cross to the other side. To view the world from the perspective of someone who is finding it increasingly difficult to navigate the systems and world that we and they once took for granted.

The following themes are the day-to-day acts that make a difference to the way an older person experiences the world of health and social care whether at home, a GP practice, hospital or nursing home.

Acknowledge me

This is the fundamental start to every encounter. Acknowledgement can be a smile, a nod of the head, a greeting. Picture if you will, a ward redesigned to be dementia friendly. An older man is sitting on a bench beside the nurse's station looking at the people walking past, they notice him but nobody smiles or greets him by name, he has become part of the background. This is an example of a 'missed opportunity' for attachment and inclusion described by Clissett *et al.* (2013). So what can be done to turn this into an 'opportunity'?

The power of a smile and a greeting is illustrated by Ms S-B.

> I attended a hospital for the first time a month ago for pain management. The lady in Receptionist greeted everyone with a brilliant 'good morning' and a smile and 'would you like a cup of tea? I can get you one'. I said to her: 'Oh! that is a very warm welcome' and that continued throughout the morning . . . I said to her: 'I don't feel I am in a hospital when I am here' and it was true because of the way she greets you and speaks to you. She was like that with everyone, no one was different, just making you feel comfortable in the space you are sharing.

Mrs FC agrees PCC is:

> Somebody who took the trouble to smile and say 'Hello Mrs [name]' and appear to be available for a question. To be acknowledged 'Hello Mrs [Name]' is really important. . . Some of the patients I talk to feel that nobody is paying that much attention to them, them as a person.

Use the name I prefer

The use of a person's name is very powerful, but this can also be misused. Modern society has become informal, where the use of a person's first name, even if only a recent acquaintance, has become a normative convention. Ms S-B reminds us that every individual has a right to decide how she/he wants to be addressed and it is part of a respectful partnership to first establish what this is and gain the person's consent.

> Ms S-B: Yes, addressing people properly is very important . . . when this youngster was calling out to me . . . bawling down the corridor [using just her first name] and I said to

her, 'I don't recall going to school with you' [i.e. not an old friend], so she apologized. Conversely there was another youngster who called out 'Ms S-B'. So I complimented her. 'Thank you for not calling me by my first name, obviously you have been well brought up'. She said 'Oh! My Grandmother would never have it any other way'. You know, two sides of the same coin.

Give me your time

An important feature of a person who works in a person-centred way is someone who takes the time to talk to a person and the family or carer.

> Mrs FC: Taking the time to talk to you, nurses so often were in a rush and when I did [hospital name] 'In Conversation' last year talking to patients and nurses, one of the things patients frequently said was: 'I didn't like to ask the nurses they are so busy, they are very good the nurses but they are so busy, I don't like to ask them this query or that query.'

> Ms S-B: The time factor, they are focusing on getting their rota completed (I am just using rota loosely) trying to get that completed rather than spending a lot of time with one person. . . . When I had my second hip operation I had a team of people coming into do the necessary like wash my feet. There were some who when they came they were always in a hurry, they couldn't do things if I asked them to; they couldn't do it because they had to get to another appointment. There were two who came and they were not watching the time, they just did everything possible to make me comfortable. So coming from the same unit, the same pool but those were the differences, you know, some who would stay with me, give me quality time to make sure that I was comfortable before they left and others who were just anxious to get away. They were meant to be seeing me for 45 minutes, 15 minutes and they were gone. . .

These experiences highlight the competing pressures healthcare staff experience and with increasing demand and fewer staff this is difficult to balance. However, these stories illustrate how a sense of 'perpetual busyness' undermines people's confidence to approach us seeking help and emotional support.

Help me to navigate the system

Many of the experiences of older people are of being part of a system that makes no allowances despite their reduced physical or mental capacity or recognizes how difficult ordinary things have become due to illnesses.

Ms S-B tells of a GP who said she must return to hospital because of suspected complications following her hip surgery but shrugs his shoulders when her son asked how she will get there. They ended up walking, Ms S-B in a lot of pain. An eight-hour wait in casualty followed, only to be told return on Monday for an ultrasound and an outpatient appointment but they were not told what for. She was also left for over an hour in a wheelchair waiting for an ultrasound because they forgot she was there.

Mrs FC recounts visiting an older person as an advocate to help her with a housing concern but instead

> Sitting down with the lady sorting out which hospital she was going to and when and for which ailment, she certainly had two and I have a feeling she had three different hospitals to get to and that if you are old, not very well and getting confused, it is extremely difficult.

There are individuals who help the older person navigate this system because they recognize the person is not coping or is in difficulty, for example, the porter who finds the wheelchair when Ms S-B cannot walk any more and tells her son to register his mother quickly before the office closes, otherwise there would be an even longer wait, or to take another example, the receptionist who realized Ms S-B had to have the ultrasound before going to the clinic:

> Ms S-B: That saved a lot of time, otherwise I would have to walk to the new suite in a new block and then walk back to the old block to get the ultrasound, then back to the new block. I don't know how I would have fared.

These are examples of healthcare staff seeing the person first rather than the task and treating the person as an individual.

Ms S-B describes the staff in the specialist clinic she was eventually referred to with the pain in her legs.

> The way they spoke to me; they addressed me with an element of care, she [the doctor] looked at the legs and all that. . . . it was as if she was caring for someone she knew, like a relation and I appreciated that.

As people with increasing levels of frailty continue to live in the community and access day, outpatient, GP and acute services there is a need for a broader appreciation of what constitutes a barrier. Fragmented services and environmental barriers strain the reserves of older people to cope and maintain independence. Person-centred care is seeing beyond the immediate task, especially tasks we regard as routine, and recognizing how the behaviour of healthcare staff impacts on the individual.

Reader activity

Can you describe an incident where you had an opportunity to help someone navigate the system, to make the journey less fragmented and easier to cope with?

> How did you recognize the person needed that extra help?
> Based on your experience can you describe what happens when the older person does not get this help?

Listen to me

A related theme to navigating the system is being listened to and included in decisions both as a patient and carer.

> Mrs FC: My husband who had diabetes, he had a very bad heart and he had colon cancer. He was in a bed and opposite him was a patient with MRSA, and the nurse had said to me he has MRSA, he has to stay in his area, this was in the ward. I was there on the Sunday and this chap got up and was wandering around going to the general bathroom. And I said to one of the nurses 'I thought he was meant to stay in a protected environment' and the nurse said 'Oh! No it is all right'. The next day I spoke to the staff nurse: 'my husband is very vulnerable to MRSA and this chap is going into the loos [toilet]' and she said 'Oh! He is not meant to do that' and by the afternoon they had moved him. The nurse on Sunday did not pay any attention at all.

Mrs FC relates a more poignant experience and illustrates the central role of the carer in the life and wellbeing of an older person

> Mrs FC: On the third day after an operation for colon cancer my husband was vomiting constantly and extremely unwell. He had been diagnosed with heart failure three years before and had been into hospital several times. I was his carer, I knew his breathing, it was not the same, I knew it was different. As I left the ward at 7.30pm I said to the sister that there was something wrong with his breathing. She replied that she would ask the physiotherapist to look at it in the morning. He was found blue at 6.30 the next morning and rushed to intensive care where he died later that day; he had inhaled vomit into his lungs and the infection from there had spread to all his other organs.

Mrs FC did not need early warning scores or oxygen saturations to know that her husband, who she had cared for and about whose health she knew every detail, had deteriorated. As healthcare professionals we can dismiss this intimate knowledge carers have which can be to the detriment of an older person. A person-centred partnership with an older person is also a partnership with the family or carer.

Involve the carers

The carer partnership is centred on communication and taking the time to discuss treatment plans and realistic outcomes. When this happens it leaves a lasting positive legacy and when it does not there is a breach of trust which can influence future encounters with healthcare professionals.

> Mrs FC: When my husband was ill with several things wrong with him . . . he was too ill to take in what was happening to him and he used to say to the consultant to come back when my wife is here and tell her because she will understand what you are saying and they did, they did come back . . . I was very impressed and thanked them very much, I was very pleased and thought it was very good of them to come to explain it to me.

I have known other people in hospital where the wife or family member has not been told what is happening because they are not there when the doctors come round and nobody bothers to tell the family member even when the person is very ill and unable to communicate to the wife or family what is happening. . . . It's complicated, the person doesn't want you just to talk to the carer they want to be talked to too, but the carer needs to know.

Effective communication between healthcare staff, patients and family carers is based on feelings that information is shared and that they are being included in decision-making, feeling there is someone you can contact when you need to and feeling the service is responsive to your needs (Walker and Dewar 2001). This is reiterated in the NHS commitment to 'No decisions about me, without me' (DH 2012). On a day-to-day basis effective communication between an older person and the care team is informed by understanding what is important to an older person, who the important people are in an older person's support network and what their roles are. Healthcare staff working with older people should be able to use their communication skills to mitigate against barriers to communication such as sensory impairment, cognitive decline or high levels of frailty. Documents such as 'This is me' promote staff and family collaboration to identify the important information about a person including his or her everyday preferences and meaningful activities. In turn this information should be reflected in PCC plans and staff interactions with the person and the family.

Reader activity

Reflect on a recent conversation you had with an older person's family member or carer.

Would you describe it as a person-centred conversation?
Did you know what the person's role (not just their relationship) was in the older person's support network?
What did the person already know before you started giving information?
Did you ask what the person's view was of his/her relative's condition?
Did you ask what was the person's concerns were at that time?
What did you record about the conversation and hand over to other members of the team?

Treat me with respect

Older people often describe being invisible and powerless to influence the care system they are in. Ms S-B echoes this view: '[I am]not the same as the one in the next room. . . just a number, here comes another one, I am just a number and it makes me feel uncomfortable.'

Ms S-B: When I had my first operation I had my right hip done, the consultant came into the ward and said to me, 'Oh Ms S-B. I have had a look at your X-rays, they look OK but you are going to be here for another day or two'. About an hour or so later, somebody, a lady, came along . . . she stood in the front of these two suites and bellowed out [my name]. So I just raised my head and said 'This is she'. From her position [outside the door] she said, 'You are going home, you are going home today'. So I said 'Today?' Just an hour before the consultants had said I'd be there another day or two. So she said, 'Yes today, do you have keys?', and I said 'no I don't, and I will have to phone around to find where my son is'. I was still experiencing the effects of the anaesthetics and I thought well that is pretty bad. So I had to phone around, make contact with my son. He rang them and said 'No, I am coming to get my mother, you are not sending my mum home like that. . .'

Encounters like this diminish an individual's sense of control. A lack of involvement in decisions that impact care and wellbeing causes stress and leaves the person feeling vulnerable and that they or the family have to fight to regain control. Planning and intelligent communication can achieve the same outcomes while maintaining respect for the individual.

Lack of consideration or prejudice

Ms S-B makes the point that older people often have to fight against more than one prejudice: 'I am a woman, I am black and I am old'. All too frequently a petty lack of consideration results in an older person using scarce reserves of energy to maintain his/her dignity as illustrated in the following story.

Ms S-B went for a hip X-ray after her surgery. She was wearing a girdle with metal hooks but nobody realized, so the X-Ray had to be repeated. The female radiologist assisting Ms S-B to undress asked the young male radiographer to leave the X-Ray suite. Ms S-B takes up the story:

Ms S-B: He said 'no I am not going anywhere' and he started going off 'This is the NHS and in the NHS you don't have choice, you can't ask for a Muslim doctor, you can't ask for a female doctor. . .' he went on at a rate.

When the X-ray was finished I said to him. 'Now look here young man. I know all about the NHS and I do know I have choice'. . . He stood there like a log, he didn't move, he didn't say a word and I said to him 'you would not have your mother lift her skirt in front of a strange man would you?' He did not know where to look. . .

My culture and my personal preference

Some of the stories illustrate cultural dimensions and sensitivities to care. The authors both emphasized the use of a person's name as a matter of individual as well as cultural respect. Other important areas that emerged in the conversations with the co-authors were sensitivity toward modesty; privacy and gender considerations in personal care; awareness of personal and cultural food preferences when helping people, especially with cognitive decline, to select from food menus; and the barrier to communication strong accents can cause especially if people are already weak or have sensory impairment.

Planning for person-centred care in practice

The experiences shared by the co-authors in this chapter illustrate the complexity and diversity of factors that shape people's experience and perception of care and interactions with caregivers. The experience of care is unique to each individual, but for nurses to plan and deliver dignified and PCC in practice, there are a number of important considerations and transferrable principles that can be applied. These relate to approaching care as a partnership, establishing communication, listening to the person and family carers, and respecting their knowledge and choices. Professional nursing for older people is based on delivering a compassionate, partnership approach and requires highly trained and motivated people. Working with older people requires the skills and knowledge to recognize and manage issues that negatively impact on quality of life. These include physical decline leading to frailty; symptoms such as chronic pain, reduced mobility, incontinence, cognitive or sensory impairment; low mood, social isolation or environmental barriers. It also requires the practitioner to see beyond these conditions to the person's capability, resilience and preferences and to work in ways that promote quality of life as well as dignified end of life care. Person-centred care planning is a mechanism to promote partnership with the older person and the family/carer, but it requires sensitive and skilled communication with multi-disciplinary teams working across acute, community and social care boundaries.

Summary

Older people, within wider society and health and social care, battle indifference, stereotypical images, inflexible systems and individual ideologies that undermine their independence and dignity. Along the way they encounter individual professionals and non-professional health and social care staff who take an interest in them as an individual and help to smoothe their journey. At times this requires little more than a smile, the correct use of their name and the time to listen and ask them what they want. However, this is overly simplistic; it also requires highly trained, motivated and collaborative teams working across organizational boundaries to lessen the impact of physical, social, economic and environmental barriers to support quality of life and individual identity throughout older adulthood.

As an individual practitioner the enormity of delivering highly skilled PCC to an increasing older and more complex population can be overwhelming. This chapter has emphasized the impact that the individual can have in one-to-one interactions. It is the quality of the presence and communication that makes a difference to the older person's and the family's sense of control and 'value' within large health and social care systems. It is the one-to-one encounters between practitioners and older people that are the essence of PCC.

The final words of wisdom in this chapter are from the co-authors who have shared their experiences. They provide a practical insight into developing and sustaining a person-centred philosophy within everyday practice.

Personal touch

Miss S-B: Young health care professionals . . . must take their job seriously and their focus must be providing care for the people in their charge. . .. There is one thing between text book and coal face experiences, they are not the same. You can have all the book knowledge you can take in but if you do not have that personal touch and that life experience your job will not be complete, you have to marry the two together.

Cross to the other side

Mrs FC: Try and imagine for a minute what it is like to have lost your abilities to walk, perhaps to talk all that fast . . . to be unwell in a world that is becoming difficult for you to manage and is shrinking around you.

Try and put yourself into the head of an older person and to see their illness might be making life very difficult for them and how they can do things and communicate with you. You've got to kind of get across to the other side to see how difficult the world had become for the ill person. . .. There is still a person even if their capacity is limited.

References

Ball, J., Murrells, T., Rafferty, A.M. *et al.* (2014) 'Care left undone' during nursing shifts: associations with workload and perceived quality of care, *British Medical Journal Quality & Safety*, 23(2): 116–25.

Bridges, J. (2009) *Best Practice for Older People in Acute Care Settings (BPOP): Guidance for Nurses*. Available at: http://rcnpublishing.com/userimages/ContentEditor/1373367366877/Caring-for-older-people.pdf (accessed 17 January 2015).

Bridges, J. and Nugus, P. (2010) Dignity and significance in urgent care: older people's experiences, *Journal of Research in Nursing*, 15(1): 43–51.

Bridges, J., Flatley, M. and Meyer, J. (2010) Older people's and relatives' experiences in acute care settings: systematic review and synthesis of qualitative studies, *International Journal of Nursing Studies*, 47(1): 89–107.

Bridges, J., Nicholson, C., Maben, J., *et al.* (2013) Capacity for care: meta-ethnography of acute care nurses' experiences of the nurse-patient relationship, *Journal Advanced Nursing*, 69(4): 760–72.

British Geriatric Society (BGS) (2014) *Fit-for-Frailty*. Available at: www.bgs.org.uk/campaigns/fff/fff_full.pdf (accessed 17 January 2015).

Brooker, D. (2003) What is person-centred care in dementia? *Reviews in Clinical Gerontology*, 13(3): 215–22.

Brown, P. (2008) Trusting in the new NHS: instrumental versus communicative action, *Sociology of Health and Illness*, 30(3): 349–63.

Calnan, M., Badcott, D. and Woodhead, G. (2006) Dignity under treat? A study of the experience of older people in the United Kingdom, *International Journal of Health and services*, 36(2): 355–75.

Calnan, M., Calnan, T., Hillman, A. *et al.* (2013) 'I often worry about the older person being in that system': exploring the key influences on the provision of dignified care for older people in acute hospitals, *Ageing and Society*, 33(3): 465–85.

Care Quality Commission (2013) Time to listen in NHS hospitals. Dignity and nutrition inspection programme 2012. Available at www.cqc.org.uk/ (accessed).

Clissett, P., Porock, D., Harwood, R. and Gladmann, J. (2013) The challenges of achieving person-centred care in acute hospitals: a qualitative study of people with dementia and their families, *International Journal of Nursing Studies*, 50(11): 1495–503.

Commission on Dignity in Care (2012) *Delivery Dignity*. Available at: www.nhsconfed.org/Publications/reports/Pages/Delivering-Dignity.aspx (accessed 12 November 2015).

DH (Department of Health) (2012) *Liberating the NHS: No Decision About Me, Without Me*. Available at www.gov.uk (accessed 17 January 2015).

Edvardsson, D., Fetherstonhaugh, D. and Nay, R. (2010) Promoting a continuation of self and normality: person-centred care as described by people with dementia, their family members and aged care staff, *Journal of Clinical Nursing*, 19(17–18): 2611–18.

Francis, R. (2013) *Report of the Mid Staffordshire NHS Foundation Trust Public Inquiry*. Available at: www.official-documents.gov.uk.

Fried, L.P., Tangen, C.M., Walston, J. *et al.* (2001) Frailty in older adults: evidence for a phenotype, *Journal of Gerontology: Medical Sciences*, 56: M146–56.

Kitwood, T. (1997) *Dementia Reconsidered: The Person Comes First*. Buckingham: Open University Press.

Maben, J., Adams, M., Peccei, R. *et al.* (2012) 'Poppets and parcels': the links between staff experience of work and acutely ill older peoples' experience of hospital care, *International Journal of Older People Nursing*, 7(2): 83–94.

Meiner, S. (2015) Theories of aging, in S. Meiner (ed.) *Gerontologic Nursing*, 5th edn. Missouri: Elsevier.

Nicholson, C., Meyer, J., Flatley, M. and Holman, C. (2013) The experience of living at home with frailty in old age: a psychosocial qualitative study, *International Journal of Nursing Studies*, 50(9): 1172–9.

Nilsson, M., Ekman, S. and Sarvimäki, A. (1998) Ageing with joy or resigning to old age: older people's experiences of the quality of life in old age, *Health Care in Later Life*, 3(2): 94–110.

Nolan, M. (2001) Successful ageing: keeping the 'person' in person-centred care, *British Journal of Nursing*, 10(7): 450–4.

Phillips, J. (2010) Ageism, in K. Ajrouch and S. Hillcoat-Nalletamby (eds) *Key Concepts in Social Gerontology*. Los Angeles, CA: SAGE.

Prorok, J., Horgan, S. and Seitz, A. (2013) Health care experiences of people with dementia and their caregivers: a meta-ethnographic analysis of qualitative studies, *Canadian Medical Association Journal*, 185(14): 669–80.

Rockwood, K. and Mitnitski, A. (2011) Frailty defined by deficit accumulation and geriatric medicine defined by frailty, *Clinical Geriatric Medicine*, 27: 17–26.

Tadd, W. and Calnan, M. (2009) Caring for older people: why dignity matters – the European experience, in L. Nordenfelt (ed.) *Dignity in Caring for Older People*. Oxford: Wiley-Blackwell.

Tadd, W., Hillman, A., Calnan, S. *et al.* (2011) *Dignity in Practice: An exploration of the care of older adults in acute NHS Trusts.* Available at: www.netscc.ac.uk/hsdr (accessed 17 January 2015).

Taylor, I. and Kelly, J. (2006) Professionals, discretion and public sector reform in the UK: re-visiting Lipsky, *International Journal of Public Sector Management*, 19(7): 629 –64.

Walker, E. and Dewar, B.J. (2001) How do we facilitate carer's involvement in decision making? *Journal Advanced Nursing*, 34(3): 329–37.

Person-centred approaches to carers' experiences

Dr. Julia E. Pelle

Introduction

According to the last United Kingdom (UK) Population Census in 2011, there are an estimated 5.8 million people providing unpaid care in England and Wales (ONS 2013). This number has increased by 600,000 since the last UK Population Census in 2001. In addition, the increase is significant in the highest unpaid category, of fifty or more working hours per week (ONS 2013). When you consider that there is a greater demand for this form of care, within the UK population living longer, unpaid care has become not only a socio-political and financial concern (Colombo 2011), but will also impact on how nurses and other health professionals engage with the diverse range of carers now providing informal care across the lifespan.

This chapter will focus on how nurses can apply more person-centred approaches to working with informal carers in health and social care, in the UK. A definition will be provided which encompasses a description of the informal carer role. Particular attention will be given to how carers (which refers to family carers or friends) gained recognition through the UK Population Census (ONS 2001; 2011) and health and social care policy.

An overview of the different groups of informal carers as identified by the UK Population Census of 2011 will be discussed. Furthermore, the role of the nurse in developing a partnership approach to working with informal carers will be reviewed considering a diverse group of carers. An important part of partnership working with informal carers is paying attention to their personal health and psycho-social needs, life goals, social networks, caregiving practice and appreciation of the social environment in which they deliver care. This also forms a core aspect of person-centred approaches to nursing care (Draper and Tetley 2013).

LEARNING OUTCOMES

Reading this chapter should enable the reader to:

- Identify the informal carer within the context of care provided
- Understand the role of informal carers and the impact of health and social care policy on caring
- Appreciate the requirement of personalization when working with carers
- Review and develop the role of the nurse in carer assessment

Definition of informal carer

The following definition of 'informal carer' comes from the Department of Health, Social Services 2002:

> Carers are defined as people who, without payment, provide help and support to a family member or friend who may not be able to manage without this help because of frailty, illness, or disability. Carers can be adults caring for other adults, parents caring for ill or disabled children or young people aged under 18 caring for another family member.
>
> (DHSSPS 2002)

The case of Malcolm described below illustrates how individuals may not immediately define their role:

Reader activity

Conduct a database search using the search term 'informal carers' in health and social care.

What other 'terminology' is used to describe 'informal carers' in the literature?

Recognizing carers in UK health and social care policy

Since the inclusion of the word 'carer' in the 2001 UK Population Census, there is clear acknowledgement of the contribution of family carers and friends (also referred to as care-givers and informal carers) in the health and social care of individuals, most of whom have long-term social, physical and mental health problems (DoH 2000; Pinquart and Sorensen 2011; Rowe 2012).

There has also been a number of health and social care policies recognizing the value of unpaid carers. These included the Carers Recognition and Services Act (DoH 1995) and the Carers and the Disabled Children's Act (DoH 2000). The introduction of the Carers Equal

Opportunities Act (DoH 2004) signalled a focus on looking at the socio-environmental issues, which influenced caring including a commitment to supporting carers to have more balanced social leisure and working lives.

Although UK government policies have now acknowledged carers, some carers may not always be able to recognize their caring role and often see this role as an important part of their familial duty to their sick relative. The case study below gives some further insight into a family carer's perception of their caring role.

Malcolm

Malcolm is 24 years old and helps his mother Jackie, care for his father Ben, who lives with Huntington's Chorea.

"You don't really acknowledge yourself as a carer, because he's (Ben) my Dad and of course I would care for him when he is ill! I see this as what being a family is really about, when Mum gets tired with caring for Dad, I take over and she does the same for me, but however tired we get, we do this as a family. . ."

Establishing a strategy for carer support

The Labour government brought in a National Strategy for Carers in 1999 (DoH 1999) with recommendations of a second pension for unemployed carers or those on low income. As a result, local authorities were given a Carers Grant to provide respite care for carers.

In 2006, in the White Paper *Our Health, Our Care, Our Say* (DoH 2006), the government introduced a 'New Deal for Carers' which established the Standing Commission on Carers in 2007. This commission set up training for carers called 'Caring with Confidence' (DoH 2008b) and launched an information a helpline and website to support carers (DoH 2009).

Before the change of government in 2010, the Labour Party carried out a major review of the National Carer Strategy of 1999 and brought in a new carer strategy, *Carers at the Heart of the 21ˢᵗ Century: Families and Communities* (DoH 2008a). This strategy promised more financial investment (in addition to the Carers Grant) into statutory and voluntary organizations. Emphasis was placed on additional awareness training for staff in statutory services and an increased carer premium on income-related benefits. A carer-specific programme was introduced at Job Centre Plus and a Skills Health Check and careers advice service. Finally the strategy contended that it would support carers to remain physically and mentally well.

In 2010, under the UK coalition government, a new carer strategy was launched, *Recognised, Valued and Supported: Next Steps for the Carers' Strategy* (DoH 2010). This document relayed the need for health and social care services to focus on carers' health needs (Burrows and Gannon 2013) through carer assessments and supporting carers' involvement in decision-making around care. This strategy repeated the need for carers to have respite care and more access to paid work opportunities. In a bid to support patients and their carers to become more independent and attend to their wellbeing, the 'personalization agenda' was re-invigorated in this carer strategy (Glendinning *et al.*, 2014; DoH 2014c).

Personalization and the focus on more person-centred care

'Personalization' was a concept that emerged in the 1970s when a number of community groups lobbied for better service provision of those with mental and physical disabilities and mental health problems. The idea fostered the need for independent living, social participation (inclusion), control, choice and empowerment. Part of this process led to the development of self-directed support and personal budgets, the aim of these being to reform social care systems (Social Care Institute for Excellence 2012).

An outcome report was also published along with the new coalition government's carer strategy, *Recognised, Valued and Supported: Next Steps for the Carers Strategy* (DoH 2010), which emphasized the benefits of 'personalization' for carers, and allowed for more person-centred care (self-care) and perceived the carer as an 'expert' on their own needs. A final conclusion of this report was that more *'whole family based approaches'*, should be considered in developing partnerships between carers and statutory health and social care services (DoH 2010).

Reader activity

Read the definition of personalization below and answer the questions that follow. The Department of Health (2008c) provide the following definition:

'. . . every person who receives support whether provided by statutory services or funded by themselves will have choice and control over the shape of that support in all care settings.'

How does personalization

- support family carers and friends in their care of a relative/friend with a long-term healthcare problem?
- pose a challenge to the relationship between
  - the carer and the cared-for person?
  - the carer and statutory services?

Within each of the UK carer policies developed since 1995, there was not only recognition of the value of carers, but also a growing awareness of the diverse range of carers living in the UK.

Identifying informal carers in the UK

Initially, the UK Population Census (ONS 2001) highlighted more female carers carrying out unpaid work as informal carers. They also tended to be carers for sick children and elderly relatives. However, the most recent UK Population Census (ONS 2011), provided a detailed overview of the typology of informal carers. These included Child/Adolescent carers who may be caring for a parent; carers from the Black, Asian and Minority Ethnic (BAME) communities (DoH 2009); carers from the Lesbian, Gay, Transgender and Bisexual (LGTB) communities (Willis 2014); and spousal carers with acknowledgement of the number of men who are actively involved as carers of their wives, siblings, parents, children and elderly relatives. When identifying informal carers, there needs to be recognition of not only their role in the family and the community, but of the formal carer as a 'person'. The term 'double-duty carers' refers to individuals who maintain a role as both a health professional and informal carer, which presents a number of quite unique challenges when trying to work in partnership with statutory services.

The different long-term health and social problems also bring with them a diversity of carers' caring experiences because of the varying nature and the range of physical health problems, mental health problems, end of life care and care of the person with dementia care.

The full 'typology' of carers living in the UK population is complicated by the fact that individual carers often perceive their carer role as a natural part of being a relative or friend and therefore 'their duty' to care; as such they do not necessarily acknowledge the label of carer, caregiver or informal carer as important (Jegermalm and Sundstrom 2014).

Consider the following case of Jenny as an example of a person who realized that it was 'the right thing' to be identified as a carer.

Jenny

Jenny is a 56–year-old who lives on her own and works as a secretary of a small carpet firm. She recently started caring for her next door neighbour Maisie, who lives with rheumatoid arthritis and finds it hard to get about.

'I do her shopping every Thursday and get her the healthy foods her district nurse recommends. I had no idea that I could get some financial support for the things I do for Maisie. To be honest, it did not cross my mind, as I was not family and well, we have been neighbours for ten years and she always cheers me up when I'm down, so it was the least I could do, but then the nurse mentioned Maisie having a choice in who she wanted to care for her, and the kind of support you could get, it felt strange at first, but Maisie has no contact with her niece and nephew, who live up North, so it seemed the right thing to do. . .'

A brief typology of carers

In the sections that follow we briefly consider the different situations of carers, giving examples.

Reader activity

Compare and contrast the advantages and disadvantages of being

a non-professional carer
a professional carer

Young carers: children and adolescents

The 2011 Census indicated that almost 178,000 under 18 years of age have caring responsibilities. The vast majority are providing less than twenty hours of care a week; however thousands provide higher levels of care. Emerging definitions of 'young carer' place carer numbers at about three million. It is important, however, to recognize differences between a young carer who is part of a group of family carers looking after a sick relative and a young carer supporting a lone parent with, for example, an enduring mental health problem (Huddleston and West 2011). In the example Alan is 14 and is a young carer for his younger brother Nathan (who is 10 years old) and lives with Spina Bifida.

Alan

'Nathan needs help with getting washed and dressed in the morning, so I usually help him, as he has the room next to mine in our house. When I was younger, I helped Mum and Dad care for him. I remember he was always in hospital a lot whilst I was at school. We would swap stories about school and hospital, he's my best friend and we do quite a lot of things together!'

Working age carers and older adult carers

Three million people combine caring for a loved one with paid work. Over two million people have given up work at some point to care for loved ones. Three million have reduced working hours (Carers UK and YouGov 2013). As part of Caring and Family Finances Inquiry UK Report (Carers UK 2014) the peak age of caring also often coincides with a time when an individual starts to develop their career. Seventy per cent of carers were over £10,000 worse off as a result of reduced earnings (Carers UK 2014). Every year over 2.1 million adults become carers and almost as many people find that their caring experiences come to an end. The peak age of caring is 50–64 years, which is still considered working age. Carers that manage to juggle work and informal care find they forgo promotion or miss out on job opportunities because they cannot increase their working hours or move location to take up a better position. Almost one in four say they have changed their working pattern to care and some remain anxious that caring would reduce their capacity to work in the future (Carers UK 2011).

The impact of caring responsibilities and ability to work is a growing economic challenge for employers and the UK economy as well as families. Age UK estimates that there is a cost of £5.3 billion a year to the economy in lost earnings and tax revenue and additional benefit payments. In more recent years, employers have also reported on the adverse effects of caring on their workforce. This places more pressure on employees, causing physical and mental health problems and leading to declined productivity, as well as a loss of valuable staff members (Age UK 2012). In the over-65 age group there is a notable rise in the number of carers compared to the general carer population.

Reader activity

Compare and contrast the differences between young carers (children and adolescents) and adult carers (to include young adults and working age adults).

1   Discuss the benefits and challenges of being an older age carer.

Gender and the caring experience

Women are more likely to be carers then men. Females comprise 58 per cent of carers, while males comprise 42 per cent of the carer community in the UK (ONS 2011). The percentage of carers who are female rises to 60 per cent for those who are caring for 50 hours or more a week (NHS Information Care for Health and Social Care 2010). At present women make up 73 per cent of the people receiving carers' allowance for caring 35 hours or more a week. Caring also tends to affect men and women at different times. Women are much more likely to care in middle age. One quarter of women aged 50 to 64 years have caring responsibilities, compared to one in six men (ONS 2011). Women have a 50:50 chance of providing care by the time they are 59, compared to men who have the same chance by the time they are 75 years old. Women are more likely to be 'sandwich carers' (combining elderly care and child care). They are also more likely to give up work in order to care. This imbalance reduces among older carers, where men are most likely to provide care among retired people. The following case study describes the challenges of a woman who tries to balance both her family role as a wife and mother with the caring role she has for her mother:

Andrea

Andrea is 43 years old, married with two teenage sons and also cares for her mother Mary, who was diagnosed with Alzheimer's disease at the age of 71.

'The first time I noticed a change in Mum was when she got up to make us all a cup of tea in the kitchen then came back into the living room and asked who we all were and demanded we leave her house! I was really scared then and I just burst into tears. I knew we had to get her to the doctor. The worst part of this illness is when Mum just doesn't know who we are, you never really get used to that and it has taken a long time for us to readjust as a family, but we are getting there . . .'

Reader activity

Review the UK Census information of 2011 provided in Table 16.1.

What differences do you notice between the male carers and the female carers in the UK Census 2011?

Lesbian, gay transgender and bisexual (LGTB) carers

As well as experiencing the pressures of caring common to all carers, LGBT carers may experience additional issues and challenges in their carer role. They may feel out of place in traditional carer support groups or uncomfortable about who can help. They may also be anxious about accessing services for fear that they are going to be judgemental and not LGBT friendly. For LGBT carers of a parent, they may feel their own identity is pushed to one side, particularly when living with the parent, and they may no longer feel free to enjoy intimate relationships. Furthermore, they may experience complex personal issues, family or discriminatory challenges (Willis *et al.*, 2011). LGBT carers caring for a partner may feel under pressure to 'come out' about the nature of their relationship with the cared-for person, each time they meet a different practitioner. The lack of recognition and acceptance of the LGBT relationship (be it friendship or intimate) and identity can be an added stressor for carers.

Table 16.1 Percentage of men and women in selected economic positionsproviding unpaid care, and ratio of percentages of those in *'Not in good health'* if providing 50 hours or more unpaid care per week to those providing no care

Gender	Employment Status	1–19 hours	20–49 hours	50+ hours	Ratio
Men	Works full time	7.14%	1.13%	1.07%	2.4
	Works part time	9.01%	1.78%	1.74%	1.9
	Unemployed	5.92%	1.54%	1.49%	1.8
	Student	3.38%	0.55%	0.39%	4.6
Women	Works full time	9.6%	1.4%	1.3%	2.7
	Works part time	11.7%	2.0%	2.5%	1.9
	Unemployed	7.2%	1.9%	2.1%	1.8
	Student	4.1%	0.8%	0.8%	4.4

Source: Office for National Statistics (2011).

Joyce

Joyce is 38 and a lesbian who cares for her partner Ali. Ali, who enjoyed work as a personal trainer, suffered a heart attack two years ago at 40 years of age and struggles with not being as active as she once was.

'Mostly I go with Ali to the GP and her hospital appointments. It's hard to see her not being as active as she was when we first met, but every so often, you see the glint in her eye that she wants to do more – I try and make sure she paces herself and although she does the cooking, I do most of the housework, because Ali can easily get tired. Sometimes, I feel bad, but I find myself monitoring her diet and making sure she follows the doctor's advice in healthy eating. . .'

Carers of people with long-term/physical health problems

Carers may be in a temporary carer role because the person receiving care may regain his or her independence. Other care receivers may need more long-term care. Carers may experience shock and fear when the care receiver is first diagnosed with a long-term physical health problem. Carers may feel excluded during the early stages of professional care. Having to wait for an operation and procedure can be difficult. Carers may feel unable to plan the future and get on with life. Carers can become anxious around the life-threatening nature of the long-term physical health problem, when there is a relapse of the long-term condition or if there needs to be further tests or investigations (Clark *et al.*, 2008). For some carers the impact of the long-term condition on family life can mean missed opportunities to go on holiday, and a lack of ability to work or gain employment. Within carers' personal relationships, there may be a loss of intimacy and problems having sexual intercourse or experiencing pleasure during intimacy. The commitment to caring for a sick person can be unexpected for some carers who can become physically and emotionally exhausted. The mixture of emotions can range anywhere between feeling genuine love and concern, sadness and anger to feelings of frustration, isolation and fear for the future. Carers may find it hard to ask for help and when help is offered, they may find it hard to accept. At the same time, the experience of caring can be rewarding, educational and instil a sense of personal discovery alongside patient recovery.

Carers of people with severe/long-term mental health problems

Up to 1.5 million people care for a person with a mental health problem. These mental health problems can include a diagnosis of schizophrenia, bipolar disorder, clinical depression and personality disorder. Although statutory community care was provided by health and social care professionals, there was an increasing move towards the transfer of care to family members and friends. The signs and symptoms associated with severe and enduring mental health problems can also include sudden changes in behaviour, mood and thought, and impact on physical health. As informal carers have the most contact with the care recipient, this can lead to a high degree of burden. Shah *et al.* (2010) describe two types of family burden which carers experience in their caring role –objective and subjective. Objective burden refers to carers' experience of social-related problems, for example education/employment and economic difficulties, loss of close social and leisure activities and poor attention to personal physical health and wellbeing. Subjective burden focuses more on the carers' emotional response to their caring role – the stress, anxiety, guilt, frustration and anger – and significant for many carers is the change in persona of the care recipient which surmounts to carers' grief or feeling of loss. Albert and Simpson (2015) in a phenomenological study exploring carers' experience of caring for a relative during a mental health crisis, found that carers felt a 'double deprivation' which they described as a) not receiving adequate support from health and social care professionals and b) having to protect their social network from the trauma of the mental health crisis. Caring was interspersed with feelings of guilt and loyalty for carers, which made it difficult for them to discuss their experience of aggression in the relationship with the care recipient. This made caring a terrifying experience and was further compounded by feelings of being abandoned by statutory services.

The case of Brian below provides an example of the impact of subjective burden:

Brian

Brian is a 54–year-old man who works part time at the John Lewis Partnership as a Section Manager. Five years ago, his wife Jane was diagnosed with clinical depression, following the death of their youngest son in a car accident.

'The days when Jane feels well and is happier in herself seem to be getting less and less and she drinks more. Sometimes I come home and find bottles of red wine on the dining room table. It's got to the point where I feel alone in this marriage and I know this sounds horrible but it's like living with a perfect stranger. I've turned into her carer and not her husband, but I won't give up on her. The thing is, I'm still grieving for our son too . . .'

Carers of people with learning disabilities

Willis (2014) states that one of the consequences of the NHS and Community Care Act 1990 was that the responsibility for the health of people with learning disabilities was devolved from nurses within statutory services to the primary care services and paid carers with the help of the new Community Learning Disability Teams (CLDTs). These teams include psychiatrists, community learning disability nurses and occupational therapists. However, for most family carers, problems occur at the transition phase where the individual with a learning disability moves from children's services to adult services. Family carers find they are forced to adapt to changes in the philosophy of health and social care in adult services where there is less monitoring and less collaboration around care planning and decisions on treatment. In addition, family carers are less likely to be acknowledged for having a particular knowledge of the health and wellbeing of their relative and lose their partnership status, which they had when working with child health services.

About 840,000 carers care for people with a learning disability and autistic spectrum disorders in the UK. The Personal Social Services Survey of Adult Carers in England (2009/2010)

(The NHS Information Centre for Health and Social Care, 2010) reported that the majority of carers of an adult with learning disabilities had been caring for more than 20 years. Some of these carers reported not being in paid employment due to their caring responsibilities. Carers of people with learning disabilities have higher levels of dissatisfaction with support or services received from social care service, compared to other carers, a point illustrated by the case of Ruth:

Ruth

Ruth is a 52-year-old single mother of three and a full-time carer for her youngest daughter, Sarah. Sarah is 17 years old and has multiple learning disabilities.

'Sarah needs help with every aspect of her daily life. She loves being around the family and has an infectious laugh, which really endears her to you! When she was younger I felt as though me and my family had all the help from health and especially social care services, but now that Sarah is 17, it's like all the services have been pulled away from us. No matter how much I ask for more help, it is an uphill struggle to get it! My partner left us last year, saying he couldn't cope with it any more, so I lost that emotional and physical support to care for Sarah. Although my other two daughters help as much as they can, I worry that they need to have their own independence. . .'

Black and minority ethnic (BAME) carers

Carers UK (2011) carried out a review of informal care in the UK and found that BAME carers faced a number of problems in terms of accessing support. They were less likely to be consulted about any impending hospital discharge or receive additional support from their GP about their carer role. Carers were also more likely to miss financial support or receive practical support. Therefore, despite the acknowledgement of BAME carers in UK health and social care policies, both research studies and health and social care service provision reveal a low uptake of services from these communities (Carers UK 2011).

Previous studies have found that BAME carers do not readily identify themselves as 'carers' and tend to see caring as part of the customary or familial role. In 1998, the Social Services Inspectorate suggested that there exists a common assumption that BAME communities like to 'look after their own' (DHSSI 1998). The notion that they should be identified or considered separately from the person they care for can be perceived as 'alien' and more likely to damage familial relationships. There may be other reasons why BAME communities are perceived as 'looking after their own'. Yeandle and Buckner (2007) found that when affected by poor health and financial difficulty BAME communities sometimes face particular difficulties which include i) concealing ill health; ii) experiencing lower levels of employability; iii) being held back by reduced opportunities for social participation; iv) lacking the type of support they need as individuals and v) being hampered by limited coping skill. However, inter-generational differences may foster a perception of care and caring and being a carer that is very similar to their white counterparts for third and fourth generations of BAME communities.

Reader activity

How does culture and ethnicity impact on the informal carer role?

Parental carers

Within the carer role, the experience of 'familial obligation' or 'duty' is different for each carer. Parental carers often feel a strong obligation to continue or extend their parenting role for the cared-for person from childhood/adolescence into adulthood. There may be difference in how mothers and fathers as parents develop their caring role, where fathers may access more pragmatic approaches and mothers see caring as an extension a natural maternal role (Jones and Morris 2012). Parental obligation can give way to overprotectiveness in the caring role. Some pressures on the marital relationship may be experienced and at the same time parents also see more closeness in their marital relationship as a result of their caring roles.

Sibling carers

Like parental carers, sibling carers can feel a familial duty to care for their relatives, particularly when parental carers are absent. As in the case of all carers, sibling carers can become frustrated, embarrassed and angry within their caring role. They also experience a change in the relationship with the cared for sibling, as they take on more of an advocacy role. Some siblings become less close and less warm in their relationships with the cared for sibling. Those siblings still in school or college may experience problems with attendance, completing study or broken peer relationships. They may also be concerned about whether the cared for sibling receives public and social acceptance (Sin *et al.*, 2015). When sibling carers partner with other family members in the caring role, they may have reduced recreational time as a family. Concerns about whether they will develop illness like the cared for sibling can also be present (Forrest *et al.*, 2015). For adolescent young adults, adult carers may express their worries, not only about the future of the cared for person, but also the future of the sibling carer. Conversely, sibling carers in some studies report feeling very proud of assisting in the care of their relative, experience low conflict, warm relationships and have lots of fun with the cared for sibling. Some sibling carers develop a pragmatic approach to coping with the caring role and can sometimes adapt more quickly than parental carers. When included in the process of caring siblings demonstrate clear responsibility in the caring role, which is supported by a general protectiveness towards their relative (Angell *et al.*, 2012).

Spousal carers

Marital obligation was important for the spousal carers who feel an obligation to be there for their spouse as part of a commitment to their marital vows. However, the onset and diagnosis of chronic illness may leave spousal carers experiencing loss in different ways. Cheung and Hocking (2004), in a study exploring experience of spousal carers of people with multiple sclerosis, found that carers may feel the loss of a partner, loss of self, loss of companionship/partnership, loss of support, loss of income and lifestyle and missed opportunities for future planning. However, spousal carers also found that they had learnt new hobbies and discovered personal strengths and confidence in overcoming the obstacles and challenges in their caring role. This afforded them the time to reflect on their achievement and feel hope for their future.

The role of the nurse in fostering partnership with informal carers to deliver person-centred care

The role of the nurse in supporting informal carers in twenty-first century UK encompasses a number of 'steps' to partnership. This invariably begins with a focus on patient care, which includes a perspective on family and social supports through the assessment process. The introduction of the 1995 Carers (Recognition and Services) Act meant carers were entitled to an assessment of their needs and their ability to continue caring. Further legislation in 2000 (Carers and Disabled Children) Act and the 2004 Carer Equal Opportunities Act extended carers' rights, suggesting that all statutory organizations should work together to tailor services in support of carers' needs.

Recommendations within assessments take into account the type and volume of caring activities, carers' coping strategies, other responsibilities and the relationship with the care recipient. More recently the Care Act (DoH 2014b) and the Children and Families Act (DoH 2014c) further strengthened the rights of all carers along with the person they cared for to have an assessment of their needs regardless of their income, finance or level of need. Both acts came into effect in April 2015. Young carers and the parents of disabled children are also included in the new system.

Reader activity

Reflect on the different types of 'informal carers' you meet in your practice placement experience.

1 What are some of their requests from health and social care services?
2 What are some of their main concerns about their relative or friend as a carer?

The role of the nurse in carer assessments

The most recent carer strategies for England and Wales (DoH 2010) identify timely, holistic assessments as key to delivering carer support, where individuals are a) recognized for the work they do in caring; b) involved in the decisions that affect them; c) engaged to maintain as normal a life as possible outside their caring role; and d) supported to maintain their health and wellbeing.

The Care and Support Bill for England (Secretary of State for Health 2012) gave carers rights to an assessment without having to formally request one, as a local authority's duty to assess will be triggered where it appears an individual may or will have needs because of their caring role. This removed the previous eligibility criteria, which required carers only to receive an assessment if they were providing substantial care on a regular basis.

Under the new legislation carers will have the right to a support plan that is regularly reviewed and to services to meet their eligible needs. However, there are some problems with statutory services carrying out carer assessments. Research studies indicate that practitioners do not recognize the value of separate assessments and also failed to prioritize the completion of carer assessments, focusing predominantly on patients and the cared for person. Some of the practical challenges of conducting such an assessment are illustrated by Sue:

Sue

Sue is a Senior Staff Nurse working in the local Accident and Emergency department.

'The majority of family carers who identify themselves to us as a department tend to provide very helpful information. I have found that they can give context to how the symptoms of an illness developed in their relative or friend. However, sometimes, because they are so worried, they may interrupt or take over when I am trying to gain more individualized information from the patient. At times, like this, I often suggest that they 'grab a coffee' from our hospital cafeteria to give me more time to focus on the patient. While this may seem dismissive, it is not the intention. I try to put myself in their shoes; often they see all the effects of an illness on family life, which can be very stressful . . .'

Carers themselves appear to have low expectations and do not appear to understand the purpose of carer assessments having contributed to the assessment of the person they are caring for. There is little evidence to suggest that information from the carer assessment informs service user planning. There is great variation between local authorities when operationalizing the eligibility criteria, as well as the different approaches to carrying out the carer assessment, where carers are either assessed independently or jointly with the cared for person. There are only a limited number of validated carer assessment tools and where the carer assessments are carried out, they are often not reviewed in a timely way.

Assessment can be an important first step in successfully supporting individuals in and beyond their caring role. Carer assessments can be carried out via face-to-face meetings, by phone or by online contact. Local councils can also carry out a supported self-assessment, which may involve filling in a self-assessment questionnaire, or local organizations may be asked to carry out the assessment. Carer assessments should be carried out by a social worker or another trained professional. The carer assessment will consider whether or not a carer's role impacts on their health or prevents them from achieving outcomes. A carer assessment covers the following topics: the specific aspects of the caring role and its impact on carers and their social well-being; the carer's physical and mental health; the carer's feelings and choices about caring; the carer's work life, study/education attainment, training and leisure activities; the carer's relationships, social networks and life goals; the carer's accommodation status and what if any, emergency plan the carer has in place (DoH 2014a).

Using a family-based approach to understanding the care experience

Research into the strength and resilience of families and family networks has been carried out for several years. When the nurse is really working in partnership with both patient and carers their assessment of health and social care needs can be enhanced by using a family-based approach to care which not only centres on 'personhood' for the patient and carer, but can help the nurse to develop trust and build engagement with both patient and carer (Skerrett 2010). Personhood refers to the way in which an individual communicates with their social environment and how they develop their self-awareness and self-identity. When the nurse has an understanding of personhood for both patient and carer, there is an opportunity to look at motivation to self-care and capacity to care and enter into discussion about sharing care.

The nurse's role in assessing the immediate health and social care concerns of patients could also include an assessment of the family or friends supporting the patient. An important role for the nurse in assessment of patient and carer is whether the assessment needs to be carried out individually or jointly or both. This aspect of the nurse's role can only be ascertained by knowing both carer and cared for person. Part of this assessment should include the relative strengths and resilience of the family relationships. For example, two of the conceptual approaches, which closely resemble the carer experience and which include both patient and their relationship with professional carers, are a) the Family Strengths Framework which has been developed by many different researchers, spanning a period of forty years, however, the work of Stinnett and Defrain will be the focus of this section (Sittner et al., 2007); and b) the Resilience Model of Stress, Adjustment and Adaptation (RMSAA) by McCubbin and McCubbin (1996).

The Family Strengths Framework by Stinnett and Defrain stems from their research in the 1970s, which involved more than three thousand families and more than 30 separate investigations over a twenty-year period. In 1985, Stinett and Defrain conducted another national research study, which specifically explored the characteristics of what were considered

Table 16.2 Family Strength Qualities

Commitment	Promoting family welfare and happiness; balancing relationships
Appreciation	Positive recognition in a positive environment to enhance personal self-worth
Positive communication	Respectively using listening and conversational skills to discuss family issues without attacking each other
Enjoyable time together	To enhance relationships and establish family identities
A sense of spiritual wellbeing	A unifying force that brings meaning and purpose to guide lives
The ability to cope with stress and crisis	Uniting the family through good communication skills, adding humour to the situation, keeping things in perspective

Source: Stinnett and Defrain (1985).

'strong families'. As part of their study findings six family strength qualities were revealed which could be linked to the caring experiences of family carers (see Table 16.2).

The Family Strengths Qualities noted in Table 16.2 could be used by the nurse to focus the discussion in assessing carer experiences of their carer role and how this impacts on health and illness for both patient and carer.

The RMSAA model, which relates more directly to family carers' caring experience, has two phases. These are i) the adjustment phase where carers only make minor changes in their day-to-day lifestyle in response to the 'stressor' (this can refer to any aspect of the caring experience, e.g. receiving diagnosis of a long-term physical health problem) related to caring for their relative or friend; and ii) the adaptation phase where carers make major changes to their day-to-day lifestyle and this can often follow a period of disorganization within a family or close relationship and/or crisis which is described as 'maladjustment' to the caring experience.

Summary

The number of families and friends who deliver unpaid care in the UK continues to increase across the lifespan in the UK. The nurse's role encompasses a series of steps to understanding the carer experience.

Helping carers recognize the type of caring they do and how often, and giving them time to discuss the impact of caring on their mental, physical, social and spiritual wellbeing is an important start in the partnership with statutory services. Sustaining a clear role definition of engaging with both patient (cared for person) and carer together and separately presents an ongoing challenge for nurses and other health professionals. However, the work that goes into understanding the personhood of the care recipient and the personhood of the carer and the family culture social environment they mobilize in is both a necessary and important part of the nurse's role. Nurses need to keep an updated and evidence-based knowledge of the different carer policies and strategies for supporting carers in the UK, most of which refer to and give guidance on the different typology of carers and how to tailor services to their needs. Regular reviews of the 'partnership' relationship with carers should consider how carers are perceived by nursing staff: as another pair of hands or a person in their own right who has equal shares in all aspect of care.

Severity of any illness can also have a significant negative impact on carers, which leaves them emotionally drained or physically worn out from their caring role. The nurse has a role in assessing family carers' and friends' strength and resilience to continue caring, receive more help with caring or opt out of caring altogether. In acknowledging the different carers within a family, the nurse can discover the inter-relationships between the cared for person and their immediate caring network, which can offer new ways of working/caring and reveal adaptive and maladaptive coping strategies. Early intervention and the use of education and health promotion should not be ignored – information and knowledge shared with carers can go some way to helping carers develop a positive regard for their caring role and attend to their own self-care, which is vital to them being able to maintain an effective caring role.

References

Age UK (2012) *Improving Later Life Together: Annual Review 2011/2012*: London: Age UK.

Albert, R. and Simpson, A. (2015) Double deprivation: a phenomenological study into the experience of being a carer during a mental health crisis, *Journal of Advanced Nursing*, DOI: 10.1111/jan.12742.

Angell, M.E., Meadan, H. and Stoner, J.B. (2012) Experiences of siblings of individuals with Autistic Spectrum Disorders, *Autism, Research & Treatment*, (949586), DOI: dx.doi.org/10.1155/2012/949586.

Burrows, A. and Gannon, K. (2013) An evaluation of health and well-being checks for unpaid carers, *Journal of Integrated Care*, 21(3): 148–56.

Carers UK (2011) *Half Million Voices: Improving Support for Black Asian Minority Ethnic Carers (BAME) Carers*. London: Carers UK.

Carers UK (2013) *Supporting Working Carers: The Benefits to Families, Business and the Economy*. London: Carers UK.

Carers UK (2014) *Caring and Family Finances Inquiry UK Report*. London: Carers UK.

Carers UK and YouGov (2013) *Supporting Working Carers: The Benefits to Families, Business and the Economy*. London: Carers UK.

Cheung, J. and Hocking, P. (2004) The experience of spousal carers of people with multiple sclerosis, *Qualitative Health Research*, 14(2): 153–66.

Clark, A.M., Reid, M.E., Morrison, C.E. *et al.* (2008) The complex nature of informal care in home-based heart failure management, *Journal of Advanced Nursing*, 61(4): 373–83.

Colombo, F. (2011) *Help Wanted? Providing and Paying for Long Term Care*. Paris: OECD Publishing.

DHSSPS (2002) *Valuing Carers: Proposals for a Strategy for Carers in Northern Ireland*. Belfast: DHSSPS.

DHSSI (Department of Health & Social Services Inspectorate) (1998) *'They Look After Their Own, Don't They?': Inspection of Community Care Services for Black and Ethnic Minority Older People*. London: HMSO.

DoH (Department of Health) (1995) *Carers Recognition & Services Act*. London: HMSO.

Department of Health (1999) *Caring about Carers: A National Strategy for Carers*. London: HMSO.

Department of Health (2000) *Carers and Disabled Children Act*. London: HMSO.

DoH (2004) *Carers Equal Opportunities Act*. London: HMSO.

DoH (2006) *Our Health, Our Care, Our Say: A New Direction for Community Services*. London: HMSO.

DoH (2008a) *Carers at the Heart of the 21ˢᵗ Century – Families and Communities*. London: HMSO.

DoH (2008b) *Caring with Confidence*. London: HMSO.

DoH (2008c) *Putting People First: Personalisation Toolkit*. London: HMSO.

DoH (2009) *Delivering Race Equality in (DRE) Mental Health Care: A Review*. London: HMSO.

DoH (2010) *Recognised, Valued and Supported: Next Steps for the Carers Strategy*. London: HMSO.

DoH (2014a) *Carers Strategy: The Second National Plan 2014 to 2016*, London: HMSO.

DoH (2014b) *The Care Act (Part One) 2014*. London: HMSO.

DoH (2014c) *The Children and Families Act 2014*. London: HMSO.

Draper, J. and Tetley, J. (2013) *The Importance of Person-centred Approaches to Nursing Care*. London: The Open University.

Forrest Keenan, K., McKee, L. and Miedzybrodzka, Z. (2015) Help or hindrance: young people's experiences of predictive testing for Huntington's disease, *Clinical Genetics*, 87(6): 563–9.

Glendinning, C., Mitchell, W. and Brooks, J. (2014) Ambiguity in Practice?: Carers' roles in personalised social care in England, *Health and Social Care in the Community*, DOI:10.1111/hsc.12123.

Huddleston, M. and West, D. (2011) The hidden young face of care, *Practice Reflexions*, 6(1): 39–45.

Jegermalm, M. and Sundstrom, G. (2014) Stereotypes about caregiving and lessons from the Swedish panorama of care, *European Journal of Social Work*, DOI:10.1080/1361457.2014.892476.

Jones, L. and Morris, R. (2012) Experiences of adult stroke survivors and their parent carers: a qualitative study, *Clinical Rehabilitation*. DOI: 10.1177/0269215512455532.

McCubbin, M. and McCubbin, H. (1996) Family coping with health crises: The Family Resiliency Model of family stress, adjustment and adaptation, in H. McCubbin, A. Thompson and M. McCubbin (eds) *Family Assessment: Resiliency, Coping and Adaptation – Inventories for Research and Practice* Madison, WI: University of Winconsin System.

ONS (Office of National Statistics) (2001) *Census UK*. London: ONS.

ONS (2011) *Census UK*. London: ONS.

ONS (2013) *More than 1 in 10 Providing Unpaid Care as Numbers Rise to 5.8 Million*. London: ONS.

Pinquart, M. and Sorensen, S. (2011) Spouses, adult children and children-in-law as caregivers of older adults: a meta-analytic comparison, *Psychology and Aging*, 26(1): 1–14.

Rowe, J. (2012) Great expectations: a systematic review of the literature on the role of family caregivers in severe mental illness, and their relationships and engagement with professionals, *Journal of Psychiatric and Mental Health Nursing*, 19(1): 70–82.

Shah, A., Wadoo, O. and Latoo, J. (2010) Psychological distress in carers of people with mental health disorders, *British Journal of Medical Practitioners*, 3(3): 327–34.

Sin, J., Jordan, C.D., Henderson, C. and Norman, I. (2015) Psychoeducation for siblings of people with severe mental illness, *The Cochrane Library: Intervention Review*, DOI:10.1002/14651858.CD010540.pub2.

Sittner, B.J.; Brage Hudson, D. and Defrain, J. (2007) Using the concept of family strength to enhance nursing care, *The American Journal of Maternal/Child Nursing*, 32(6): 353–7.

Skerrett, K. (2010) Extending family nursing: concepts from positive psychology, *Journal of Family Nursing*, 16(4): 487–502.

Social Care Institute for Excellence (SCIE) (2012) Report 55: *People Not Processes: The Future of Personalisation and Independent Living*. London: SCIE.

Stinnett, N. and DeFrain, J. (1985) *Secrets of Strong Families*. New York: Berkeley Books.

The NHS Information Centre for Health and Social Care (2010) *Personal Social Services Survey of Adult Carers in England: 2009–2010*. London: The Health and Social Care Information Centre.

Willis, D.S. (2014) Inconsistencies in the roles of family – and paid – carers in monitoring health issues in people with learning disabilities: some implications for the integration of health and social care, *British Journal Learning Disabilities*, 43(1): 24–31. DOI: 10.1111/bld.2015.43.issue-1/issuetoc.

Willis, S., Ward, N. and Fish, J. (2011) Searching for LGBT carers: mapping a research agenda in social work and social care, *British Journal of Social Care*, 41(7): 1304–20.

Yeandle, S. and Buckner, I. (2007) *Carers, Employment and Services: Time for a New Social Contract? Report No.6*. London: Carers UK/University of Leeds.

Index

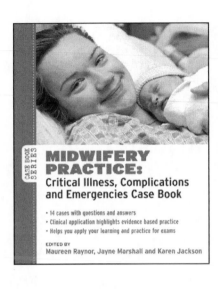

MIDWIFERY PRACTICE
Critical Illness, Complications and
Emergencies Case Book

Maureen Raynor, Jayne Marshall and Karen
Jackson

9780335242733 (Paperback)
May 2012

eBook also available

Part of a case book series, this book contains 14 common pregnancy and
childbirth emergency scenarios to help prepare student midwives for life in
practice. Each case explores and explains the pathology, pharmacology and care
principles, and uses test questions and answers to help assess learning.

Key features:

- Covers the principles, pathology and skills involved in a range of birthing
  scenarios
- Each chapter includes Q&A's, further resources, pre-requisite learning,
  summaries, boxes and learning tools in order to track and further learning
- The practical cases will help you link theory to practice

www.openup.co.uk

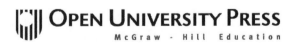

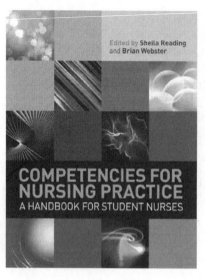

COMPETENCIES FOR NURSING PRACTICE
A Handbook for Student Nurses

Sheila Reading and Brian James Webster
(Eds)

9780335246748 (Paperback)
August 2013

eBook also available

Achieving the NMC Competencies is an ongoing requirement that nurses work towards across all three years of pre-registration study. This book illuminates what students need to understand about each of the competencies and illustrates how best to achieve them in training and practice.

Key features:

- Each chapter tackles a different competency
- Uses activities and examples to help readers get to grips with the competency and relevant NMC requirements
- The book is very interactive and offers lot of portfolio activities for students to try, and use to demonstrate competency as they build a portfolio evidence

www.openup.co.uk

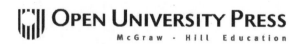 OPEN UNIVERSITY PRESS

McGraw · Hill Education